HEARING-IMPAIRED CHILDREN IN THE MAINSTREAM

Edited by
Mark Ross
with special assistance from Helen Ross

Parkton, Maryland

YORK
PRESS

This book was manufactured in the United States of America. Typography by Brushwood Graphics, Inc., Baltimore, Maryland. Printing and binding by McNaughton & Gunn, Inc., Ann Arbor, Michigan. Cover design by Joseph Dieter, Jr.

Library of Congress Catalog Card Number 90-71342
ISBN 0-912752-22-X

Contents

Contributors

Dorothy Boothroyd-Turner, M.E.D.
Program Coordinator
Special Education-Itinerant
Toronto Schools
43 Millwood Road
Toronto M4S IJ6
Canada

Diane Brackett, Ph.D.
Director
Communication Department
New York League for the Hard
of Hearing
71 West 23rd Street
New York, NY 10010

Laraine C. Conway, M.S., M.E.D.
Educational Specialist for the
Hearing Impaired
Boys Town National Research
Hospital
555 N. 30th Street
Omaha, NE 68131

William E. Castle, Ph.D.
Director
National Technical Institute for
the Deaf
1 Lomb Memorial Drive
Rochester, NY 14623

Carol S. Flexer, Ph.D.
Associate Professor
University of Akron
Department of Communication
Disorders
Akron, OH 44325

Ann Geers, Ph.D.
Director of Clinical Services
Central Institute for the Deaf
818 South Euclid
St. Louis, MO 63110

Ruth R. Green, M.A.
Executive Director
New York League for the Hard
of Hearing
71 West 23rd Street
New York, NY 10010

Patricia J. Heller, Ph.D.
Director
Psychological/Social Work
Services
New York League for the Hard
of Hearing
71 West 23rd Street
New York, NY 10010

Jane R. Madell, Ph.D.
Director
Audiology Department
New York League for the Hard
of Hearing
71 West 23rd Street
New York, NY 10010

David Manning, Ed.D
Director
Mainstream Center
Clarke School for the Deaf
Round Hill Road
Northampton, MA 01060

Antonia B. Maxon, Ph.D.
Associate Professor
Communication Sciences
Department
University of Connecticut
Storrs, CT 06268

Donald McGee, Ph.D.
Program Specialist, Hearing-
Vision Impaired
Fairfax County Public Schools
2831 Graham Road
Falls Church, VA 22042

Winifred H. Northcott, Ph.D.
Consultant and Lecturer
Educational Programs for the
Hearing Impaired
4510 Cedarwood Road
Minneapolis, MN 55416

Mark Ross, Ph.D.
Director
Research and Training
New York League for the Hard
of Hearing
Adjunct Professor, City
University of New York
71 West 23rd Street
New York, NY 10010

Sue Schwartz, Ph.D.
Parent Coordinator
Montgomery County Public
Schools
850 Hungerford Drive
Rockville, MD 20850

Denise F. Wray, Ph.D.
Assistant Professor
University of Akron
Department of Communication
Disorders
Akron, OH 44325

Elizabeth Ying, M.A.
Clinical Supervisor
Children's Programs
Communication Department
New York League for the Hard
of Hearing
71 West 23rd Street
New York, NY 10010

Preface

The New York League for the Hard of Hearing sponsored a conference entitled "Mainstreaming Revisited" in October 1989. This book is an expanded version of the proceedings of that conference. The New York League has encouraged and supported hearing-impaired children in the mainstream for over 50 years. Our experiences over that time have led us to believe that mainstreaming is a legitimate educational option for most hearing-impaired children.

There is, nevertheless, a widespread belief that mainstreaming became a serious educational option in this country in 1975, with the passage of Public Law 94-142, the Education for Handicapped Children Act, but this simplifies the actual situation existing prior to that time. "Mainstreaming" has alway been an educational practice: the rationale was described as early as 1815 and it has not changed significantly over the years. What has changed is our recognition that mainstreaming is not, and should not be, considered an end in itself. The challenge in educating hearing-impaired children in the mainstream is the same as it is in any other setting: to ensure that the children receive an appropriate education. Advocates of mainstreaming point to the potential advantages of educating hearing-impaired children alongside normal-hearing children. Skeptics worry that this placement may provide few if any educational advantages; they fear the costs to the child's psycho-social status and self-image, if the process is not accomplished carefully. Both points of view will be expressed in this book and both have merit.

The contributors to this book work in various settings and have different professional responsibilities vis-à-vis the children. The content of their chapters reflects this diversity. Where does the "truth" lie? In none and all of the viewpoints and experiences reflected in the various chapters.

Five of the contributors in the book are my colleagues at the New York League for the Hard of Hearing. Their participation in the conference and in the book is not an example of professional nepotism. They were selected because of their professional stature and skills; they bring different points of view and backgrounds to their chapters.

The first chapter, by Winifred H. Northcott, is based upon the keynote presentation at the conference. It brings to bear a unique personal and professional perspective. As the hearing daughter of deaf parents, Dr. Northcott literally has been in the field all her life. She has seen, and shares with us, the immense changes that have taken place in the education of hearing-impaired children in this country. She associates the more successful mainstreaming efforts with skill in oral communication, but cautions us to be aware that it is individual children we are mainstreaming and not some general category. A distinction she has emphasized over the years is the difference between *integration* (the old term for mainstreaming) and *assimilation*. Integration is the physical presence of a hearing-impaired child in a regular classroom. This is easy to arrange. It is much more difficult to ensure that the child is an accepted and respected member of the group, or fully "assimilated" in the classroom.

The next section of the book deals with assessment considerations. In this section, Jane R. Madell explains the basics of the audiological assessment. As a number of authors remind us throughout the book, we are concerned with these children because they have a hearing loss. This is their primary condition; all others (and there may be many other problems) are either derivative or secondary. Without a complete audiological evaluation to guide us, it is not possible to plan a coherent management program for a child.

The following two chapters in this section relate to the possible consequences of a hearing loss, from a communication and a psychoeducational point of view. Elizabeth Ying, in her chapter on speech-language assessment, reminds us that in a communication evaluation, *listening* factors are a fundamental concern. Without knowing the precise speech perception capacities of a child, it is impossible to determine if the results of a communication evaluation reflect peripheral (message reception) or more central (linguistic) deficiences.

This same concern can be seen in the chapter by Patricia J. Heller. A child may be labeled psychologically deviant because of behaviors that are direct consequences of the hearing loss. As in the communication evaluation, it is necessary to ensure that test responses attributed to the hearing loss are separated from the child's fundamental psychosocial status. In a psycho-educational evaluation, we are concerned not only with a child's weaknesses, but with his or her strengths and learning style.

Finally, in this section, Diane Brackett shows how the results of all the assessments are used to formulate an Individualized Education Program (IEP) for a child. The goals set must reflect a realistic appraisal of the child's capacities; these goals must be sufficiently rigorous to be challenging, but not so advanced as to be frustratingly unrealistic. As Dr. Brackett shows, there is a direct relationship between the assessment results and the management plan.

In the next section, management considerations are described in detail. As before, we lead off with audiological management, by Jane R. Madell, in recognition of the fact that the best way to minimize a child's problems is to head them off at their source, the hearing loss itself. Appropriate audiological management can substantially minimize the development of academic and communication deficiencies produced by the hearing loss. The need to ensure a favorable listening environment is stressed, as is the need to employ FM auditory training systems effectively.

We would like to believe that effective and appropriate audiological management will eliminate secondary problems and, therefore, no other management focus will be necessary. Unfortunately, this is a rarely achieved dream. Almost always there remain communication, academic, and psycho-social problems that must be addressed. Diane Brackett discusses the general organization and procedures of a speech and language management program. Her focus on communication competency, in addition to the more traditional speech and language therapies, reflects much of her own work over the years and her recognition that the communication needs of children are more complex than had heretofore been realized.

The core of any management program of the mainstreamed hearing-impaired child must be the regular classroom. It is the classroom teacher who is faced with the child for most of the school day. The chapter on classroom management was contributed by Laraine Conway, who brings to it many years of experience as a regular, special, and resource room teacher. Hers is a practical response to "What do I do now?", the frequent plaint of regular classroom teachers confronted with a hearing-impaired child for the first time.

Finally, in the management section, Sue Schwartz discusses the psycho-social implications of mainstreaming. At the conference on which this book is based, her presentation and her topic elicited more intense responses from the audience than any other. As I interpret the relevant literature, there is little doubt that mainstreaming appears to have favorable academic and communication implications; children who are mainstreamed score higher on academic achievement and linguistic measures than comparable children who are not mainstreamed. But this is not the entire story. We must not ignore the psycho-social implications of mainstreaming. To achieve superior scores on academic and linguistic measures at the cost of a negative self-image and an unhappy childhood is not a good trade. Dr. Schwartz discusses this issue and suggests what can be done to improve the psycho-social status of mainstreamed hearing-impaired children.

The five chapters on exemplary programs include more than simple descriptions of the programs. Each of the authors in this section describes different approaches, problems, and issues in the mainstreaming process. The programs represent a range of options, within each of which the educational challenge is different and involves variations in the degree of actual mainstreaming.

The Toronto program, described by Dorothy Boothroyd-Turner encompasses the regular schools in the city of Toronto. Her focus is on the *appropriateness* of a particular placement for a specific child. She describes several mainstreamed children, and discusses their performance and ability to function within a regular classroom. As she rightly points out, mainstreaming is not for everyone. Any educational placement for a child, and particularly any shift in a current placement, must be justified and rationalized in objective terms.

Donald McGee describes a program in Fairfax, Virginia that explicitly recognizes that hearing-impaired children do not constitute an undifferentiated homogeneous mass. Although successful *individual* mainstreaming can most easily be effected when a child demonstrates the necessary oral skills (as Dr. Northcott points out), in the Fairfax program a number of mainstreaming options are provided. Children who utilize modes other than oral communication can benefit from the increased offerings in a regular school, and learn and profit from the interactions with normal-hearing students. In this program, we see the economies of scale. The children have opportunities for selective mainstreaming, combining both access to the regular program and the support of other hearing-impaired students.

A different approach is described by David Manning. In his program at the Clarke School for the Deaf, Dr. Manning describes the intense preparation for mainstreaming offered to their graduates, and the gamut of support services provided to these children. Some of these services are directed toward the children, and others focus on the regular school staff. Both foci are necessary in a support program. The direct services are time-limited, no more than several hours a week, whereas the in-service component has management implications throughout the child's school day. The telephone and the computer are used liberally for follow-up purposes. Not the least of the noteworthy aspects of this program is the organized and comprehensive data collection system by which performance of the children is described and continuously tracked.

The next two chapters remind us that the hearing-impaired children we see in preschool, elementary, and high school eventually grow up and that many go on to higher education. William E. Castle, Director of the National Technical Institute for the Deaf (NTID), describes the relationship of NTID to the Rochester Institute of Techology (RIT) and how this relationship permits and fosters the integration of the hearing-impaired students at NTID with normal-hearing students of RIT. NTID is a school for severely and profoundly hearing-impaired students who use sign language as the major mode of class communication. For these students to take advantage of the offerings and atmosphere of RIT, it is necessary to provide interpreters, notetakers, and other support personnel in the regular classrooms. Dr. Castle describes how this can be accomplished effectively. He also makes another point that deserves restating: the value of the relationship between NTID and RIT students goes in both directions; the education and experiences of normal-hearing students are also enriched by this association (as evidenced by the superior offerings of the Theatre Department at NTID).

Carol Flexer and Denise F. Wray are concerned with functionally hard-of-hearing college students. They report on the program they organized at the University of Akron. What is particularly interesting is that the need for such a program became clearly apparent only *after* it was organized. As professors in the Communication Disorders department, they were aware that some hard-of-hearing students were having problems in college. The extent of their difficulties became clear after these authors began working closely with students. When I first read their publications on the program, I was both horrified and elated. Horrified that in the late 1980s our hard-of-hearing college students were so ill-served, and elated that a focused remediation program could be so successful. We *can* make a difference and this chapter describes just how it can be done.

A prerequisite for making a difference with hearing-impaired students, at any level of education, is knowledgeable and informed professionals. Antonia B. Maxon reviews the rationale and content of in-service training programs. She develops the concept of the "Individual In-service Plan" (IIP) wherein the informational content necessary to manage a specific child's needs serves as the training mechanism to teach general management principles, and she outlines a multilevel modular approach to in-service training. The likelihood of a successful mainstream program for any particular child must relate to the training, knowledge and skill of professionals dealing with that child. Without an ongoing in-service training program, a successful mainstreaming program is questionable.

Ann Geers provides us with some of the pay-off information. She reports on a study that evaluated the academic and communication performances of 100 orally educated, profoundly hearing-impaired children. Most of these children are currently being educated in mainstream settings. She relates their performance to the ages at which they were mainstreamed, and to the performance of children in special settings and to normal-hearing children. For those of us familiar with the "expected" accomplishments of profoundly hearing-impaired children, their scores are a revelation. And what they were able to do should be even more possible for children with lesser degrees of hearing loss.

We can look at a child's accomplishments in academic and communication areas and conclude that the placement was (or was not) a successful one for a particular child. Just looking at test scores, however, does not tell us the human cost of the mainstream experience. In her chapter, Ruth Green reviews the responses of three parents and three mainstreamed students to questions that she posed. No one who is in a position to make educational recommendations regarding hearing-impaired children can afford to ignore the kind of information these respondents provide. The parents tell us about their anxieties, their fears, and their uncertainties, and how these continued, ebbing and flowing, for years and years.

The former students, all articulate and clearly successful academic products, tell us about the battles and distress they felt over the years in reaching their present level. None of them was sorry they went through the process although several had some doubts about whether they would want to go through it again, knowing what they know now. Their challenge to us, in the interests of future generations of children, is that the advantages of the mainstream process be realized for them without the penalties of social isolation and personal unhappiness. We must learn from the past.

My charge, in the last chapter, is to provide a perspective about the past, present, and future. I briefly review some of the highlights in the history of mainstreaming, in the early nineteenth century and in our pre-P.L. 94-142 modern era. I also take the opportunity to review some interesting research studies and some of the outstanding issues to reinforce and extend some of the ground covered earlier.

I close with what I term the "Mainstreaming Bill of Rights," composed of ten statements and principles that, in some form or other, have been discussed and presented in the preceding chapters. I make no claim to offer original insights. Rather, these points represent a distillation of what, in my judgment, are the most significant conclusions, cautions, and recommendations that can be made about the process of mainstreaming hearing-impaired children. I elaborate on each chapter and, in this way, present my own point of view and suggestions to our successors. One thing we can be sure of, however, is that the "last word" on the topic of mainstreaming has yet to be written.

Acknowledgments

This book could not have been written without the active cooperation and support of the personnel of the New York League for the Hard of Hearing. Beyond the specific contributors to the book who are associated with the League, there was the staff in the Development office who helped organize the conference on which this book is partially based. Manuel Cuenca, Joe Brown, and Caroline Johnson, professionals all, took the inevitable glitches and problems in stride and ensured that the proceedings went smoothly. The assistance of the Metropolitan Life Insurance Company, who supported and hosted the conference, is gratefully acknowledged. Their unstinting help reminds us that human faces do reside behind the facade of large corporations.

My special thanks to Ruth Green who, besides being a contributor to the book, is the Executive Director of the New York League for the Hard of Hearing. She has fought for the rights of hearing-impaired children for all the years she has been associated with the League. Her insistence that the welfare of the children is our foremost reponsibility permeates the working atmosphere of the League.

In many books, one sees an acknowledgment to the spouse for the support given the author during the laborious task of editing or writing the book. In my case, my appreciation extends much beyond keeping the home fires burning smoothly while the book was being worked on. My wife Helen, an experienced professional in her own right, was an active partner in the editing of the book. She edited the chapters and tried to ensure that the authors met her high standards in content and writing. Any deficiencies in these areas occurred only when we ignored her advice.

Mark Ross

Chapter • 1

Mainstreaming:
Roots and Wings

Winifred H. Northcott

The political climate of the early 1970s was volatile. A groundswell of outrage and protest by civil rights protesters highlighted the reality of discrimination against handicapped individuals in every aspect of daily living. The eloquence of personal testimony by the victims and advocates for reform captured front page headlines and editorial support in the media. There were poignant scenes of protesters grouped on the steps of the Capitol in Washington and in front of barrier-laden university and corporate buildings. "I am a human being: do not spindle, fold or multilate," read the sign borne by a demonstrator in a wheelchair.

The issue of civil rights for the disabled, including the handicapped, led to a studied analysis of society's prevailing attitudes, stereotypes, and myths about the handicapped. In the instance of deafness, certain oft-repeated generalizations became themes with variations presented to the public, to state legislatures, and to the Congress of the United States:

Hearing-loss equals deafness, which implies sign language.
When a deaf child is born, he is part of two families: his nuclear family and the deaf community.
Deafness is absolute—irreversible.
The deaf child or youth requires a critical mass of other deaf persons to feel comfortable and supported.
To speak and to be educated in regular classes is to deny one's deafness.

In the 1970s the identified goal of public school education was world citizenship: encouraging self-control, open-ended discussion, and questioning time-honored tenets by which the world was governed. John Dewey, acknowledged leader of the progressive movement in education a half-century earlier, would have applauded. As a philosopher and advocate of "child-centered education" and the "student-centered classroom," he warned that we cannot seriously reform our schools without substantial reform of our society (Gummere 1988).

LEGAL GUARANTEES FOR HANDICAPPED PERSONS

In not-so-rapid succession, Congress responded to the appalling evidence of discrimination by passing three historic pieces of legislation that describe a philosophy as well as a specific "bill of rights" for the disabled. This legislation assures every handicapped person the earned right to equal opportunity in every dimension of activity: education, social services, training and employment, and government benefits.

Public Law 94-142: The Education for All Handicapped Children Act (1975)

Addressing the unmet need for individualized services and programs for all handicapped children and youth, Congress legislated and described the procedural safeguards governing the *process* of determining educational placement for each individual child based on a *difference,* not a *deficit* model. It requires state and local education agencies (LEAs) to submit formal written plans and written procedures for approval in order to:

> . . . assure that to the maximum extent appropriate, handicapped children, including children in public or private institutions or other care facilities, are educated with children who are not handicapped, and that special classes, separate schooling or other removal of handicapped children from the regular educational environment occurs only when the nature or severity of the handicap is such that education in regular classes with the use of supplemental aids and services cannot be achieved satisfactorily (20 U.S.C. 1401 et seq.).

The burden of proof shifted to the local district of the child's residence to demonstrate that he or she could not be "appropriately" programmed in the mainstream, either in a neighborhood school with support services or by means of contract with a local community agency or institution.

Under the 1978 amendments to Title II of the Elementary and Secondary Education Act, which address *human rights, oral communication* is formally identified as the fourth basic skill in addition to reading, mathematics, and written communication. "It is the declared right of every child in the public schools of America to receive formal instruction in the basic skills of *speaking* and listening" (Dublinske 1979). Nowhere does it proclaim, "Except for the deaf."

Section 504 of the Rehabilitation Act of 1973

Early in 1977, after immense pressure from consumers and advocates, regulations were published and assigned to the Office of Civil Rights for prosecution in cases of discrimination against the handicapped by recipients of federal Health, Education, and Welfare (HEW) funds. These regulations forbid discrimination against otherwise qualified handicapped individuals.

A portion of the regulations implementing Section 504 deals exclusively with preschool, elementary, secondary, and postsecondary education. They are formula grant programs under which local school districts receive money for education of the handicapped; funds can be withheld in cases of demonstrated discrimination (Northcott 1984; Tucker 1984). State and local plans describe the continuum of alternative educational settings and the procedures to follow in case of parent-school-team disagreement. The monitoring teams of state and federal officials are interested in the *process* by which parents and staff are informed of educational alternatives rather than in the statistics of how many children are integrated into regular classes.

A Comprehensive Position Statement: CED

The Executive Board of the Council on Education of the Deaf (CED) affirmed by unanimous vote on June 23, 1986 the principles that are central to P.L. 94-142. The CED is composed of the membership of the Alexander Graham Bell Association for the Deaf, the Conference of Executives of American Schools for the Deaf, and the American Instructors of the Deaf. The Resolution was reaffirmed on December 10, 1979, published in professional journals and newsletters, and distributed to the membership of the three participating organizations.

The Resolution on Individualized Educational Programming for the Hearing Impaired (Deaf and Hard of Hearing) (1976) formally recognized the legal mandate to administrators of public education programs to provide individualized instruction and services to hearing-impaired students of school age without exclusion, and stated that "no single method of instruction and/or communication (*oral* or *total communication*) or educational setting can best serve the needs of all such children." The resolution identified these major aspects of such instruction and services:

the educational setting ranging from partial or full-time regular classroom placement to partial or full-time educational programs of-

fered in a special class in public/private day schools or public/
private residential schools,

the method of instruction and instructional strategies which shall be
employed during the school day, and

the need for continuing monitoring, assessment and modification/extension
of each school age child's program including method of instruction and educational setting as his or her changing personal, social
and instructional needs dictate.

Public Law 99-457: Early Intervention Program for Infants and Toddlers with Handicaps: Final Regulations

The Final Regulations for P.L. 99-457 were established under the 1986
amendments to the Education for the Handicapped Act of 1969. They
assure that states that apply for funds are mandated to:

Integrate infant/preschool programs, 0–5, in the continuum of case
management and coordinated services for children and youth of
school age—0–21.

Require by 1993 a current Individual Family Service Plan (IFSP) in place
for every eligible child and the child's family.

Interact with medical and health providers in a multidisciplinary approach to integrated and coordinated services.

Contract or arrange for services with medical, health, and education
providers.

Replace the term "handicaps" with the term "children eligible for this
part."

Shift from remediation to prevention of developmental delay in one or
more of the following basic areas of behavior: cognitive development; physical development, including vision and hearing; language and speech development; psycho-social development; self-
help skills.

MAINSTREAMING: AN HISTORICAL PERSPECTIVE

"Those who cannot remember the past are condemned to repeat it."
George Santayana, *The Life of Reason* [1905–1906], vol. 1

Impressions in Retrospect

In order to understand the roots of *mainstreaming* as we interpret it today as a concept, a philosophy, a direct service option, and a legislative
reality, it is necessary to take a backward glance at what was euphe-
mistically called "the field of education of the deaf."

The decades of the 1930s, '40s, and '50s were considered halcyon days, although there were few innovations in education. There were creative teachers of the deaf, group hearing aids, and supportive parents. The sureness of the etiology of deafness (congenital or childhood illness) gave comfort to parents and teachers; it was later documented by Jensema (1974) that in those days there was a significantly lower incidence of additional handicapping conditions.

The audiogram was the major basis for educational placement of a deaf child in a detection, labeling, and sorting process in which remnants of residual hearing were ignored. Hearing aids were often sold in drugstores or in the "notions" section of department stores. Hearing aid evaluations were conducted in private and community clinics, and the prescription for an individual hearing aid was hand-carried to a local hearing-aid dealer (Ross 1986). The generic term, *hearing-impaired* (*deaf* or *hard of hearing*), gained gradual acceptance in the 1970s; its neutrality carried no automatic prediction as to the educational setting or mode of communication in which a child or youth would communicate. Throughout those decades, educational alternatives were few: public and private oral schools for the deaf, oral classes housed in a regular public elementary school, or enrollment in a state-supported residential school as a daily commuter ("day pupil") or boarding pupil. In the last instance, the oral method of communication and instruction was common for all entering children until they reached the second or third grade, when a two-track program—either *pre-vocational* or *academic*—went into effect on the basis of individual assessment. Children in the former program communicated via the *simultaneous* (*combined*) method of instruction, which added fingerspelling and American sign language to speech and speechreading.

Children generally stayed in the same school setting from kindergarten through 12th grade. Adventitiously deafened and many hard-of-hearing students generally received their education in classes for "the deaf" and often became the natural leaders and proponents of the separate entity of the deaf community with sign language as its unifying force (Meadow 1975).

Following World War II, many of the superintendents of these state-supported residential schools were recruited from the ranks of engineering and industry. A majority of these well-educated men ("the Old Guard," with a token woman or two among them), had been awarded honorary doctorates by Gallaudet College (now Gallaudet University) and used the title, Doctor. An eminent colleague observed in a formal address at a convention of the Alexander Graham Bell Association for the Deaf that many were "long on political acumen and short on administrative skills" (Connor 1986).

Within the traditional nuclear family, the expectations of deaf and of hearing parents ran high. Alumni of oral schools spoke about these expectations at assembly meetings of the entire school body. One distinguished graduate, Dr. Edwin W. Nies[1] (Lexington '07; Gallaudet '11; University of Pennsylvania Dental School '14), said in part in 1934:

> You all know the importance of preparation in any kind of test. Athletes prepare for a race. A team prepares for a big game. You prepare for examinations by reviews, extra study, etc. My preparation for eight years of college and a doctor's diploma came from this same school as you now attend, and with fewer advantages. There was no rhythm work then although one teacher of speech had begun to use a guitar to help in her work. Speech takes many years to learn, the only place to learn it is in school. An employer's attitude is important. He knows you come from an oral school. He expects you to speak and read the lips. In this busy age, there is no time to write. Learn to speak as well as you possibly can. Keep your mind alert, receptive and retentive (Nies 1934, commencement address).

In the traditional pattern of those decades, mothers stayed at home and reinforced the work of the schools as it was conveyed at parent-teacher-alumni meetings that served as social events as well. Fathers went to work but attended PTA meetings routinely. Together with alumni, as volunteers in sports, scouting, or church-related activities, they assured the active acceptance of many deaf children and youth in integrated play and learning environments outside of the school day. In the absence of early psychological support to parents, they realized the truism: "Parents learn from each other."

Certification

Prior to 1965, certificates were issued for various *classes* of teachers and related to professional preparation as *academic* or *vocational* teachers, with or without a degree. The "one size fits all" concept prevailed (e.g., K–12). The "goodness of fit" between an individual teacher's competencies and vacancy(ies) was in proportion to the size and resources of the school district or the public or private residential and day school.

Each teacher of the deaf was also a speech teacher by virtue of having completed one three-credit course at an established teacher training program, a course entitled, The Teaching of Speech to the Deaf. In traditional schools formal lipreading lessons (speechreading) were commonplace, and a vocabulary of nouns and action verbs was presented to nursery age children still in the play-learning stage of de-

---

[1]Edwin Nies, D.D.S., is the late father of the author. He served concurrently, for 37 years, as the school dentist at Lexington School for the Deaf, New York City, (an oral school) and at the New York School for the Deaf, White Plains, New York (a manual state school). "Wasn't he schizophrenic?" asked a young graduate student recently. "No, he was a truly integrated individual," was the reply.

velopment. The cardinal principle of adult-child interaction was "Wait until the child looks at you and then begin to speak." "Diagnosed as deaf . . . and trained to remain so" is the predicted outcome for many children, observed Michael Reed, former Director of the Inner London Authority.

Amplification

When I began teaching, amplification in the classroom consisted of group headsets and hearing aids mounted on a wooden frame. Each child was "wired for sound" and also anchored to his seat, except for special speech work at the teacher's side. A pupil could always disrupt the current lesson by exclaiming, "I hear nothing!" Sound engineers made only periodic visits for repairs, except in well-established centers where they enjoyed resident status.

A HOLISTIC APPROACH TO LANGUAGE LEARNING

"Take care of the sense, and the sounds will take care of themselves."
Lewis Carroll, *Alice's Adventures in Wonderland*

Children gradually acquire functional receptive and expressive language in a global way when teachers weave life experiences of children into active language learning that challenges higher level thinking. Consider these verbal demands: "How can we find out? What do YOU think happened? What does it remind you of?"

Alexander Graham Bell, a teacher of speech to the deaf, understood this and wrote his own stories for seven-year-old Georgie Sanders (Bell 1873). These stories demonstrate how his pupil could learn to modulate his voice by attending to the heavier script writing and closely spaced phrases in portions of full, descriptive sentences (e.g., in this instance, about the *Bear and her Cubs* [see figures 1 and 2]).

Open-ended questions encourage reading for comprehension; they help children make inferences and use solid reasoning. For Dr. Bell and Georgie, oral communication was natural and so was turn-taking, cooperative discussion, and formal speaking, each of which fell into place naturally. Gerogie was taught to *see* it (through speechreading), *say* it, *write* it, *refine* it (with help), *read* it, and *think*—a progressive way to learn in 1874.

Master Teachers and Conceptual Thinkers

Edith Buell (1934), Mildred Groht (1958), and Edith Fitzgerald (1923), who developed the key for grammatical correction, were the triad of

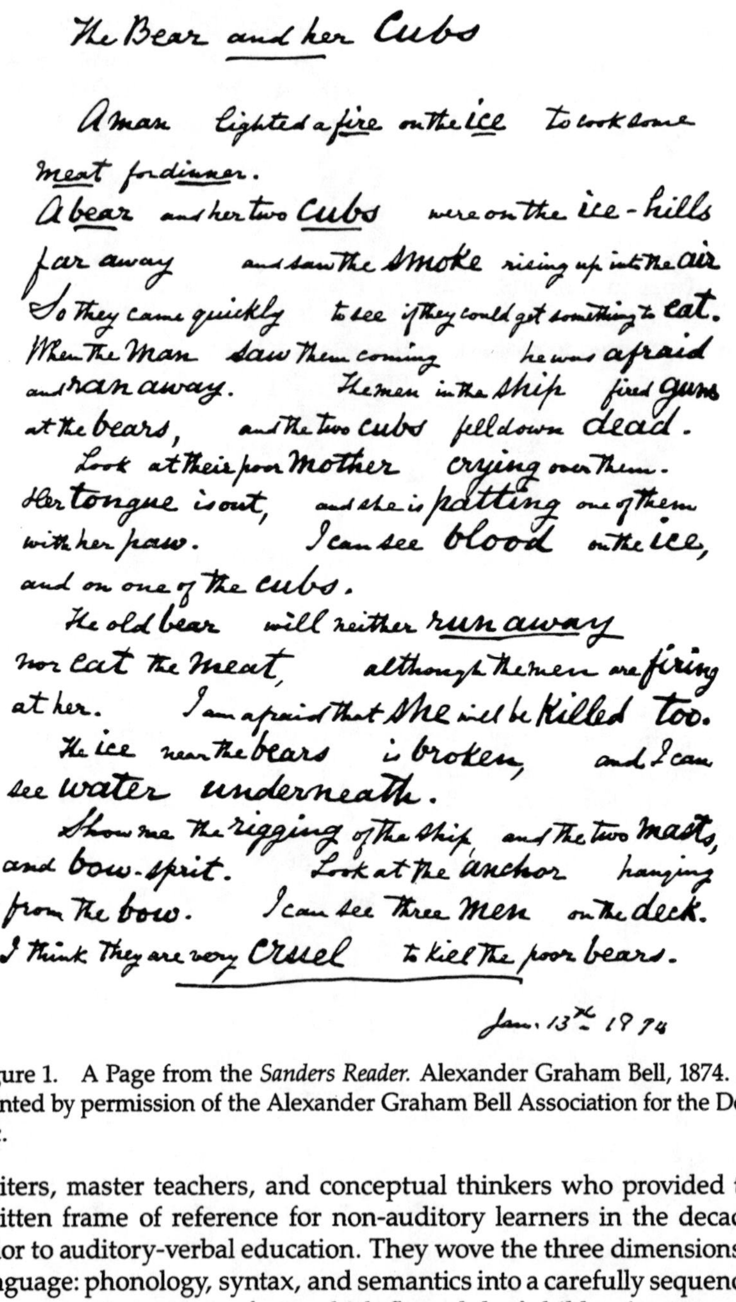

The Bear and her Cubs

A man lighted a fire on the ice to cook some meat for dinner.

A bear and her two Cubs were on the ice-hills far away and saw the smoke rising up into the air. So they came quickly to see if they could get something to eat. When the Man saw them coming he was afraid and ran away. The men in the ship fired guns at the bears, and the two cubs fell down dead.

Look at their poor Mother crying over them. Her tongue is out, and she is patting one of them with her paw. I can see blood on the ice, and on one of the cubs.

The old bear will neither run away nor eat the meat, although the men are firing at her. I am afraid that she will be killed too.

The ice near the bears is broken, and I can see water underneath.

Show me the rigging of the ship, and the two masts, and bow-sprit. Look at the anchor hanging from the bow. I can see three men on the deck. I think they are very cruel to kill the poor bears.

Jan. 13th 1874

Figure 1. A Page from the *Sanders Reader*. Alexander Graham Bell, 1874. Reprinted by permission of the Alexander Graham Bell Association for the Deaf, Inc.

writers, master teachers, and conceptual thinkers who provided the written frame of reference for non-auditory learners in the decades prior to auditory-verbal education. They wove the three dimensions of language: phonology, syntax, and semantics into a carefully sequenced language arts program, from which flowed deaf children's mastery of academic subjects and increased interest in reading independently for information and pleasure. Repitition and refinement of functional spoken language for active living, laced with ingenuity, was woven around

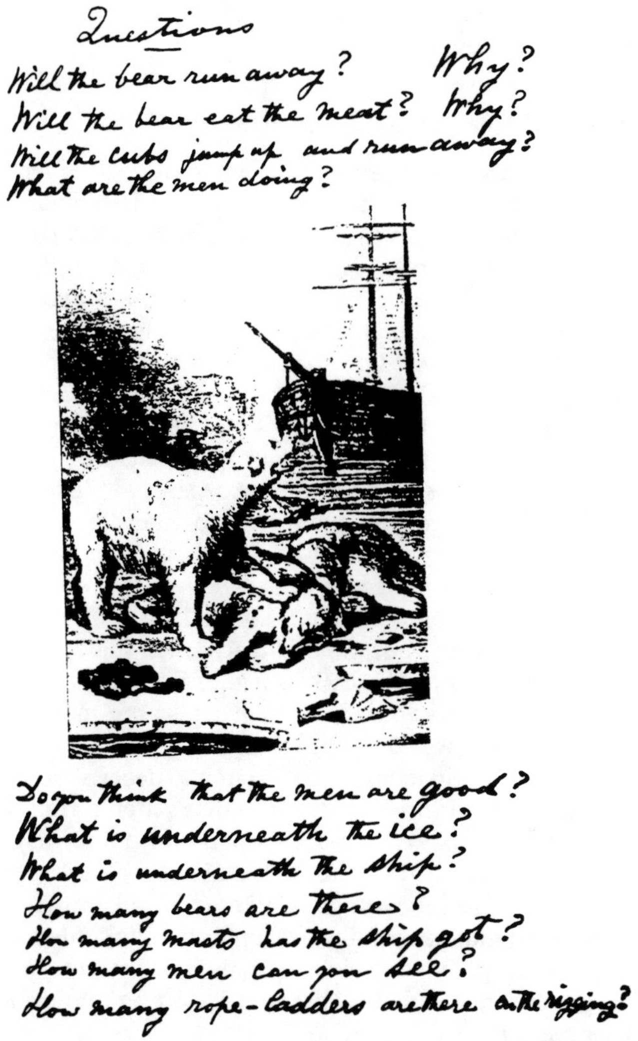

Questions

Will the bear run away?   Why?
Will the bear eat the meat?   Why?
Will the cubs jump up and run away?
What are the men doing?

Do you think that the men are good?
What is underneath the ice?
What is underneath the ship?
How many bears are there?
How many masts has the ship got?
How many men can you see?
How many rope-ladders are there in the rigging?

Figure 2. A Page from the *Sanders Reader* by Alexander Graham Bell. Reprinted by permission of the Alexander Graham Bell Association for the Deaf, Inc.

children's experiences. The process meant that a structured teacher and an unstructured child could enjoy true communication, sharing thoughts and feelings in a natural, spontaneous, individual way as modern as the holistic method of approaching language learning today.

Woodward (1988) points out that these visual-oral children with profound hearing losses were the mainstay of oral classes until the middle of the 1960s when auditory-verbal techniques for language learning started to become commonplace and "many of them are oral education's conspicuous successes."

Parents and Oral Deaf Adults: A Powerful Team

Beginning in 1964 a series of national and international conferences addressed the educational needs of hearing-impaired infants (Davis 1965). The National Advisory Committee on the Education of the Deaf, whose Chairman was Homer Babbidge, insisted that an adequate system of public school education must include "programs to facilitate language and speech preparation for children as young as one to two years of age" (*Education of the Deaf* 1965, p. 2).

The charge was issued in 1967, at the National Conference on Education of the Deaf, that "the 0–3 group should be considered a special entity within the preschool category with specialists for this subgroup actively recruited and specialized training organized" (*Education of the Deaf* 1967, p. 77). However, it was noted that for many of the children in existing preprimary programs, ages three to five, the curriculum generally consisted of "simplified versions of elementary school practices or of unstructured free play" (*Education of the Deaf* 1967, p. 7).

In response, project directors and teachers in the Demonstration Home Projects, funded by the U.S. Office of Education, convened in 1968 to discuss current educational practices in the management of deaf infants. Nowhere was the dimension of support to parents in the *affective* domain addressed: that is, counseling to deal with the tension, anger, and emotional barriers that prevented parents from bonding with their hearing-impaired children upon the initial diagnosis of hearing loss (Northcott 1971; McConnell 1968).

The process of having parents of older children and youth guide young parents of audiometrically deaf infants highlighted the overarching philosophy of Dr. Althena Smith, the late psychologist at John Tracy Clinic, Los Angeles, who observed, "Getting into *motion* takes the E out of *emotion.*"

Formal self-help groups of parents were highly visible for several decades prior to the passage of P.L. 94-142. Oral hearing-impaired adults who were well educated, well spoken, and confident—with a wide variation in speech intelligibility—participated in joint planning of workshops and retreats for new parents grappling with the problem of coping with hearing impairment in their children. Their differences in life style, social and economic status, and their wry humor were an inspiration; their effectiveness as role models was invaluable in helping re-shape parental ambition and expectations for their young children as auditory-verbal candidates for assimilation in the mainstream in later years (Findore 1984).

Professional specialists—audiologists, speech pathologists, social workers, and teachers—participated in the many conferences held. They and other participants began to examine the system of delivery of educational services: the absence of role specialization in the schools; the impact of myths and stereotypes about deafness on educational placement of children and youth; the sanctity of the audiogram in educational decision making; and standards for certification of teachers and administrators. Oral deaf adults spoke from experience about family adaptations, sibling relationships, career choices, and social isolation/integration.

Many parents showed confusion, grief, and anger. "There's nobody to go to." "For years I sought answers from experts. Then my child went to school and I discovered I was the resident expert." There was a groundswell of outrage: "We demand partnership in educational decisions made unilaterally for our children." At home, the consequences of mismanagement were borne by families in restless silence. "For the common good" of all hearing-impaired children was the underlying philosophy of self-help groups. *Options* and *choices* were the premises, including the mode of communication best suited to each child's demonstrated abilities and preference. Reasonable compromises were possible in those decades; organized political pressure was not yet a contributing factor.

Gradually, national coalitions of parents and advocates, working across single disability lines, drew up a geneal blueprint for educational opportunity for all children and youth with special needs (an improvement over the label "handicapped"). A new era was dawning. P.L. 94-142 had become a reality.

MAINSTREAMING: PHILOSOPHY . . . PRACTICES . . . PROBLEMS

"For parlor use, the vague generality is a life-saver."
George Ade, *Forty Modern Fables, The Wise Piker*

"General notions are generally wrong."
Lady Mary Wortley Montagu,
A letter to Wortley Montagu, March 28, 1710.

Webster's *New Collegiate Dictionary* defines *mainstream* as a "prevailing current or direction of activity or influence." As P.L. 94-142 is interpreted today, mainstreaming is a goal, a concept, a philosophy undergirding the principle of educating all children with disabilities in regular schools. A synonym is *integration,* whose operational definition in this instance is physical placement with children and youth in regular classes: to integrate into a large unit. The missing link is the concept of *assimilation:* to absorb into the cultural tradition of a population or group; to take in and absorb as nourishment, which implies that children with disabilities have the right to the greatest amount of integration appropriate to their unique needs.

The Cascade of Special Education Services

The original hour-glass model by Deno (1970) was appropriate as it indicated that the largest number of hearing-impaired children and youth required the least number of special services and thus constituted Level I (see figure 3). Today, this vertical figure would be turned horizontally to indicate a smorgasbord of options and alternatives for an individual child according to his or her unique academic, social, and emotional needs. Fluidity of movement from one setting to another with appropriate support services resulted in two basic classifications of children leaving nursery and preschool programs: *coming back* to regular classes via the IEP in later years, following initial kindergarten placement in special classes; and *never leaving:* those who progressed into regular kindergarten and first grade for all or part of the school day.

Access to or opportunities for participation in activities in the school environment may be *physical,* in terms of placement in a regular class; *social,* with the help of teachers, aides, and non-disabled peers; *academic* or *community,* in sites that offer opportunities for learning practical life skills.

Why Integration? Why Mainstreaming?

Administrators, teachers, and parents recognize the heterogeneity among children with an educationally significant hearing loss. Due in part to the low incidence of deafness in the school age population and to the fact that only limited alternatives can be maintained in many small cities or single school districts, regionalization of services via a county or intermediate school district has become an increasingly practical and political expedient. A comprehensive regional delivery system assures the availability of two separate methods of instruction in two separate but equal "tracks," designed to meet the individual needs of all pupils enrolled: (1) students learning by the *auditory-verbal* or *visual-oral* method under the philosophy of oralism and (2) students learning via the *combined* or *simultaneous* method of communication (a form of sign language and finger-spelling in addition to speech, audition, and speechreading) under the philosophy of *total communication.* In a national questionnaire across educational settings, an analysis showed clearly that children, teachers, and parents do not use both

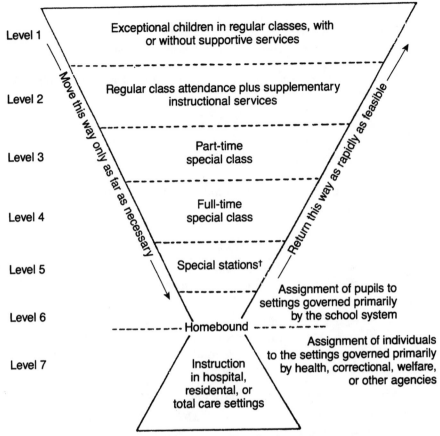

†Special schools in public school systems

Figure 3. The cascade system of special education services (Deno 1970). Reprinted by permission of the Council for Exceptional Children from *Bulletin, Exceptional Children* March 1973 39:495.

speech and signs at the same time in communication with each other (Jensema and Trybus 1978). When the use of speech is high, the use of signs is low—and vice versa. One channel furnishes linguistic information, the other becomes so much "noise" (Carson and Goetzinger 1975; Gaeth 1967; Gates 1970; Goetzinger 1974; Goetzinger and Proud 1975; Titus 1978).

When asked why students with hearing impairments should attend regular schools, one parent replied, "It's a hearing world." The TAPP Project, Technical Assistance for Parent Programs, Massachusetts, (Taylor et al. 1987, p. 29) has identified seven major goals in response to the hypothetical question:

Why Integrate?

To prepare for life in society: "the real world."

To learn from others: children learn from observation and motivation to imitate.

To have normal experiences: the vibrancy and excitement of regular schools.

To change attitudes; overcome prejudices, increase frequency of contact.

To teach democracy: the best way is to practice it.

To make friends: the bonds of commonality can foster natural relationships.

To challenge exclusions: "are special schools merely a form of societal prejudice?"

The Advantages . . . from the Point of View of:

The hearing-impaired student him or herself: (Northcott 1973; Connor 1986; Schildroth and Karchmer 1986; Luterman 1986; McCartney 1987; Atkins 1987; Stoker and Spear 1984)

I am a person first, and then I have a disability.
I learn to take risks . . . to contribute in discussion.
I talk to my peers as equals . . . I think big and we dream together.
I know who I am and where I stand.

Parents of hearing-impaired children and youth:

I have a clearer picture of my child's abilities and limitations through comparative observation.
He is not further handicapped by abnormal surroundings.
Friendships with hearing peers develop in an unselfconscious way.
Friendships with parents of hearing classmates are based on common problems and satisfactions related to age and interests.

Hearing peers of hearing-impaired students:

I've figured out that labels about deafness are "pretty far out."
It's a two-way street. I get help in math as a swap for my help in their tough subjects.
Perfect speech doesn't "cut it"; ignoring frustration and taking advantage of opportunities to work and socialize does.

Parents of hearing classmates:

Greater appreciation of individual differences.
Advantageous role for my child, as a helper and friend.
Casual or intense association with parents of special needs children is of mutual benefit.

Teacher in a regular classroom:

In-service training has helped me gain confidence and competence in relating positively to my hearing-impaired students.

Gain an aide who helps special needs students hold their own.

Increase in my range of competencies in creative teaching.

Richness of class discussion due to diversity of experience and backgrounds.

Satisfaction in seeing student(s) meet or surpass Individualized Education Program (IEP) objectives.

Some Predictors of Success in the Regular Classroom

In the early years, oral education was seen as the key to later regular class placement. Infant-preschool programs routinely included placement in regular nursery schools for many youngsters. The ability to speak for one's self and be understood was central to the prediction of assimilation for a majority of children in the neighborhood school with hearing peers (Northcott 1971; Simmons-Martin and Calvert 1979; Jensema, Karchmer, and Trybus 1978; Connor 1986). The characteristics of students assimilated in the regular classroom include:

Higher percentage of college-educated parents
Higher income families
Attendance in family-oriented infant/preschool programs
Higher proportion of white students.

The characteristics of the students include:

Early fitting of hearing aids (binaural, when recommended)
Early family-oriented infant/preschool programming
Auditory-oral approach to language learning (dynamic use of aided residual hearing), in contrast to *visual-oral*
An inductive approach to rule learning (e.g., holding out a cookie and cracker and offering a phrase for modeling, "That one, please.")
Regular nursery school placement, around the age of three, with special education support
Speech as the primary method of communication (Jensema 1974, 1977; Jensema, Karchmer, and Trybus 1978; Jensema and Trybus 1978; Luterman 1986; McCartney 1987; Stoker and Spear 1984).

Comments

Public Law 94-142 mandates the process of individualized educational programming for hearing-impaired (deaf and hard-of-hearing) children. Homogeneous grouping in special classes is a vital option: children may be taught by the *oral* method or the *simultaneous* method. "In the mainstream" to the extent appropriate, is a major goal for every child—for some children however, the special class or school may be the least restrictive alternative.

Deafness today is not absolute or irreversible. Deafness does not automatically equate with an uncoupling from the world. The dimensions of deafness are several, and each is significant:

Medical—audiometric deafness
Educational—a functional definition
Social—where one finds one's identity
Economic—stereotypes enter in
Political—improved and expanded services for the members of the deaf community.

This is the formal definition of the term *deaf* as reported to the President and Congress of the United States:

> We also use the term deaf to refer to all persons with hearing impairment, including those who are hard of hearing, those deafened in later life, those who are profoundly deaf, etc (*Toward Equality* 1988, xi).

This definition makes it easy to overlook the need for heterogeneity in treatment and placement for the population of hearing-impaired students. In addition, one finds children enrolled in the public state schools with one, two, and three additional educationally handicapping conditions beyond their deafness (Schildroth and Karchmer 1986).

THE SERVICE DELIVERY SYSTEM: SURPRISES AND SETBACKS

Public Law 94-142 mandates an appropriate education for a hearing-impaired child or youth—not the best education possible as court cases show. Schools are heavily involved in procedural issues related to parent involvement in special education planning for the child. An Individualized Education Program (IEP) is developed at a team meeting to which parents are invited, with an advocate if they wish. They are then required to sign the plan if they concur.

The steps in the Parent Appeal process are a second, torturous sequence of interaction between parent and school staff; when differences cannot be resolved locally, suit is brought in federal district court because of the federal law involved (P.L. 94-142).

A Summit Meeting

In the fall of 1989, President Bush convened his Cabinet and the state governors in Washington to address reform goals for the country's schools (*Time* 1989). The concensus goals included:

The need for more federal support for the prekindergarten education process.

Identification of stringent regulations to facilitate disbursement of federal funds for creative programming.

Open enrollment for parents to choose which public schools their children may attend.

Alternative certification for specialists in subject matter areas (e.g., biology, mathematics, vocational skills) for those moving into a teaching career from the workplace.

Most vital to parents and hearing-impaired students in school, President Bush and the governors agreed on "restructuring" the educational system via more local control: specifically, letting individual schools be run by a triad of teachers, parents, and administrators rather than by consultants and bureaucrats in the less personal, regional state Departments of Education, or legislative capitals.

Implications for Local Direction

The establishment of national priorities for educational reform in the public schools of America is invaluable in helping to shape the nature of state reform, as well. Review of the professional competencies required of today's special education consultants in State Departments of Education will lead to significant modifications in certification standards in the near future. Too often the state consultant on speech-language and hearing conservation is a speech pathologist, with minimal preparation or experience in individualized programming for the hearing-impaired school-age population.

Pre-service education of special education teachers will be expanded to include required courses in curriculum and instruction related to normal child growth and development, language acquisition, and practicum in integrated settings. The demand, in some states, by superintendents of public residential schools, that their schools become centers for the diagnosis, assessment, and referral for all children with hearing loss in the state will be subsumed within the larger question across disabilities. Can a statewide diagnostic/referral center render objective decisions while continuing to operate a direct-service educational program as well?

In earlier decades, a Rainbow Coalition forced civil rights legislation for the disaffected; now, expanded local control will permit the exploration of talents and the redesign of curricula to benefit students of diverse cultures and educational settings. Mathematics and science fairs, increasingly popular, are illustrations of equal opportunity for approval through achievement of hearing-impaired students.

Support Specialists

The teacher of the deaf no longer "owns" the deaf child nor is he or she in charge of the student's comprehensive program; in team staff meetings for an individual child, this education specialist is just one member of the multi-disciplinary team.

The regular classroom teacher is a vital member of this team. He or she requires in-service orientation to the presenting characteristics of varying styles and abilities of hearing-impaired students. The professional growth experiences (e.g., lectures, workshops, observation) should be provided by special education teachers and support specialists who believe in mainstreaming and recognize that not all hearing-impaired students require all the special education services available. They will describe ways in which the special teacher may visit in the regular classroom with minimal disruption to all. I am reminded of a cartoon showing two school boys reporting on the content of their box of Valentines. "I got a Valentine from my speech therapist, my psychologist, my behavior mod specialist . . . " and the other boy remarked, "Gee, I wish I lisped."

Orientation of the regular classroom teacher can change attitudes and stereotypes and alter initial impressions. "I can't understand him and he can't understand me. He never takes his eyes off me." We do not always hold people accountable for inappropriate behavior: administrators and hearing-impaired students themselves are included.

The interpreter is the newest support specialist. The assumption is that some students in part- or full-time regular classes may require the services of an *oral interpreter* or a *sign language interpreter* for a portion or all of the school day.

The hearing-impaired student will determine whether *transliteration* (a literal repetition of the speaker's remarks) or *interpretation* (the incidental or substantial re-wording of an original spoken message) is preferred (Northcott 1984; Brill 1981; Castle 1984).

The membership of the Registry of Interpreters for the Deaf (RID), the national evaluation and certification organization, voted at its 1989 Convention that the certification for oral interpreters, at all levels of competence, is a separate certification process and not a specialty certificate requiring sign langue proficiency and sign language transliteration as prerequisites. There have been no formal evaluations by the RID of candidates for oral interpreting certification since 1986; professional preparation of oral interpreters is currently limited to a single course in a few federally funded training centers that specialize in sign language interpreter preparation. Short-term workshops for parents and teachers of oral children and youth are growing in popularity. On regular college and university campuses, hearing classmates of hearing-impaired students are similarly prepared as paraprofessionals to assist in seminars and academic classrooms, convocation, and mediated lectures, as requested. The accommodation is to the hearing-impaired consumer; the problem lies with speakers who diminish speechreading potential because of an immobile upper lip, full beard, blackboard presentations, or classroom habits like pacing.

Regular classroom teachers, administrators, and often the hearing-impaired student and his or her hearing classmates are not necessarily familiar with the process of integrating the oral or sign language interpreter into daily classroom activity. This unfamiliarity can limit cooperation. Fall orientation week is a logical time to help teachers and administrators understand the use of interpreters.

In the development of an Individualized Education Program (IEP), written guidelines are required to determine the role and function of an interpreter as a member of the multidisciplinary team jointly involved with parents in the development of an IEP. Can service be given at a social school-related function? Is the oral or sign language interpreter formally listed among available support specialists in the school system? Can an interpreter testify about a student's daily functioning in the classroom in that individual's absence? Perhaps most critical of all—in addition to holding national or state certification by a formal interpreter evaluation/certification body—is the interpreter professionally certified as a teacher or tutor of academic subjects?

The Missing Links

The current system of educational management of the hearing-impaired infant, child, and youth is based on a *difference* and not a *deficit* model of direct service. Parents know their "rights" that take the form of procedural safeguards in joint parent-staff development of the IEP mandated by P.L. 94-142: parental approval and sign-off are safeguarded. The parental appeal process is a vital part of each state's written plan.

How foreign to the general informality of earlier years when a parent and teacher exchanged opinions, sought advice, and drew fresh thoughts about the child they cared about jointly. Parents today face at times a multidisciplinary team of many members. When an uncertain parent adds a parent advocate to the planning meeting, it can compound the adversarial atmosphere. Federal laws can catapult a case into Federal district court. P.L. 94-142 rulings in court say that placement does not need to provide the best education, but must be of educational benefit and include appropriate support services. An open-ended listing of links that are lost or altered in the current system might include:

Close to home:

The pivotal role of the teacher of the hearing impaired, who no longer "owns" the child

The special class or resource room for the *visual-oral* child within the neighborhood school

The oral or sign language interpreter in the classroom: lacking teacher certification to function as a tutor or notetaker.

At the State level:

The "persuasion" of the state consultant for the hearing impaired

The federally funded statewide in-service workshops for teachers of the hearing impaired

The regulations and policies governing the certification, position responsibilities and salary range of the oral or sign language interpreter.

At the National level:

The public residential school, facing declining enrollment and changing nature of students, many of whom can be classified as multi-handicapped, is desperately seeking a new role as the center for statewide assessment, diagnosis, and referral for all hearing-impaired children

The Office of Demographic Studies of Gallaudet University: The Annual Survey of Hearing-Impaired Children and Youth in special classes and schools is no longer reflective of achievement test scores and performance levels of most children in the mainstream; these children are generally lost to the special education count

Networking and Justice Advocacy. The action role of advocate for the common good is increasingly assumed by formal technical assistance projects underwritten in whole or part by federal funds: e.g., Parent Advocacy Coalition for Educational Rights, Minnesota (PACER); Parent Education and Assistance to Kids, Colorado (PEAK); Technical Assistance for Parent Programs, Syracuse University, New York (TAPP).

PARENTS AND FAMILIES

"All had rather it were well for themselves than another."
            Terence, *Andria*, Act II, Scene 5, Line 15, *c*. 185–159 B.C.

Families today are in transition, and commitment takes different forms. There is a convulsive change in moral and social values in our society. Families face the reality of separation and divorce; two career parents; single parents; POSSLQs (People of opposite sex sharing living quarters); the WOOPIES (Well-off older people who may shrug off the role of grandparent). In other families, the pervasive influence of alcoholism and drug abuse may render some families dysfunctional. For many children, an impersonal home atmosphere places enormous stress, beyond deafness, on their shoulders.

In earlier decades, prior to the passage of P.L. 94-142, families of hearing-impaired children joined state organizations to press for educational change through workshops and retreats. They identified priorities to be met through lobbying of state legislators on behalf of their deaf and hard-of-hearing children. Today, the delivery of educational services is individualized and support specialists are available to supplement classroom instruction for children identified as having special needs in various academic subject areas. Parents, in turn, have reverted to a concentration on their own family and child/children who have special education needs. "For the Common Good of All Hearing-Impaired Children" is no longer the rallying cry. Options and choices of educational settings and curriculum content are available in the public schools. As one parent stated in an IEP staff meeting, "Lady, tell me what your specialty is and I will tell you what you can do for my child and for me."

Parents today aren't just looking for solutions, they want *energy* to guarantee some kind of helpful relationship with teacher and school, to guarantee some kind of continuity in traditional, mutual support. They know a multidisciplinary team is no substitute for effective parenting. Yesterday's surety about the known etiology of hearing loss has frequently given way to the reality of "unknown" cause today. It jars the confidence of parent and teacher alike: predictability for the pure, "deaf-only" child is gone.

WHERE DO WE GO FROM HERE?

Open Enrollment Expands Family Choices

Open enrollment in public schools is a reality in an increasing number of states, gaining advocates and visibility today. Minnesota was the first state to legislate an open enrollment policy that allows students and families to select the best school experience from kindergarten through 12th grade. The opportunity to visit schools outside the district, to ask questions and compare, and to select a match between an individual child's interests, abilities, and needs and the best array of support services for a hearing-impaired child, means greater freedom of choice, options, and opportunities.

Alternative Means of Acquiring Credentials

New Jersey is opening up a new avenue for thousands of men and women with "real world" experience in the corporate world and the general marketplace to become teachers at the high school level. Chemists in manufacturing, for example, can take equivalency examinations to demonstrate their range of competencies, which means breaking the monopoly of the traditional teacher-training institutions. It is an exciting forward direction in teacher certification.

The Neighborhood School Itself

The age-old partnership of the family and the school has returned; once again it embraces the local school board, the local Parent-Teacher-School Association and the neighborhood school. The principle that parents, working together, can improve their own lives and the quality of education in the local system, is a democratic one.

The academic achievement of hearing-impaired children well placed in the regular school and classroom is not in question. Subsequent chapters will document this carefully. Creative approaches to programming for children in rural areas are needed: models are available that involve Sunday through Thursday night foster-home placement, with social, medical, and health agency help available.

Hand Over the Reins to Students—
ALL Students—in the Mainstream

Through their own creative ideas in student council and lunchroom encounters comes practice in cooperation and joint planning and added self-respect. The hearing-impaired student may function as a peer or a cross-age tutor, or be tutored in turn: acquaintances on the next block or same bus route can become friends.

Only when the hearing-impaired student finds out where he or she looks for self-esteem as an individual, finds ways to feel secure within, and learns to separate his or her identity from the physical setting in which learning takes place, only then will he or she truly have the freedom of choice P.L. 94-142 promises. Let us stop measuring the value of education by the degree of integration it offers. Ask, instead, "Where is one particular child finding his identity, being curious, competitive, and turned on by school? Where is his best friend? And a bunch of other friends? Where, indeed?"

SUMMARY[2]

Mainstreaming is the act of being in the flow of life: an active process of learning to cope with the whirlpools, the eddying currents and the tranquil moments that are found in daily living among a cross-section of humanity. Whether an interlude or an enduring environment for *hearing-impaired children and youth*, it will help to shape their dreams, knowledge, and understanding and they will never be the same again.

We lose the integrity of education of the hearing-impaired through deliberate separation of children who are capable of functioning in the mainstream in varying degrees. It is society's loss, as well.

We can restore that integrity. We can restore it through honest and united efforts to end the physical exclusion from their neighborhood school. Hearing-impaired children, youth, and adults capable of challenge *can* be assimilated into equal membership in society. The degree of deafness is no longer a barrier.

It is our challenge to provide the way through application of advanced educational practices. The enabling laws exist; the regulations are in place.

REFERENCES

Ade, G. 1901. The Wise Piker. *Forty Modern Fables.* New York: Harper.

Atkins, D. V. (ed.) 1987. Families and their hearing-impaired children. Monograph. *The Volta Review* 89:5.

Bell, A. G. 1873. *The Sanders Reader.* Washington, DC: Alexander Graham Bell Association for the Deaf, Inc.

Brill, R. G. 1981. The mythology of interpreters for deaf elementary pupils. *The Deaf American* 33:17–18.

Buell, E. M. 1934. *Outline of Language for Deaf Children.* Book 1. Washington, DC: The Volta Bureau.

Carroll, L. 1960. *Alice's Adventures in Wonderland.* New York: New American Library, Penguin.

Carson, P. A., and Goetzinger, C. P. 1975. A study of learning in deaf children. *Journal of Auditory Research* 15:73–80.

Castle, D. L. 1984. Effective oral interpreters: An analysis. In *Oral Interpreting: Principles and Practices*, ed. W. H. Northcott. Baltimore: University Park Press. (Distributor: Washington, DC: Alexander Graham Bell Association for the Deaf, Inc.)

Connor, L. E. 1986. Oralism in perspective. In *Deafness in Perspective*, ed. D. M. Luterman. San Diego: College Hill Press.

Davis, H. (ed.) 1965. The young deaf child: Identification and management. *Acta Oto-Laryngologica:* Supplement 206.

Deno, E. 1970. The cascade of special education services. Bulletin. *Exceptional Children* 39:495.

---

[2]This Summary is the blend of thoughts of two friends, in harmony: LaFawn Biddle and Winifred Northcott.

Dublinske, S. 1979. Standards for effective oral communication programs. *Language, Speech, and Hearing Services in Schools* x:195–202.

Education of the Deaf. 1965. A report to the Secretary of Health, Education, and Welfare by his Advisory Committee on the Education of the Deaf. Washington, DC: The U.S. Department of Health, Education, and Welfare.

Education of the Deaf: The Challenge and the Charge. 1967. A Report of the National Conference of Education of the Deaf, April, 1967, Colorado Springs, CO.

Findore, M. 1984. Self-help in the mainstream. *The Volta Review* 86:99–107.

Fitzgerald, E. 1923. Technical language work in the primary department. *The Volta Review* 25:203–214.

Gaeth, T. H. 1967. Learning with visual and audiovisual presentations. In *Deafness in Childhood*, eds. F. McConnell and P. J. Ward. Nashville: Vanderbilt University Press.

Gates, R. R. 1970. The differential effectiveness of various modes of presenting verbal information to deaf students through modified television format. Unpublished doctoral dissertation. University of Pittsburgh.

Goetzinger, C. P. 1974. Psychological considerations of hard of hearing children. In *The Speech Clinician and the Hearing-Impaired Child*, ed. R. L. Cozad. Springfield: Charles C Thomas Co.

Goetzinger, C. P., and Proud, G. D. 1975. The impact of hearing impairment upon the psychological development of children. *Journal of Auditory Research* 15:1–60.

Groht, M. A. 1958. *Natural Language for Deaf Children.* Washington, DC: Alexander Graham Bell Association for the Deaf, Inc.

Gummere, R. M. 1988. He's back. *Columbia* April:223–27.

Jensema, C. J. 1974. The relationship between academic achievement and the demographic characteristics of hearing-impaired children and youth. Monograph: Series R, Number 6. Office of Demographic Studies. Washington, DC: Gallaudet College.

Jensema, C. J., and Trybus, R. J. 1978. *Communication Patterns and Educational Achievements.* Monograph: Series T, No. 2. Washington, DC: Gallaudet College.

Jensema, C. J., Karchmer, M. A., and Trybus, R. J. 1978. *The Rated Speech Intelligibility of Hearing-Impaired Children: Basic Relationships and a Detailed Analysis.* Series R, No. 6. Washington, DC: Gallaudet College, Office of Demographic Studies.

Luterman, D. M. (ed.) 1986. *Deafness in Perspective.* San Diego: College Hill Press.

McCartney, B. 1987. Factors contributing to the lives of the hearing impaired: Perspective of oral adults. *The Volta Review* 89:325–39.

McConnell, F. 1968. *Proceedings: Current Practices in Educational Management of the Deaf Infant (0–3 Years).* Nashville, TN: Bill Wilkerson Hearing and Speech Center, Vanderbilt University Press.

Meadow, K. P. 1975. The deaf subculture. *Hearing and Speech News* 43:16–18.

Nies, E. W. 1934. Commencement address. Lexington School for the Deaf, New York, NY.

Northcott, W. H. 1971. Infant education and home training. In *Speech for the Deaf Child: Knowledge and Use*, ed. L. E. Connor. Washington, DC: Alexander Graham Bell Association for the Deaf, Inc.

Northcott, W. H. 1973. *The Hearing-Impaired Child in a Regular Classroom: Preschool, Elementary, and Secondary Years.* Washington, DC: The Alexander Graham Bell Association for the Deaf, Inc.

Northcott, W. H. (ed.) 1984. *Oral Interpreting: Principles and Practices.* Baltimore:

University Park Press. Distributor: Washington, DC: Alexander Graham Bell Association for the Deaf, Inc.

Ross, M. 1986. A perspective on amplification: Then and now. In *Deafness in Perspective*, ed. D. M. Luterman. San Diego: College Hill Press.

Santayana, G. 1905. *The Life of Reason*, Vol. I. New York: Scribner.

Schildroth, A. B., and Karchmer, M. A. (eds.) 1986. *Deaf Children in America*. San Diego: College Hill Press.

Simmons-Martin, A., and Calvert, D. R. (eds.) 1979. *Parent-Infant Intervention: Communication Disorders*. New York: Grune and Stratton.

Stevenson, B. (ed.) 1956. *The Home Book of Quotations*, 8th ed. New York: Dodd, Mead and Co.

Stoker, R. G., and Spear, J. H. (eds.) 1984. Hearing-impaired perspectives on living in the mainstream. Monograph. *The Volta Review* 86, 5:1–107.

Taylor, J., Biklen, D., Lehr, S., and Searl, S. J. 1987. *Purposeful Integration: Inherently Equal*. Syracuse: Center on Human Policy, Syracuse University.

Terence. *Andria*. Act II, Scene 5, Line 15.

Titus, J. R. 1978. The comparative effectiveness of presenting spoken information to postsecondary oral deaf students through a live speaker: An oral interpreter and an interpreter using signed English. Unpublished doctoral dissertation. University of Pittsburgh.

Toward Equality: Education of the Deaf. 1988. A Report to the President and the Congress of the United States. The Commission on Education of the Deaf. Washington, DC: U.S. Government Printing Office.

Tucker, BL. P. 1984. Interpreter services: Legal rights of hearing-impaired persons. In *Oral Interpreting: Principles and Practices*, ed. W. H. Northcott. Baltimore: University Park Press. Distributor: Washington, DC: Alexander Graham Bell Association for the Deaf, Inc.

Woodward, H. 1988. What about non-auditory learners. *Interchange* 4–6. International Organization of Educators of the Hearing Impaired.

Chapter • 2

Audiological Evaluation of the Mainstreamed Hearing-Impaired Child

Jane R. Madell

The audiologist has several responsibilities in managing hearing-impaired children in addition to the obvious one of evaluating the degree and type of hearing loss. The most important may be the provision of appropriate amplification. Regardless of the educational system in which a child is placed, optimum use of residual hearing is critical for maximizing a child's functioning. The audiologist is responsible for providing the hearing-impaired child with sufficient acoustic information so he or she can maximize auditory perception. This is accomplished through the appropriate fitting of personal and classroom amplification and assisting the child, parents, and school personnel in managing the amplification.

THE BASIC AUDIOLOGIC EVALUATION

Every audiologic evaluation has as its first goal the determination of degree and type of hearing loss. Even if a child has had many previous hearing evaluations, the basic information needs to be obtained again at each evaluation. For some children, hearing changes over time as the result of hereditary factors, disease, or unknown causes. For others, ear infections may cause a temporary hearing loss that requires medical care to be resolved. In any case, changes in hearing status need to be identified so that appropriate medical and habilitative services can be provided.

Pure Tone Tests

The basic evaluation includes air and bone conduction testing. For very young children, techniques need to be used that will encourage the child's cooperation. (This book deals with school age children so techniques for children under age three are not discussed. For further information on younger children refer to Madell [1988], Hodgson [1978], and Northern and Downs [1984].) Play audiometry is a useful technique for children aged two to five or six years. Because the child would probably be uninterested in raising his or her hand when a sound is presented, the audiologist makes a game of the task by asking the child to put a toy in a bucket, a ring on a ringstand, or to build a tower with blocks when a sound is heard. By changing toys frequently, it is possible to keep a child's attention and obtain the required information.

Air conduction testing reveals the degree of hearing loss. This is determined by averaging the thresholds obtained at 500, 1,000, and 2,000 Hz. Audiograms with thresholds falling between 25–40 decible hearing level (dBHL) are considered mild hearing loss; thresholds between 40–55 dBHL are considered moderate hearing loss; thresholds between 55–70 dBHL are considered moderately-severe hearing loss; thresholds between 70–90 dBHL are considered severe hearing loss, and greater than 90 dBHL indicates profound hearing loss (see figure 1).

Type of hearing loss is determined by the relationship between test results obtained with earphones (air conduction) and with a vibrator placed behind the ear on the mastoid bone (bone conduction). If bone conduction testing is in agreement with air conduction testing, the hearing loss is sensorineural (caused by damage to the inner ear). If bone conduction testing indicates normal hearing and air conduction testing indicates that there is a hearing loss, then the hearing loss is conductive (caused by damage to the outer or middle ear). It is possible to have a mixed hearing loss—a hearing loss that has both conductive and sensorineural components. Most conductive hearing losses are treatable medically, and most sensorineural hearing losses are not. All hearing-impaired children need medical evaluation as part of the evaluation process to determine if any part of their hearing losses are treatable medically. For children with temporary or permanent conductive components to their hearing losses, ongoing otologic treatment is indicated.

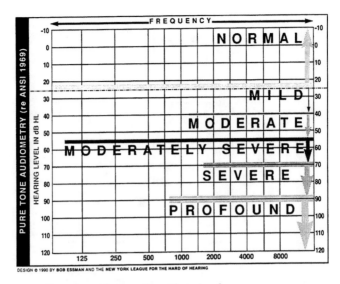

Figure 1. Audiogram with severity of hearing loss.

Immitance Testing

Immitance testing is a part of every basic audiologic evaluation. It pro-vides information about the functioning of the middle ear and about the possible presence of fluid, a retracted eardrum, or a break in the ossicular chain, to name a few possibilities. This information, along with pure tone testing, is of great assistance to physicians in diagnos-ing and treating hearing-impaired children and adults. The two major components of the immitance test battery are tympanometry and acoustic reflex testing.

Tympanometry is an objective technique for measuring the mobil-ity of the tympanic membrane as a function of variations in air pressure in the external auditory canal. The changes in air pressure are plotted on a graph called a tympanogram. An eardrum is most mobile when the air pressure on both sides of the eardrum is equal. In this case the tympanogram will show a Type A curve (see figure 2). A cold or a throat infection may block the air flow through the Eustachian tube causing the pressure on both sides of the eardrum to become unequal. If this continues for an extended period of time, fluid can build up in the middle ear resulting in a Type B curve. A type B curve is also found in ears of patients with otitis media, congenital malformations of the middle ear, perforations in the eardrum, ventilating tubes in the ear-drum, and ears clogged with cerumen. When a Type B tympanogram is present, otologic evaluation is indicated. Type B is an advanced form of Type C (see below).

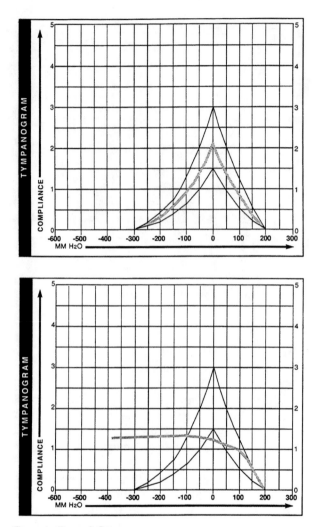

Figure 2.   Type A, B, and C tympanograms.

Type C tympanograms are found when the pressure on both sides of the eardrum is unequal. The eardrum may be mobile, but the peak movement of the drum is at a negative pressure of −200 deca Pascal (daPA) or greater rather than at the normal pressure of 0 daPA. This situation is present when a child is developing or recovering from a cold, or when Eustachian tube functioning is poor. A child with a Type C tympanogram should be retested within a few days to monitor the progress of middle ear functioning. If the Type C tympanogram con-

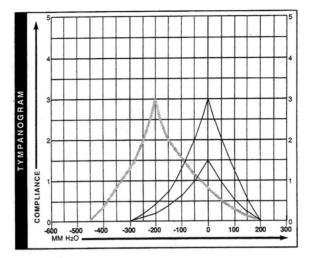

Figure 2. *continued*

tinues for an extended period of time or a Type B tympanogram develops, otologic evaluation is indicated.

The second component of the immitance test is a test for the acoustic reflex. The acoustic reflex is the contraction of the stapedius muscle in the middle ear that occurs when a loud sound is present. It normally acts to protect the ear from loud sounds. In normal ears, an acoustic reflex is present between 70 and 100 dB above the normal threshold for tones. Reflexes are not likely to be present with sensorineural hearing losses greater than 60 dB or when active middle ear pathology is present. Reflex levels may change with certain disease processes such as growth of an acoustic tumor. Acoustic reflex testing is used to confirm pure tone test results as well as to assist in diagnosis of certain neurological conditions.

Speech Audiometry

Speech audiometry provides the most critical information about a hearing-impaired child's functioning and ability to use audition. How much speech a child is able to understand is more critical in terms of everyday functioning than the ability to hear pure tones. It is essential that every attempt be made to tax a child's listening skills by measuring auditory functioning in a variety of different ways. Only by fully diagnosing a child's speech perception skills are we able to select appropriate amplification, as well as to provide the information needed by the speech-language pathologist, teacher of the hearing-impaired child, and classroom teacher for the planning and provision of habilitative services.

Frequently, audiologists, speech-language pathologists, and teachers of hearing-impaired children assume that a child will not be able to perform a difficult auditory task simply because of the child's degree of hearing loss. These professionals may not test speech perception or may use tests that are too simple for the child's capabilities. As a result too few demands are placed on the child's listening skills resulting in a child who does not maximize his or her auditory functioning. This assumption may have a more negative effect on the child's functioning than does the degree of hearing loss.

Speech Awareness Threshold: The initial task in speech audiometry, especially for very young chlidren, is the speech awareness threshold (SAT). The question asked is "at what hearing level does the child first respond to sound." We are not asking if the child understands it—simply does he or she hear it. Most speech stimuli are acoustically broad band frequency stimuli. When a child responds to "Hi, David" at 45 dB, we only know that he or she has heard some part of that acoustic message at 45 dB. We do not know what part it is. The child may have heard the low frequencies of the vowels or the consonant /d/, or the higher frequencies of /h/. In order to get a better picture of the contour of a child's hearing loss, it is helpful to use speech stimuli that assess awareness at specific frequency bands. Using low and high frequency phonemes can help do that. Obtaining thresholds for /ba/ or /bu/ will provide information about low frequency hearing. Thresholds for /ʃ/ will provide information about mid-high frequency hearing, and /s/ will provide information about high frequency hearing. Even in the absence of other speech test information, these types of responses make it possible to know whether or not speech information is received at a loud enough level to be useful for speech perception. Ling (1978) suggested using the phonemes [/a/, /i/, /u/, /ʃ/, and /s/] to determine if a child is receiving auditory information throughout the frequency range required for perception of speech. The test can be performed by the audiologist, speech-language pathologist, classroom teacher, or parents as a way of checking on a child's functioning. The clinician says the sounds in random order and asks the child to repeat them. The child's ability to repeat them demonstrates that he or she has heard them. Testing at different distances allows the clinician to know at what distance the child is able to hear each sound.

Speech Reception Threshold: The next speech audiometry task is the Speech Reception Threshold (SRT). The SRT is the lowest level at which a child can understand 50% of spondees (two syllable words with equal stress on both syllables). The test words should be familiar to the child. In preparing for this test, the audiologist may tell the child which words are going to be used or may ask the child to point to pictures. The SRT should be close to the child's average pure-tone hearing level. If the child has a sloping hearing loss, the SRT will be closer to the best threshold (the frequency at which the softest threshold is found) than to the pure tone average. If the child does not have the language to use standard spondees, a nonstandard test can be performed using familiar words, familiar objects, or body parts. The fact that a child cannot do the standard task does not eliminate the need to obtain some information about the child's threshold for speech.

Word Recognition Testing: Word recognition testing (i.e., speech discrimination, the ability to understand speech) provides the most useful information in determining how well a child will function in following normal conversational speech. If the goal of the evaluation is to assess a child's functioning in a regular classroom, it is necessary to make the listening task as close to normal as possible. If we can test with the recorded word lists used for adults we should do so. This may not be possible for several reasons: the child may not have the vocabulary, the child's speech may not be sufficiently clear to allow the tester to understand it, or the child may not have the speech perception skills necessary to perform the task. Therefore, it will be necessary to modify the procedure in order to obtain the required information.

If the test limitation is simply one of inadequate vocabulary, then using a test with a simpler vocabulary, such as the Phonetically Balanced Kindergarten Test (PBK) (Haskins 1949), or use of the word lists from the Word Intelligibility for Picture Identification (WIPI) (Ross and Lerman 1970) or Children's Hearing in Pictures (CHIPS) (Elliot and Katz 1980) would solve the problem. If the child's poor articulation is the problem, the child can write down the words if he or she has that ability, use the words in sentences, or the tester can employ a picture pointing test such as the WIPI or the CHIPS. Modifications, however, change the interpretation of the test results. Writing errors may be confused for perception errors. Language problems may affect the child's ability to make up sentences. A picture pointing task, while eliminating some of the other problems, is a closed-set task (there is only a limited number of choices), as opposed to an open-set task in which the stimulus may be any word. We can expect, therefore, that the child will obtain a much higher score than would be obtained in an open-set task. The Isophonemic Word List (Boothroyd 1984) is useful for assessing and identifying specific perception errors. Words are read to the child who is asked to repeat them. The child's responses are recorded phonemically. Evaluation of the errors allows the clinician to identify areas needing remediation, either by modifying the amplification or through therapy.

Table I lists the available word recognition tasks from the easiest to the most difficult. If a selected task turns out to be too difficult, an easier one can be attempted. On the other hand, if the child does very well on a task, the audiologist should attempt a more difficult one in an attempt to come closer to assessing the child's functioning in normal conversation. Figure 3 shows test results for a particular child on a number of different word recognition tasks. This figure shows that test selection has a significant effect on how the child performs. It is frequently necessary to use more than one test to get the full picture of a child's abilities.

Table I.   Speech Audiometry Tasks in Order of Difficulty from Easiest to Most Difficult

Awareness/Detection
   Voice
   Music
   Ling 5-sound test (/a/, /i/, /u/, /ʃ/, /s/)
   Syllable Identification (1 vs. 2)
Thresholds
   Numbers
   Body Parts
   Familiar Objects
   Spondee Objects, Pictures, or Words
Word Recognition
   Closed Set Discrimination
      Numbers (vowel recognition)
      Body Parts
      Familiar Pictures
      NU Chips
      WIPI
      Alphabet Test
   Open Set Discrimination
      NU Chips Words (without pictures)
      WIPI Words (without pictures)
      PBK
      W22 or NU6 Monitored Microphone Voice
      W22 or NU6 Recorded
      Isophonemic Word Lists (Boothroyd) (Phoneme recognition)
      Sentences
      Connected Discourse

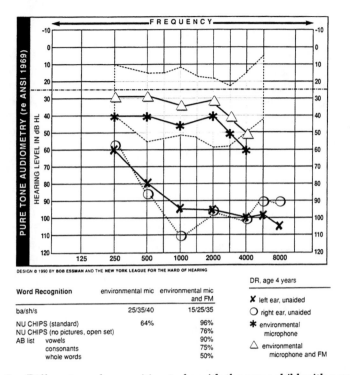

DESIGN © 1990 BY BOB ESSMAN AND THE NEW YORK LEAGUE FOR THE HARD OF HEARING

DR, age 4 years

Word Recognition	environmental mic	environmental mic and FM
ba/sh/s	25/35/40	15/25/35
NU CHIPS (standard)	64%	96%
NU CHIPS (no pictures, open set)		76%
AB list vowels		90%
consonants		75%
whole words		50%

✗ left ear, unaided
○ right ear, unaided
✳ environmental microphone
△ environmental microphone and FM

Figure 3.   Different word recognition tasks with the same child with a severe to profound hearing loss.

Test Conditions: Speech audiometric testing should be conducted under earphones to determine the functioning of each ear. Word discrimination should be performed at a comfortable loudness (usually 40 dB above the SRT). It is sometimes necessary to test at several different loudness levels to find the level that provides the best results (known as the phonetically balanced [PB] max). In addition, it is necessary to test the child without earphones in situations more typical of every day functioning. To accomplish this, testing is performed in the sound-field. In this condition, the speech signal emanates from a loudspeaker located in a sound-treated room.

Testing should be performed at a normal conversational level (50 dBHL) to determine how the child will function under ordinary listening conditions. If the child does well at the normal conversational level, testing should be repeated at a soft conversational level (35 dBHL) to assess the child's ability to hear when the speaker is at a distance or speaking softly. Next he or she can be tested at a normal conversational level with competing noise present to simulate functioning in a classroom setting. (Four talker complex noise is a good stimulus to use as a noise source because it makes a difficult listening situation.) Testing can be conducted with speech and noise equally loud (signal-to-noise [S/N] level of 0 S/N) or with speech slightly louder than noise (+ 6 S/N). If the child has no hearing aids or if the child has a mild or moderate hearing loss, testing will be attempted without amplification.

If the child has amplification (a hearing aid or FM system), word recognition testing needs to be repeated at normal and soft conversational levels in each amplification condition—that is, with the hearing aid worn monaurally, binaurally, and with the FM system. By testing each ear separately, it is possible to determine whether both hearing aids are functioning well, whether one needs to be modified, or whether the child performs better with only one aid than with two. (While this latter occurrence is extremely rare, it sometimes happens.)

Test results at soft conversational levels in quiet and with competing noise are useful in predicting how well a child will function in a classroom. If a child scores poorly at quiet levels and in the presence of noise, it is fairly certain that the classroom will be a difficult listening situation. The testing will demonstrate the need for amplification in general and the need for an FM system specifically (see figure 4). Repeating the testing, with an FM system, will demonstrate the advantages that such systems can offer.

AMPLIFICATION

Selecting Amplification

Ling (1984) has stated that the selection and use of appropriate amplification may be the single most important habilitative tool available to a hearing-impaired child. With that in mind, there are certain basic assumptions about amplification for children that assist in forming our procedures for selection.

1. Any child whose unaided hearing evaluation (including speech recognition testing in quiet and in the presence of competing noise) indicates less than optimal functioning in any listening condition should be considered a candidate for amplification. This includes children with mild and unilateral hearing losses (Bess, Tharpe, and Gibler 1986).
2. The main purpose of amplification is to permit the hearing-impaired child to use his or her residual hearing for perception of speech. Therefore, ability to perceive speech needs to be the major consideration in the selection of amplification.
3. The amplification system of choice is not dependent on hearing loss per se, but on the characteristics of the child and the communication environment in which he or she functions. Although a

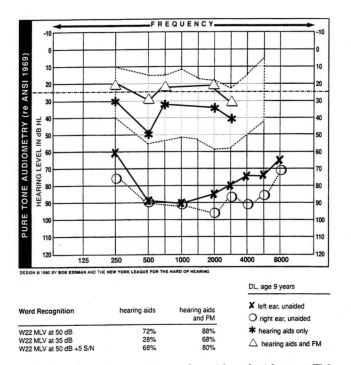

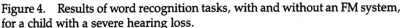

Word Recognition	hearing aids	hearing aids and FM
W22 MLV at 50 dB	72%	88%
W22 MLV at 35 dB	28%	68%
W22 MLV at 50 dB +5 S/N	68%	80%

DL, age 9 years

X left ear, unaided
O right ear, unaided
* hearing aids only
△ hearing aids and FM

Figure 4.   Results of word recognition tasks, with and without an FM system, for a child with a severe hearing loss.

child may perform well enough with a particular hearing aid in quiet at normal conversational levels, it may not be reasonable to expect that child to function that way in his or her daily living situations. In these situations noise will almost always be present and the intensity of the speech stimulus will often vary. Information about the child's listening abilities in different conditions should be part of the determination of the type of amplification system selected.

4.   Nearly all hearing-impaired children will benefit from classroom use of FM amplification in addition to personal amplification, because even the best classroom is not a good acoustic environment.

Type of amplification is an important factor to consider. Behind-the-ear (BTE) hearing aids are the most common ones selected for children. They have the advantage of being adjusted easily as information about auditory function changes, and if appropriately selected, are compatible with FM systems. However, for very small ears frequently it is difficult to increase the volume with a BTE hearing aid without getting feedback. In-the-ear (ITE) hearing aids that are popular with adults usually are not good choices for children. Children's ears grow fairly rapidly, necessitating frequent remakes (a new mold built around the electronics). This is not only expensive, but during the remake the child will be without amplification. In addition, ITE aids are usually not FM compatible, which will make it difficult for the child to use classroom amplification. Teenagers who resist using BTE hearing aids may be good candidates for ITE ones. However, the problems of compatibility with classroom amplification should not be overlooked with this population.

Body worn amplification is a good choice for some hearing-impaired children, especially for young children with severe and profound hearing losses. These are especially useful when used with FM systems. Because the microphone is on the chest rather than on the ear, it is possible to turn the hearing aid louder, thus making better use of the maximum capacity of the hearing aid without getting feedback. In addition, the body itself tends to increase the low frequency response of the aid, which is very useful for children with severe and profound hearing losses in early auditory training activities. Other advantages include an enhanced ability for the child to monitor his or her own voice, because of the location of the microphone, and enabling the child to take control of his or her amplification, because the various controls are easier to adjust. The use of an FM transmitter by the parent, therapist, or teacher increases the amount of auditory information the child can receive by eliminating the problems of distance and background noise. At the New York League for the Hard of Hearing we have been fitting FM systems as primary amplification on preschool children with severe and profound hearing losses for eight years and have been very impressed with the results (Madell 1988; Madell and Brackett 1989).

Characteristics of the Amplification System

The purpose of an amplification system is to facilitate learning by audition. It is the responsibility of the audiologist to demonstrate the value of the appropriate amplification system to the child, the family, and the school personnel. The amplification system, at a minimum, should have the ability to modify frequency response, gain, and output. Frequency response refers to the relative amount of amplification a hearing aid produces at different frequencies. Some aids have a flat frequency response, meaning that they amplify all frequencies equally, whereas others may amplify high frequencies more than mid or low frequencies. Gain refers to the amount a hearing aid amplifies a signal it receives. (If a 60 dB signal is delivered to the hearing aid and it is output at 90 dB, then the hearing aid has a gain of 30 dB.) Maximum output is the greatest sound level that a hearing aid is able to produce.

Once this is reached, the hearing aid will not amplify further, no matter how much sound is presented. As the child's function changes and as more information about a child's hearing becomes available, it should be possible to modify these dimensions to provide the child with the most useful auditory information.

All hearing aids for children should have audio-input capabilities (the ability to be directly connected to an FM system) and a strong telephone coil (the magnetic coil in the hearing aid to pick up signals from a telephone or tele-loop of an FM system to facilitate use with FM systems. See Chapter 7). In addition, the amplification system should be sufficiently flexible to accommodate varied communication styles of parents, clinicians, and teachers. It should be simple to use, durable, and free from interference from other systems. Finally, it should be cosmetically acceptable to the child, parents, and teacher. Please note that cosmetic acceptability is the last criterion listed. Although we understand that the only useful amplification system is one that is worn, our experience has indicated that if it is possible to demonstrate that one system is significantly better than another, it will usually be accepted. If the child does not use audition as a major avenue for reception of langue, or if it is not possible to demonstrate a significant difference in function between types of amplification, then cosmetics will be a major factor in a child's choice.

Selection of Appropriate Amplification Characteristics

It is critical that sufficient gain across frequency be provided if we expect a child to use audition. If the aided audiogram demonstrates that the aid does not provide sufficient gain to allow the child to receive speech, we cannot expect the child to be able to use hearing optimally. Hearing aid texts frequently caution the audiologist to limit output in order to avoid possible decreases in hearing acuity as the result of overamplification. There is evidence that this can occur, but the possibility frequently has been exaggerated. It is my contention that the hearing-impaired child is less sensitive to output than has been suggested. The best way to deal with concerns about overamplification is to monitor hearing very carefully. Should a decrease in hearing be observed, amplification should be removed immediately and hearing should be re-evaluated after allowing time for recovery of threshold shift. My experience after 25 years of testing hundreds of hearing-impaired children indicates that concern over threshold shift as the result of overamplification is overstated. The goal of amplification is to provide a child with sufficient hearing to understand speech. If amplified speech signals are insufficiently audible, then residual hearing will be of very limited use. Obviously, we must exercise caution in selecting output levels, but our caution must be tempered by our primary amplification goals.

Earmold acoustics are a significant consideration in the selection of appropriate amplification. Combining the effect of earmold acoustics and the frequency response of the hearing aid allows the audiologist to provide a better frequency response to the client. There are basically three types of earmold modifications. Venting (placing a hole in the earmold) will decrease the amplification in the low frequencies, usually below 1000 Hz (see figure 5). The use of dampers in the earmold tubing or the tone hook of a behind-the-ear aid will reduce the peaks in the mid frequencies. Gradually increasing the diameter of earmold tubing (a horn bore) will increase the response in the high frequencies. (For more information on earmold acoustics see Lybarger [1985], and Madell and Loavenbruck [1981]).

THE AIDED AUDIOGRAM

The optimal aided audiogram should provide for the maximum audibility of conversational speech. Amplification should be available between 250 and 6000 Hz at intensities sufficient to be useful for perception of speech. Figure 6 will be familiar from basic speech acoustics. It

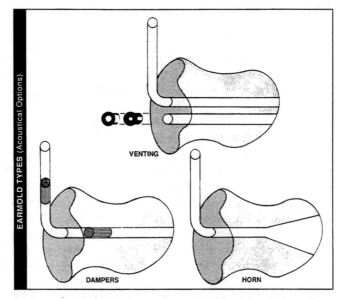

Figure 5. Earmold modifications: A—earmold with venting; B—earmold with dampers; C—earmold with a horn.

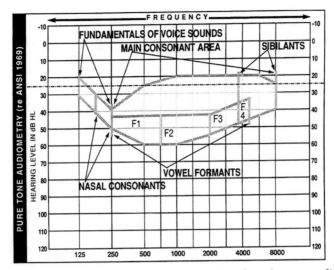

Figure 6.   General description of speech acoustics plotted on an audiogram. Reprinted with permission from Ross, Brackett, and Maxon (in press).

is shown to remind the reader of the necessity to hear throughout the frequency range if one expects to understand speech well. The suprasegmental aspects of speech (rhythm and inflection) and vowel perception are available from low frequency information. However, perception of consonants requires mid and high frequency speech information. Sibilants and fricatives require hearing in the 2,000–6,000 Hz range.

Figure 7, from the work of David Pascoe, as reported by Olsen, Hawkins, and Van Tasell (1987), demonstrates the hearing level in dBHL required for the perception of speech. Line A is the acoustic average of a speech signal. Line B indicates the level below which 90% of speech sounds fall. Line C indicates the level below which 10% of the speech signals fall. Keeping this in mind, if the aided audiogram is at the level of line C, we can expect the child to hear 10% and miss 90% of the speech information. On the other hand, if we are able to provide an aided audiogram at the level of line B, we would expect the child to hear 90% and miss only about 10%. Figure 8 takes the work of Pascoe and converts it to a standard audiogram form. By superimposing the child's aided audiogram on this form, we are able to get a better picture of what to expect from a child's aided speech perception.

It should be understood that only the lowest level of hearing, the detection level, is being represented here. This is the first step toward enabling a child to learn how to discriminate, identify, and comprehend speech optimally.

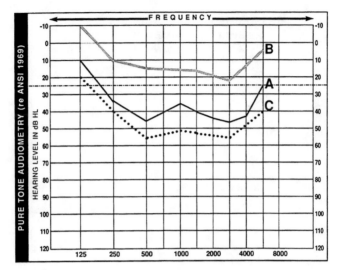

Figure 7. Speech spectrum on an audiogram form adapted from Pascoe 1980 (from Olsen, Hawkins, and Van Tasell 1987). Reprinted with permission from Olsen, Hawkins, and Van Tasell (1987).

The Amplification Evaluation

The amplification evaluation is critical in selecting the appropriate amplification to maximize a child's auditory functioning. Frequency specific information is essential. This may be obtained through sound-field warble tone or noise band thresholds and through probe tube micro-

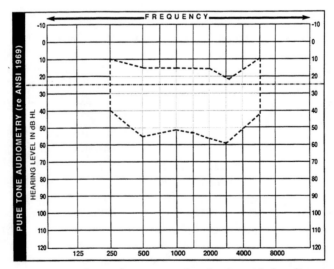

Figure 8. Adaption of speech spectrum for plotting aided audiograms.

phone measurements. This will assist the audiologist in determining if the child is receiving sufficient gain in a broad frequency range. Word recognition testing is also a critical part of every amplification evaluation. An aided SAT or SRT is not sufficient. It is necessary to obtain aided word recognition testing at normal and soft conversational levels in quiet as well as in the presence of background noise. It is not unusual for a child to obtain similar warble tone thresholds with different hearing aids and to have very different word discrimination, or to have similar warble tone thresholds and word discrimination at normal conversational levels in quiet with two different hearing aids but to have very different word discrimination scores at soft conversational levels or in the presence of background noise. The evaluation should include most comfortable and uncomfortable loudness measurements to assure that the child will be comfortable wearing the amplification. The aid should not be worn at maximum gain or maximum output. This combination of test criteria should provide the audiologist with sufficient information to select appropriate amplification.

SUMMARY

A complete audiological evaluation is a prerequisite for assessing a child's communication problems and for selecting an appropriate hearing aid and/or FM auditory training system. Amplification is critical to maximizing a hearing-impaired child's communication ability. By carefully evaluating a child's functioning with frequency specific stimuli and in a variety of speech recognition tasks, in quiet and in the presence of competing noise, the audiologist can select amplification systems that will assist the child to deal successfully with a variety of different auditory conditions. In selecting appropriate amplification for the hearing-impaired child, the audiologist provides the child with the basic learning tools for the auditory development of speech and language skills. The importance of this first and crucial step cannot be overemphasized.

REFERENCES

Bess, F. H., Tharpe, A. M., and Gibler, A. M. 1986. Auditory performance of children with unilateral sensorineural hearing loss. *Ear and Hearing* 7(1): 20–26.

Boothroyd, A. 1984 Auditory perception of speech contrasts by subjects with sensorineural hearing loss. *Journal of Speech and Hearing Research* 27:134–44.

Elliott, L., and Katz, D. 1980. *Development of a New Children's Test of Speech Discrimination*. St. Louis: Auditec.

Haskins, H. A. 1949. A phonetically balanced test of speech discrimination for children. Masters' thesis, Northwestern University, Evanston, IL.

Hodgson, W. 1978. Testing infants and young children. In *Handbook of Clinical Audiology,* Second edition, ed. J. Katz. Baltimore: Williams and Wilkins Co.

Ling, D. 1978. Auditory coding and recoding: An analysis of auditory training procedures for hearing impaired children. In *Auditory Management of Hearing Impaired Children,* eds. M. Ross and T. G. Giolas. Baltimore: University Park Press.

Ling, D. 1984. *Early Intervention for Hearing Impaired Children: Oral Options.* San Diego: College Hill Press.

Lybarger, S. F. 1985. Earmolds. In *Handbook of Clinical Audiology,* Third edition, ed. J. Katz. Baltimore: Williams and Wilkins Co.

Madell, J. R., and Loavenbruck, A. M. 1981. *Hearing Aid Dispensing for Audiologists: A Guide for Clinical Service.* New York: Grune and Stratton.

Madell, J. R. 1988. Identification and treatment of very young children with hearing loss. *Infants and Young Children* 1(2):20–30.

Madell, J. R., and Brackett, D. 1989. Assessment/management strategies for maximizing auditory functioning in hearing-impaired infants. Short Course presented at the American Speech-Language-Hearing Association Convention, November 1989, St. Louis.

Northern, J., and Downs, M. 1984. *Hearing in Children,* Third edition. Baltimore: Williams and Wilkins Co.

Olsen, W. O., Hawkins, D. B., and Van Tasell, D. J. 1987. Representation of long-term spectra of speech. *Ear and Hearing* 8 supplement:1005–1085.

Ross, M., and Lerman, J. 1970. A picture identification test for hearing-impaired children. *Journal of Speech and Hearing Research* 13:44–53.

Ross, M., Brackett, D., and Maxon, A. (in press). *Managing Mainstreamed Hearing Impaired Children in Regular Schools: Principles and Practices.* Austin: Pro-Ed.

Chapter • 3

Speech and Language Assessment: Communication Evaluation

Elizabeth Ying

INTRODUCTION

The need for an evaluation of the hearing-impaired student's speech and language performance is clearly evident, given that verbal language is the vehicle by which the regular classroom teacher instructs—and students are expected to respond. Labeling such an assessment speech/language evaluation is, however, limiting, in that it does not convey the need to assess all behaviors that directly or indirectly have an impact on the student's verbal/communicative functioning within the classroom. Given that a functionally adequate communication system is a major prerequisite for placement in a mainstream setting, the assessment of the student's communication must be comprehensive, addressing the full range of communicative demands required within the regular classroom.

While individual teaching style and classroom organization will vary from teacher to teacher, all students (as listeners) share the common need to understand a wide variety of linguistic messages, transmitted by both teachers and peers, within less than ideal listening environments. As speakers, their academic achievement and, frequently, their social acceptability are judged by their ability to convey ideas and information clearly and efficiently. The mere fact that mainstreaming is being considered for a hearing-impaired student suggests that he or she has the potential to compete within a group of normal-hearing peers in terms of both cognitive/academic preparedness and social interests. Primarily because of the reduced auditory signal they receive, however, hearing-impaired students are likely to experience more frequent communicative breakdown and social isolation than do their normal-hearing peers. The specific communicative deficits exhibited by hearing-impaired students in the regular classroom have been documented by many authors (Maxon and Brackett 1987; Ling and Ling 1978; Kretschmer and Kretschmer 1978; and Northcott 1973). These researchers, like others, advise that the choice of one test protocol over another should reflect the designated purpose of the evaluation itself. The examiner is obliged, therefore, to engage in pre-test planning and test organization in order to ensure a comprehensive assessment of the individual hearing-impaired student's communicative deficits.

RATIONALE FOR TESTING

There are essentially two reasons for conducting any communication evaluation: (1) to determine appropriate placement and (2) to determine remediation needs. Selection of the test battery as well as the interdisciplinary nature of the evaluation will depend largely upon how the findings of the evaluation process will be used.

It can be assumed that a placement assessment has already been conducted in order for a hearing-impaired child to be assigned to a regular classroom. Frequently, however, the student's academic performance, and also his or her social-communicative functioning, may dictate that consideration be given to an alternate educational placement.

Changing the recommended placement from fully mainstreamed to either a partially mainstreamed setting or a self-contained class for hearing impaired students necessitates that a placement re-evaluation be conducted. However, for the successfully mainstreamed hearing-impaired student, most communication evaluations are conducted to obtain baseline levels of performance, both receptive and expressive. The communication evaluation should not stand alone in determining either placement or remediation and support service programming. Rather, findings from the communication evaluation should be used along with information obtained from evaluations in related disciplines. Subsequent to such an analysis, it will be possible to design and implement an appropriately comprehensive management program for the fully or partially mainstreamed hearing-impaired student.

INTERDISCIPLINARY SCOPE

Critical to interpreting the findings from the hearing-impaired student's communication evaluation is the synthesis of diagnostic evaluations from the interdisciplinary team. This team is usually composed of a speech-language pathologist, an audiologist, a psychologist, and educational specialists. Specifically, from the audiological assessment one derives an objective assessment of the student's auditory potential/functioning, with and without amplification. Because such evaluations are conducted in a sound-treated test booth, only limited prognostic indicators are obtained regarding how the child functions within real-life acoustical environments.

The listening environment of most regular classrooms is considered to be a "difficult listening condition" that presents auditory barriers and obstacles for most hearing-impaired students. Ideally the student's classroom should be directly and objectively evaluated in terms of its acoustical acceptability. The educational audiologist is most prepared to conduct such evaluations. Unfortunately, however, in very few instances does this "classroom observation" occur as part of the diagnostic work-up. Audiologists, employed by either a school system or a private clinic, rarely have the time required to visit the student's classroom and take the necessary acoustical measurements.

Similarly, despite time constraints, diverse linguistic material should be used in assessing the student's aided performance. Word-level speech recognition testing, routinely administered during aided audiological testing, affords little information regarding the student's handling of lengthier material, such as sentences and paragraphs. In addition, audiological evaluations should extensively sample the extent to which additional visual and contextual cues, combined with audition, enhance the student's overall speech reception, comprehension, and/or production of spoken language.

Perhaps the more efficient way of obtaining such critically needed information is to incorporate a "functional listening evaluation" into the communication testing. (This is covered extensively below.) All levels of linguistic material (i.e., phonemes, words, sentences, and connected discourse) should be sampled, during the functional listening evaluation. It also seems logical to include the additional step of assessing the student's response to progressively varied material when presented with supplemental reception cues as well. Furthermore, because the communication evaluation usually is conducted within a naturalistic setting, as opposed to the controlled environment of an audiological booth, a more realistic picture can therefore be obtained of how the student might function, within the regular classroom.

What the student knows about the world as well as his or her full range of intellectual abilities are traditionally obtained from both the psychological and educational evaluations. Information regarding emotional/social adjustment and current academic achievement levels are also obtained through the diagnostic tasks administered by psychologists and educational specialists. Also of importance to the overall evaluation process is the assessment of the mainstreamed student's learning style and approach to a task. Previously such determinations were viewed as exclusively within the domain of psychological and educational testing. Now this information about a student is derived from the composite of his or her performance during all diagnostic evaluations. Psychologists and educators, in turn, provide valuable information regarding the student's functional communication. They can comment about what adaptations were required to convey the instructions for their testing as well as for everyday classroom activities. Their impressions of the adequacy of the student's receptive and expressive language system, in communicating about world knowledge and other "school-related content areas," should be compared with information obtained from the speech and language assessment.

TESTING CONSIDERATIONS

To obtain the most comprehensive picture of the student's communicative strengths and weaknesses, findings from the communication evaluation must be synthesized and compared with other available diagnostic information. Because "no single test samples all aspects of communication, nor does any test exclusively measure both comprehension and use" (Berry 1969), the choice of specific tests to be used in the communication evaluation should be a systematic process.

Selection of an appropriate test battery (from the vast number of available standardized speech and language assessment tools) must first and foremost respond to the communicative demands encountered by the student in instructional and social interactions within the classroom. Specific test choices are determined by the skills that are to be assessed. (To have listed this author's preferred choice of particular test material would have automatically dated this chapter—considering that novel assessment measures are developed continually.) It is therefore suggested that the communication evaluator use his or her own "best judgment" in selecting one test over another. The standard by which any test should be judged is, however, its ability to obtain the information desired appropriately and efficiently.

There is also a need to consider *how* the test material should be administered. This factor may, in fact, be even more important (in the evaluation process with a mainstreamed hearing-impaired student) than selecting the "right" speech and language assessment protocol. Individual diagnostic tools provide explicit directions regarding how they should be administered (if the standardized norms are to be used to interpret the child's performance). Obtaining a scale or percentile score may not, however, meet the primary purpose for using a particular test, or subtest, with a given student. It is not my intent to suggest that standardized tests (routinely administered during speech and language evaluations) be "modified" so that they can be administered to hearing-impaired students. Rather, it is imperative to ensure that the student has at least "received" individual test items before their response can be judged as accurate or inaccurate. To achieve this prerequisite will require some extra steps, not accounted for in the administration directions of most test manuals. A detailed list of such modifications appears in table I. The evaluator who utilizes one of these modifications should, however, be cautioned that it is his or her responsibility to describe the specific procedures used in administering any formal or informal measure. Only then can the student's performance be validly interpreted and subsequent functional changes be evaluated.

Of special concern is the issue of test validity and standardization. The fact that there are few tests normed on the hearing-impaired population is not a startling revelation to anyone involved in the habilitation/rehabilitation of children with hearing impairments. Many professionals object to using tests standardized on normal-hearing children in assessing the communication abilities of any hearing-impaired student. Such concern is however, in my opinion, unwarranted—if one operates from the viewpoint that the mainstreamed hearing-impaired student, by definition, must demonstrate sufficient communicative competence to "compete and interact" with his or her normal-hearing peers.

In addition, it has been my experience that most mainstreamed hearing-impaired students, if given a test normed on the hearing-impaired population, will score well within the top 10th percentile. Such performance scores are of little value in planning appropriate remediation programming for the mainstreamed student. More important, however, they provide no information regarding the mainstreamed student's preparation to comply with the communicative demands of the regular classroom.

COMPONENTS OF THE COMMUNICATION EVALUATION

The components of a communication evaluation are (1) reception, (2) comprehension, (3) production, (4) intelligibility, (5) conversational

Table I. Testing Strategies/Modifications (For the Hearing-Impaired Student in a Regular Classroom)

I. Select an optimal testing setting.
   - Acoustically quiet environment with child wearing amplification utilized in the classroom.
   - Visually nondistracting environment with good lighting and free of shadows or glare on the examiner's face (to permit maximum speech-reading).

II. Obtain and interpret child's performance on formal and informal test battery in various ways.
   - Analyze against evaluative data from related disciplines (including audio-logical, psychosocial, and academic).
   - Compare against performance of normal-hearing peers.
   - Compare present level of functioning against previous performance.
   - Use phonemic scoring procedures, in addition to whole word scoring, to obtain a more accurate assessment of perceptual abilities and confusions.
   - Report performance using percent-correct and percentile scores as these are frequently more informative than merely stating raw scores or age equivalents.
   - Analyze error patterns across parameters to identify the primary areas of deficit and/or the focus for subsequent remediation.

III. Ensure that the child has received the test stimulus.
   - Prior to testing, trouble-shoot amplification so that you are assured it is in optimal working condition.
   - Have the child repeat all verbal test stimuli (with the assumption that he or she will repeat what has been heard).

IV. Modify test format to obtain the most accurate assessment of the child's strengths and weaknesses.
   - Unless assessing auditory-only potential, present all verbal test stimuli full face, when the child is visually and auditorily focused on the examiner.
   - In presenting verbal stimulus, use a natural speaking rate and unexaggerated articulatory patterns to preserve standard acoustic and speechreading cues.
   - Assess auditory functioning in both ideal (i.e., close, quiet) and difficult (i.e., far, noise) listening conditions.
   - If an open-set testing format is attempted and the child is unable to respond appropriately, test stimuli might be re-administered, utilizing a closed set of possible alternatives, to obtain specific information for future training.
   - Say sentence, then show stimulus picture.
   - If the child has difficulty attending to picture stimuli (when there are several alternatives per page), show each picture frame separately, then present stimulus word or sentence.
   - Provide several demonstration models to ensure the child understands what he or she is expected to do.
   - Use visual aids to elicit desired response patterns.
   - Provide multiple repetitions of test stimuli.
   - If the child fails to respond appropriately to an isolated word, use the word in a meaningful sentence or situation to assess the effect of linguistic/non-linguistic context on comprehension.
   - In assessing written language comprehension, consider permitting the child to repeat stimuli as this might aid his or her overall understanding.

- To eliminate confusions in transcribing audio or video tapes made during evaluation sessions, write down the child's response (or test-taking behaviors) for future reference.
- Repeat child's utterance (during production tasks) to aid listener transcription and analysis at a later time.
- If the child fails to comprehend specific test stimuli, consider stressing key word or linguistic element to determine if breakdown is one of reception or comprehension.
- Insist on accurate production of stimuli (as this may affect response).

competence, and (6) written language. All of these have been documented to be problem areas for most mainstreamed hearing-impaired students. Ironically they, in turn, are the areas of greatest communicative demand within a classroom setting. The examiner's challenge is to sample the student's skills across those communicative parameters most necessary to ensure successful functioning within a classroom setting. To achieve this objective it will be necessary to utilize a range of linguistic material typically encountered by the student in his or her educational setting. Figure 1 represents one attempt to identify systematically some of the *problems* or *communicative demands* encountered by the hearing-impaired student within the regular classroom. It is also intended to afford an organizational format for selecting the areas to be assessed during the communication evaluation.

Reception

As hearing is the primary modality for receiving classroom instruction, the hearing-impaired student can be expected to experience great difficulty in reception. Factors such as the student's familiarity with the speaker and the vocabulary and language used within classroom instructional activities and social interactions will have a dramatic impact upon how much of the message is received by the hearing-impaired student. Typically, hearing-impaired students will have greater difficulty understanding multi-party conversations (i.e., following the flow of group discussions or messages not specifically directed to them), especially if presented at increased distances or in the presence of background noise. Therefore it will be important to assess these students' auditory responsiveness and to describe their auditory functioning in difficult listening conditions, such as understanding isolated words, following discourse in noise and at distances from the speaker. To assess reception comprehensively, it may be necessary to replicate the environment, by using parents, other clinicians/teachers, and/or peers to simulate a group-like situation. Tape-recorded speech babble or cafeteria noise tapes afford real-life background noise sources, for use within a clinical or educational evaluation setting.

Communicative Parameters	Linguistic Material			
	Phonemes	Words	Sentences	Discourse
Reception				
Comprehension				
Production				
Intelligibility				
Conversational Competence				
Written Language				

Figure 1.   Selecting components of the communication evaluation.

Comprehension

The comprehension demands of the regular classroom encompass both lexical and grammatical understanding, as well as accurate comprehension of more lengthy material (such as paragraphs and connected discourse). Hearing-impaired students, by necessity, rely heavily on contextual cues to follow such material, and they should not be expected to hear or identify each and every word. Therefore, the absence of extensive contextual support (frequently the case when teachers introduce novel concepts or content material) presents a special problem for the mainstreamed hearing-impaired student. The student is indeed at a great disadvantage in comparison to his or her normal-hearing peer.

The major problem in this area for hearing-impaired students is having to act upon misperceptions or partially perceived information. They are frequently observed to be unaware that they have not understood all of the intended message. In testing, it is necessary to determine whether the student is exhibiting a true comprehension problem (i.e., not knowing the words) or merely having a problem of "poor reception" (i.e., difficulty perceiving the words).

Production

As most hearing-impaired students exhibit a limited vocabulary, both receptively and expressively, they have a difficult time complying with the fast-paced production requirements of the mainstream classroom. Expressive language demands encompass both word-level and connected linguistic information. The mainstreamed student is expected to exhibit sufficient oral language to be understood. However, this requires the kind of syntactic sophistication and flexibility often lacked by the hearing-impaired student.

In assessing the student's production skills, it is critical to obtain a spontaneous as well as an elicited language sample. The fact that most commercially available production measures use an elicited format is probably an "efficiency" concern, in that it is often too time consuming to obtain a representative spontaneous language sample from a student within the specified time allotted for the evaluation. (This is, perhaps, an ideal opportunity to utilize the resources of other professionals of the interdisciplinary evaluation team. For example, the student's classroom teacher, who spends considerable time with the student, may be able to provide a comprehensive and natural spontaneous sample.)

Intelligibility

Because spoken language is the primary mode of response for routine classroom activities, the hearing-impaired student is at a serious disadvantage if his or her speech intelligibility is poor. Unfortunately, both teachers and peers are likely to misjudge the student's knowledge, ability, or interest if he or she is unable to articulate individual speech sounds clearly. Arrhythmic speech patterns, so characteristic of the speech patterns of hearing-impaired individuals, also have an adverse impact upon the student's ability to make his or her utterances readily understood, especially to the naïve listener who is unfamiliar with such patterns.

In assessing intelligibility, it is important to sample a variety of linguistic material ranging from words to sentences to paragraph material and connected discourse. Whenever possible, obtaining the judgment of a naïve listener's ability to understand the student's verbalizations adds valuable information when considering a placement change or planning a remedial program. Because the hearing-impaired student's own self-esteem may, understandably, be seriously damaged by repeated failures to make himself or herself understood, listener judgment may serve as a motivator to work harder on improving speech intelligibility. (A special note should be made that, fortunately for the hearing-impaired student, more and more formal tests are emerging that take the intelligibility factor into consideration in assessing overall articulatory functioning.)

Conversational Competence

The mainstreamed hearing-impaired student's knowledge of the social conventions that organize the conversational exchange between a speaker and a listener is frequently underdeveloped. Primarily because many of the signals that permit a smooth, efficient, and equal conversational partnership are coded auditorily, they may be unavailable or barely perceptible to any student with a significant hearing loss. The student's auditory deficit may thereby cause frequent communicative breakdown within the classroom environment.

Frequent overlap of another speaker's "turn-to-talk" and failure to relinquish the conversational floor are classic discourse deficits exhibited by hearing-impaired students. In addition, they tend to be overly passive conversational partners, who as listeners fail to provide appropriate feedback regarding what they have understood and/or their need for clarification. As speakers, hearing-impaired students dominate the conversation, in an attempt to control the topic and avoid having to resume the role of listener. They often initiate topics that are irrelevant to the immediate context or preceding utterance.

The major testing concern in the pragmatics area is, therefore, to obtain some idea of how the mainstreamed student compensates for limited awareness of specific conversational devices, such as those that signal turn-taking or topic changes. Observation of the student in as many conversational interactions as possible, with both peers and adults, while in the waiting room, on the playground, or in the classroom, affords the most comprehensive analysis of the student's discourse development.

Written Language

Deficiencies evident within hearing-impaired students' spoken language frequently are exhibited within their written language samples as well. Telegraphic constructions and deletion of grammatical morphemes typically are found in the written transcripts of these students. Also characteristic is an absence of grammatical elements that correspond to production aspects, such as ineffective use of punctuation markers and failure to establish "reader reference" through the use of clausal statements. The mainstreamed student exhibits additional difficulty when expected to write content information or test responses from verbally presented material.

Considering that writing is the most widely used response mode in almost every academic area, the importance of obtaining a written sample as part of the communication evaluation is self-evident. It is frequently necessary for the evaluator to provide the student with a versatile topic to elicit the most representative written language sample. Requiring the hearing-impaired students to read aloud what they have written affords additional information, specifically regarding their dependence on audition to self-monitor the linguistic adequacy of written language.

Functional Listening

Most of the documented communication and classroom difficulties experienced by mainstreamed hearing-impaired students are in some way related to the hearing loss itself. As stated by Maxon and Brackett (1987):

> Hearing-impaired children, due to reduced hearing sensitivity and receptive abilities, have many fewer opportunities to hear, associate and absorb the language being used around them. The impact of this "underdeveloped" communication system on academics is great (p. 393).

The importance of evaluating the mainstreamed student's functional listening skills (across the range of linguistic features from nonspeech elements to connected discourse) seems therefore clearly evident. In order to administer optimally, or to interpret subsequently, the student's performance on a variety of speech and language tasks (both receptively and expressively), it is essential to know how the student depends on, and utilizes, his or her aided residual hearing.

Factors to be considered in selecting specific test material have been listed in figure 2. These suggestions are intended to assist the communication evaluator in deciding which available tests would best sample the student's auditory capabilities for a particular type of linguistic-level stimuli. For example, at the word-level, the student's age and oral receptive vocabulary skills will have the most impact on the choice of test stimuli. While body parts might serve to give critical information regarding the vowel and consonant recognition abilities of a young mainstreamed preschooler, use of phonetically balanced consonant-vowel-consonant (CVC) word lists, such as Boothroyd's (1984) AB Lists or the CID Early Speech Perception Test (Moog and Geers 1988), would more efficiently afford information about any hearing-impaired student's phonemic perception of manner, voicing, and place features (based on the accuracy of a repeat-back response). Sentences and paragraphs from the Test of Auditory Comprehension (TAC) (Trammell et al. 1976), presented live-voice, satisfy the need to consider both contextual support and suprasegmental influences on receiving and comprehending syntactic-level material. Individual subtests of the TAC can therefore be useful in sampling the auditory skill development of hearing-impaired students, at varying ages and linguistic levels.

	Quiet			Noise	
	L&L	LA		L&L	LA

Suprasegmental Features
  Durational Contrasts
  Intensity Contrasts
  Pitch Contours
  Syllabic Number					

Words
  Familiarity
  Contextual Cues					

Sentences
  Vocabulary Familiarity
  Length
  Syntactic Complexity
  Grammatical Complexity
  Contextual Cues
  Suprasegmental Features					

Paragraph Material
  Vocabulary Familiarity
  Length
  Complexity
  Contextual Cues
  Suprasegmental Features					

Everyday Conversational Material					

L&L = Look and Listen
LA = Listen Alone

Figure 2. Functional listening evaluation. (Features listed under each assessment parameter should be considered in selecting test stimuli.)

To utilize figure 2 effectively, it is necessary to understand that auditory skill development follows a language learning schema. It has been a well-accepted fact among professionals involved in aural habilitation/rehabilitation that verbal language is learned, and is not explicitly "taught." Access to enriched and varied language within communicative interactions enables the hearing-impaired student, like his or her normal-hearing peers, to internalize the components and conventions of spoken language. Speech signals should, therefore, be the major "test stimuli" in assessing the mainstreamed student's auditory functioning. Essentially, auditory skill development can be viewed on a continuum (like the one in figure 3) moving from easy to difficult listening requirements, as follows:

EASY **DIFFICULT**

LOOK and LISTEN————————————————————LISTEN ALONE
          with:
          vibrotactile,
          cued speech,
          sign language

CLOSE————————————————————DISTANCE
QUIET————————————————————NOISE
NONVERBAL RESPONSE————————————VERBAL RESPONSE
CLOSED SET————————————————OPEN SET
SUPRASEGMENTALS——————————————SEGMENTALS
GROSS CONTRASTS——————————————MINIMAL CONTRASTS
CONTEXT BOUND————————————————CONTEXTUALLY LIMITED

Figure 3.   Continuum for auditory skill development.

Reception Modality: The easiest reception mode for the hearing-impaired student is when stimuli are presented utilizing a combination of auditory, visual, and gestural cues (i.e., both informal systems as well as cued speech or sign language). In contrast, stimuli presented listen-alone (in the absence of supplemental standard speechreading cues) places the most difficult reception demands on the student with a hearing loss.

Listening Environment: Close, quiet listening environments are better when compared to listening in noise or at increased distances.

Mode of Response: Providing a nonverbal response to verbally presented information is usually much easier for the hearing-impaired student than having the additional demand of formulating a verbal response (due to restricted or underdeveloped expressive language skills).

Nature of the Stimuli: Suprasegmental features (i.e., nonspeech features such as intensity, duration, and intonation, which carry the rhythm of the language) are readily perceived by most hearing-impaired individuals, as these features are conveyed primarily through low-frequency cues. This is the frequency range where most hearing-impaired people exhibit the greatest degree of residual hearing.

When lexical stimuli are used, the student's knowledge of the vocabulary will greatly affect ease and accuracy of reception and comprehension. Such stimuli presented within a familiar context will be easier to understand than if these same stimuli were presented within a novel context.

Figure 3 provides a schematic representation of the above considerations. Lacking in the present discussion of auditory skill development, however, is the notion that auditory proficiency develops in a systematic fashion in which *detection* (awareness of sound) is at the lowest end of the hierarchy, while *comprehension* (the ability to grasp meaning from and act upon what is said) is considered the highest level of auditory ability. In between is *discrimination*, which is defined as demonstrating awareness that two auditory stimuli are the same or different, and *identification*, which is the ability to repeat what has been received.

Including a separate category on the functional listening evaluation, for the suprasegmental features of speech, was felt to be necessary. Their assessment is especially relevant when testing younger mainstreamed children who may not have basic "pattern perception" on which to build higher level auditory discrimination and recognition skills. For example, without pitch perception, the hearing-impaired student will not be able to distinguish between questions and statements via audition alone. Suprasegmental features of duration and intensity combine to code meaning regarding changes in stress (the classic example being, "MARY hit the drum" versus "Mary HIT the drum" versus "Mary hit the DRUM").

Depending upon the nature of the material presented, the examiner can obtain a percent-correct score, thereby permitting a comparative analysis of the student's performance for several different listening conditions, as shown in figure 4.

What is most distinctly different about the communication evaluation of a hearing-impaired student as opposed to a normal-hearing student is the need to assess and/or account for factors affecting his or her *auditory functioning*. The information gathered from the functional listening evaluation enables the examiner to make a more valid statement regarding the student's *preferred modality* for formal speech and language testing. This, in turn, will provide valuable information for the support service and classroom management of the mainstreamed student.

SUMMARY

The major thrust of this chapter has been to delineate the components of a comprehensive communication evaluation for the mainstreamed hearing-impaired student. While linguistic development and speech production abilities most affect the communicative performance of any student, other factors (including cognitive development, interaction style, psycho-social adjustment, and the nature of the communicative demands) also influence overall communicative functioning. Unique to the communication evaluation of a hearing-impaired student is the

	Close/Quiet	Far/Quiet	Close/Noise	Far/Noise
Listen Alone	68	52	44	12
Look and Listen	94	80	72	44

Figure 4. An example of a functional listening evaluation using live-voice monosyllabic words.

need to assess both the acoustic environment and the adequacy of the student's aided auditory functioning (given such factors as the degree of hearing loss, listening age, and appropriateness of amplification).

It has been emphasized repeatedly that the entire interdisciplinary diagnostic team can provide the communication evaluator with critical information about the mainstreamed student's communicative functioning. The evaluator's challenge is to formulate an accurate and intuitive interpretation of the student's present level of communicative performance and/or future management needs. To achieve this, the evaluator relies primarily upon the student's responses on a selected battery of formal and informal speech and language and "functional listening" assessment tools. These test findings must also be synthesized with additional diagnostic results and impressions from related discipline and observational data, and compared against normative standards for the student's normal-hearing and hearing-impaired peer groups.

If the ultimate purpose for evaluating the communicative behaviors of hearing-impaired students is to determine their readiness to enter or remain within a regular classroom setting, some assessment must be made of the communicative demands required of these students, within their particular placements. The diversity of the communicative demands from student to student explains why specific tests used to evaluate one student may not address the evaluation needs of another. Similar individualization is required in selecting appropriate testing modifications, in interpreting the results obtained, and in designing and implementing subsequent remediation and/or support service programs for mainstreamed hearing-impaired students.

REFERENCES

Berry, M. 1969. *Language Disorders of Children: The Bases and Diagnoses.* New York: Appleton-Century-Crofts.
Boothroyd, A. 1984. Auditory perception of speech contrasts by subjects with sensorineural hearing loss. *Journal of Speech and Hearing Research* 2:134–44.
Kretschmer, R., and Kretschmer, L. 1978. *Language Development and Intervention with the Hearing-Impaired.* Baltimore: University Park Press.

Ling, D., and Ling, A. 1978. *Aural Habilitation: The Foundations of Verbal Learning in Hearing-Impaired Children*. Washington, DC: Alexander Graham Bell Association For the Deaf, Inc.

Maxon, A., and Brackett, D. 1987. The hearing-impaired child in regular schools. *Seminars in Speech and Language* 8(4):393–413.

Moog, J., and Geers, A. 1988. *Early Speech Perception Test*. St. Louis: Central Institute for the Deaf.

Northcott, W. 1973. *The Hearing-Impaired Child in the Regular Classroom: Preschool, Elementary, and Secondary Years*. Washington, DC: Alexander Graham Bell Association for the Deaf, Inc.

Trammell, J., Farmer, C., Francis, J., Owens, S., Shephard, S., Witlen, R., and Faist, L. 1976. *Test of Auditory Comprehension*. North Hollywood, CA: Foreworks.

Chapter • 4

Psycho-Educational Assessment of Hearing-Impaired Children

Patricia J. Heller

THE ASSESSMENT PERSPECTIVE

At the outset we should acknowledge the power of psycho-educational assessment in the lives of hearing-impaired children, whose futures are intimately tied to the results and interpretation of tests. To increase our sensitivity to that power, this quotation from the work of Stephen Jay Gould (1981) sets the perspective of this chapter:

> We pass through this world but once. Few tragedies can be more extensive than the stunting of life, few injustices deeper than the denial of an opportunity to strive or even to hope, by a limit imposed from without, but falsely identified as lying within (p. 28).

Psycho-educational assessment of mainstream students who are hearing impaired is conducted for the following purposes: (1) to obtain baseline information about the child and monitor progress; (2) to provide an appropriate educational program and make alterations in it as the child's needs change; (3) to predict and plan for the future; and, (4) to understand the child's strengths and weaknesses. Because human beings and environments are not static, the compatibility of the relationship between the student and the environment must be reconsidered periodically. Psycho-educational assessment can be a tool for structuring and adjusting the educational environment initially, to maintain a compatible, enriching relationship. Table I illustrates the multidisciplinary factors that have to be assessed to understand the needs of a hearing-impaired child and the continuum of educational expectations and placement options.

Figure 1 illustrates the relationship of the domains of a child's functioning to the school's curriculum and the continuum of support services. The extent of needed support services will depend on the skills the child possesses, the expectations inherent in the curriculum, and the resources available. The support services may vary along the

Table I.   Components to Consider in Assessment

Component	Skill Sampled
Degree of Hearing Loss	Speech perception and speech discrimination
Intelligence	Nonverbal cognitive ability
Verbal Functioning	Communication dependent tasks
Reading	All subject matter containing decoding/encoding
Arithmetic	Computation and word problems
Visual Motor Skills	Representation and organization of visual stimuli
Memory-Visual/Auditory	Retrieval of visual and auditory information
Multimodality Integration	All complex tasks—reading and writing
Written Language	Tasks requiring written words, content, structure, and grammar
Speech Reception (Quiet/Noise)	Ability to receive speech for social or academic purposes: words, sentences, and paragraphs
Comprehension	Ability to understand what is said: basis for reading and all language based subjects; words, sentences, and paragraphs
Expression	Ability to formulate a response that carries meaning and intent; words, sentences, and paragraphs
Speech Production Intelligibility	Ability to be understood by others
Attention	Ability to focus on relevant stimuli and maintain focus
Social/Emotional Factors	Adjustment and adaptation
Problem Solving	All areas where a solution is sought; ability to move from unknown to known
Organization	Ability to rank for priority
Use of Amplification	Willingness to wear and maintain personal and classroom amplification
Use of Sign Language	Ability to use manual communication receptively and expressively

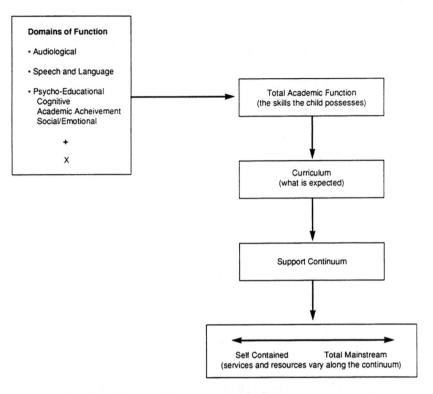

Figure 1.   Psycho-educational assessment paradigm.

continuum from a self-contained classroom to total mainstream placement.

Having a hearing handicap is stressful both for the parents and for the hearing-impaired child who tries to keep up with nonhandicapped classmates. It is also stressful for the child as it is the central focus of considerable effort and concern, and sometimes controversy. Educators, as well as parents, experience stress as they try to meet the special needs of the student and confront the question, "Are we doing the right things?" The psycho-educational assessment can help identify and resolve concerns by giving educational direction and providing reasonable expectations for everyone involved, thereby, reducing stress.

Foremost in the psycho-educational assessment of a hearing-impaired child is to discover as much as possible about how the child functions. This discovery process consists of three components. First, it is important to ascertain what the child knows. Second, it is important to explore how the child learned what is known and acquired his or her fund of knowledge. The third part of the assessment, which is central, is identification of optimal means whereby learning takes place. The learning style of the child should be clearly understood so that limitations imposed by the hearing loss can be compensated for or minimized. If there are other factors that inhibit or enhance the learning process, these also need to be identified.

PRACTICAL CONSIDERATIONS IN THE ASSESSMENT PROCESS

Initially in the psycho-educational process, a careful medical history needs to be obtained from parents or caregivers. Factors in the birth and developmental history as well as etiology of the hearing loss may relate to the learning characteristics of the child. Information about acceptance of the hearing loss is also necessary to understand how the child is viewed by his or her family members. Not all family members deal with acceptance of the hearing loss in the same way, nor do cultural communities perceive handicaps in the same way. As Garguilo (1985) and Seligman (1983) suggest, this conflict in perceptions breeds ambivalent feelings regarding the child. To understand the child's family and cultural perceptions of the child is to understand more about how the hearing-impaired child sees himself or herself, and about the character of his or her support system.

A valid assessment requires effective communication. In order to maximize communication between the child and the examiner, the child's amplification system must be in working order, and the testing must take place in an acoustically favorable location where extraneous noise is minimal and lighting is adequate. The child should be seated with his or her back to the windows to reduce glare. The examiner should be seated so the child has full view of the face, so both visual and auditory cues are available. If the child relies on sign language for reception and/or expression, determining valid estimates of the child's cognitive and educational abilities will require a psychologist who has signing skills.

In the testing session itself, it is important to note the facility of communication between the child and the examiner. Asking the child occasionally to repeat a question or word will confirm whether the child is receiving the message accurately. If the message is not received accurately, the response will not be accurate. Facility of speech/sign language reception and expression as well as the social ease with which communication occurs is central to understanding how learning takes place. An ideal listening/looking situation is not often found in the real world. Therefore, it is important for the examiner to learn how the child functions in less than ideal situations, such as the classroom. This can be achieved through classroom observation, audiological information, and functional speech testing. The psycho-educational evaluation, in other words, is part of a collaborative assessment effort.

THE PSYCHO-EDUCATIONAL ASSESSMENT PROCESS

Cognitive Assessment

To learn about the hearing-impaired child's fund of information and how he or she acquires it, the cognitive assessment should contain measures of general ability (IQ) and of specific cognitive abilities. Measures of readiness skills, reading, writing, and mathematics yield "applied" information. Assessment of the integrity of information reception, comprehension, and expression in the auditory, visual, and motor modalities, as well as memory (short- and long-term), need to be explored in many combinations. Determining strengths and weaknesses for any one or combinations of these avenues of input and output provides the foundation for understanding learning style. Moreover, skills such as reading and writing depend upon the integration of the sensory learning modalities.

Use of cognitive ability or IQ tests that have discrete verbal and nonverbal design, such as the Wechsler Preschool and Primary Scale of Intelligence-Revised (WPPSI-R), the Wechsler Intelligence Scale for Children-Revised (WISC-R), and the Wechsler Adult Intelligence Scale-Revised (WAIS-R), help to factor out the effects of hearing loss. Having a nonverbal estimate of ability can give a more valid indication of the child's ability (Sattler 1982) in areas generally unaffected by loss of hearing. The verbal portion of these instruments provides valuable information about the degree to which the hearing loss affects the acquisition of verbal information, and may serve as an index more akin to achievement testing than to a measure of innate ability.

In making an interpretation of the verbal IQ score, the examiner must ask several questions: When was the diagnosis of hearing loss made? How long has the child used amplification? Does the verbal deficit match the degree of hearing loss, the child's language age, the nature and duration of the intervention? These factors associated with the effects of hearing loss are usually reflected in and should be compatible with the language proficiency demonstrated in the Verbal IQ score. Because the Verbal IQ cannot be separated from the effects of hearing loss, use of the Full Scale IQ score with hearing-impaired children can distort and prejudicially reduce the estimate of the child's ability.

Other areas of cognitive ability addressed in the psycho-educational assessment are problem solving, attention, and concentration. The child's approach to problem solving and how he or she learns from his or her own efforts to find solutions (metacognition) are important predictors of independent functioning in a classroom. The examiner observes whether efforts are organized, if the child uses systematic attack, trial and error, or random, unsystematic, or disorganized problem-solving methods that result in frustration and defeat.

The student's attention span, concentration, and perseverence need to be noted; they are essential to effective problem solving and they allow the hearing-impaired child to compensate for his or her hearing loss. Hearing-impaired children miss some of the information presented verbally in the classroom by virtue of their hearing loss. They must concentrate harder to receive and make sense of incomplete auditory input. Amplification will not provide all the auditory information available to normally hearing children. This requires hearing-impaired children to learn to select and rank in order of importance the information they are receiving as well as to fill in the missing parts of an auditory message. Well-focussed attention and good concentration skills enhance a child's success in regular classrooms because they permit the child to take incomplete auditory information and organize it into a conceptual whole.

Achievement Assessment

Psycho-educational assessment includes achievement testing to determine what skills the child possesses and at what rate progress is made. Progress should be assessed formally every year to make sure the child is keeping pace with his or her grade mates. Achievement testing is useful to determine if knowledge gaps exist and if so, to provide qualitative, specific information to plan for filling those gaps. It is important to note the child's ability to use inference and abstract thinking in reading, and whether he or she is able to use context to understand word meanings. Having the child write a short story is especially helpful in achievement assessment. This exercise illustrates the child's ability to formulate cohesive thoughts, and his or her knowledge of syntax, spelling, vocabulary, and punctuation. Children often welcome the chance to be "writers" in a highly structured test session, bringing more of themselves into the interchange.

As the child reaches the upper grades of high school, achievement assessment becomes pertinent for planning higher education and training. Vocational skills assessment can be helpful in decision making for post-high school planning.

Social-emotional Assessment

Assessment of social-emotional development of hearing-impaired children requires special emphasis because development in these domains is dependent upon communication (see Chapter 9). Hearing-impaired children are vulnerable to delayed social skills because the hearing loss itself may reduce experiential social learning and access to the subleties of social interchange. It is not easy for a hearing-impaired child to learn social meanings in an incidental way since he or she may not overhear relevant conversation, thus reducing "experience" in the social sphere. Social skills can be assessed by using observations, and teacher and parent reports; in addition, rating scales such as the Vineland Adaptive Behavior Scale (Sparrow, Balla, and Cicchetti 1984) are useful for identifying the hierarchy of skills the child possesses and the skills that are yet to be acquired.

Hearing-impaired children tend to have more difficulty understanding and participating in group activities, which may lead them to choose social situations that do not rely on groups. This can be construed as avoidance or withdrawal when it is actually an adaptive alternative. Having close friends, not groups of friends, or preferring to spend time alone in constructive activities are not unusual. If a child seems to be following this type of social pattern, he or she might be encouraged to learn individual sports such as tennis, swimming, and golf and hobbies such as using computers, photography, painting, and astronomy, that can be enjoyed by a small group of individuals and do not require a large collective effort.

Certainly the hearing-impaired child will need to participate in groups on some levels. Learning effective social strategies for dealing with group situations is an important component of social growth. Instruction in social interaction may need to be built into the curricular design of the Individualized Education Program (IEP) (see Chapter 5).

Coping with hearing loss in the mainstream is inherently stressful no matter how successful a child may be. Therefore, the emotional status of a hearing-impaired child in the mainstream should be monitored carefully. Projective tests using drawings and storytelling can be helpful. The psychologist should also use parent/teacher reports and classroom observation to learn how the child handles the stress and frustration of everyday life. The child's view of his or her hearing loss has fundamental bearing on self esteem and adjustment and on his or her handling of the stresses that hearing loss engenders.

Development of communication strategies and their use depends on the child's acceptance of the hearing loss. A hearing-impaired child who is successful in the mainstream has learned to take responsibility for understanding others and making himself or herself understood, and is self-sufficient in the use of amplification. Learned early, these attributes not only foster satisfying social interaction but can enrich many areas of the child's life.

The psychologist should be sensitive to the parents' feelings about the hearing loss and the expectations they have for their child. Having a handicapped child generates grief and guilt that may alter the expectations parents have for their child. Moreover, the uncertainty of the future looms large for parents. Parental expectations that are lower than the child's capability permits or expectations that are too high often reflect the parent's emotional conflict regarding the hearing loss. The psychologist can help the family find balanced expectations that will allow the child the freedom to be himself or herself and to develop the feelings of mastery necessary for confidence and age-appropriate independence.

The Assessment Paradigm in figure 1 shows an X at the bottom of the domain column. The X, the unknown and rarely measurable factor, refers to the qualities inherent in the child that drive him or her to succeed in the mainstream. X refers to motivation, perseverence, fortitude, a sense of humor, flexibility, and patience—intangible personality factors that are often most responsible for a child's success in the mainstream. Gail Pflaster (1981), in her research related to identifying factors that account for success of mainstreamed hearing-impaired children, states:

> Communicative, linguistic, and personality factors interrelate with a communicative attitude as the core. In sum, we are looking for a motivated, well-adjusted child desiring to communicate and to use residual audition and spoken language (p. 79–80).

Although these intangible factors, central in predicting success in the mainstream, are difficult, if not impossible to measure in any objective fashion, they cannot be overlooked. The astute psychologist will deduce X from informal observations and interviews with the child and parents and professionals who work with the child.

Measurement and Norms

Table I lists components of functioning that should be evaluated in the audiological, the psycho-educational, and the speech and language areas. These skills are interdependent and provide multidisciplinary and holistic pictures of the child.

Should the child be compared to a hearing peer group or a hearing-impaired peer group? Because there are few tests that are normed for hearing-impaired mainstreamed children and because these children are enrolled in a regular school, it is advisable to use the norms supplied with the test instrument for normally hearing children. According to Ying and Brackett (1984), mainstreamed hearing-impaired children generally score so well on tests that are standardized for hearing-impaired children that such tests provide little usable information for designing remedial programs. Test results should indicate how well the hearing-impaired child is keeping up with his or her normal-hearing grade mates. These results can inform us of the rate at which the hearing-impaired child is progressing relative to his or her educational group. If norms are available for hearing-impaired children, these results also can be used to compare the child's skills to other hearing-impaired children.

Special testing modifications to reduce the impact of hearing loss, such as extended time limits, oral testing, or adjustment of presentation, should be considered when giving hearing-impaired children tests that were designed for normal-hearing children. If the test format penalizes the hearing-impaired individual, then other methods of obtaining the desired information may be needed. For instance, some tests require a text that is read to the child and oral presentation of questions. To ensure accurate reception, the child can be allowed to read the questions to supplement the oral presentation. Any modifications in the administration of the tests should be specified in the report.

Whereas norm-referenced tests provide information about academic progress relative to a larger group, criterion-referenced tests can be useful in pinpointing the academic skills of the child. These tests, such as the Brigance Diagnostic Inventory of Basic Skills, allow the examiner to describe the skills the child possesses rather than using a score to document progress. Based on what is or is not mastered, these instruments are useful in detecting gaps in knowledge and in planning the child's curriculum. They also provide information about the child's mastery of basic skills relative to what has been presented in the classroom. What was learned can be compared to what was taught, giving a practical index as to how well the child is learning in the regular classroom. For example, because math is a subject that builds on previously mastered skills, a criterion-referenced math test can indicate exactly which unlearned skills are responsible for breakdown in more complicated material. If the student is having difficulty understanding interest calculations, it might be that he or she did not understand decimals taught the year before.

CASE STUDIES

The following case studies were chosen because they typify common situations, and they illustrate the services that may be required at different points along the support continuum (see figure 1). They illustrate two psycho-educational assessments of hearing-impaired mainstreamed children with different areas of concern and different profiles. These evaluations were done as part of a multidisciplinary assessment; some information from related findings is included to present a total picture of each child.

Psycho-Educational Evaluation: Erin

Background Erin is a nine-year-old fourth grade student with a moderate-to-severe congenital sensorineural hearing loss in the right ear and a severe loss in the left. She was fitted with binaural post-auricular hearing aids and had an FM system for use in instructional situations. Medical and birth history were unremarkable and all developmental milestones were as expected. Erin had the benefit of early diagnosis and intervention. Her family was highly supportive and needed reassurance that they were pursuing appropriate social and educational avenues. Erin was referred for evaluation to assess her progress for program planning and determination of support services as well as to explore her social-emotional adjustment.

Erin had speech and language services ninety minutes per week and resource room help one hour per day. Her school system was concerned that she was struggling to keep up with her regular class, and was becoming more frustrated as time went on. There were no other hearing-impaired children in the local school district.

General Observations Erin initially impressed the examiner as a reserved child, but she became more outgoing and responsive as the testing session progressed, revealing herself to be socially astute and friendly. Her spontaneous conversation was intelligible but at times indicated that she had not understood the topic or question presented even under ideal listening conditions. Erin did not ask for repetitions or clarifications to signal her communication needs. She was observed to carry this pattern into her work: when she "missed" an instruction, she would withdraw, get very still, and do what she thought was asked. Erin was not assertive and compensatory strategies for coping with her hearing loss had yet to be established.

Test Results and Interpretation

Wechsler Intelligence Scale for Children-Revised:

Information	8	Picture Completion	14
Similarities	11	Picture Arrangement	11
Arithmetic	9	Block Design	11
Vocabulary	9	Object Assembly	10
Comprehension	8	Coding	10
Verbal IQ score	94		
Performance IQ score	117		

Bender Visual Motor Gestalt—2 errors—age equivalent: 9 years
Bender Recall: Above average.

Draw A Person—Koppitz Developmental Scoring: Average to high average.

Standford Achievement Test:

Primary 3 Form F

	Grade Equivalent	Percentile
Reading Comprehension	3.8	50
Mathematics Computation	6.2	70

Vineland Adaptive Behavior Scale:

Communication Domain	9 years, 8 months
Daily Living Skills Domain	8 years, 6 months
Socialization Domain	10 years, 0 months

Slingerland Test for Specific Language Disability
House-Tree-Person Drawings

Diagnostic Component	Weak	Strong
V IQ		*
P IQ		*
Reading	*	
Arithmetic		*
Visual Motor Skills		*
Auditory Memory		*
Multimodality Integration		*
Writing		*
Speech Perception		*
Comprehension	Vocabulary	Syntax
Expression	Syntax/Vocabulary	
Speech Intelligibility		*
Attention	*	
Social/Emotional	Social	Emotional
Problem Solving	*	
Organization	*	
Use of Amplification		*

The results of the Wechsler Intelligence Scale for Children-Revised indicate a Verbal IQ at the average range and a Performance IQ at the high average range. Because of the effects of hearing loss on the natural acquisition of verbal information, the Verbal IQ score should be viewed as an index of Erin's achievement rather than an estimate of her innate verbal ability. The Performance IQ can be considered a more valid indication of intellectual functioning. Erin's score at the average range for the Verbal IQ is a significant accomplishment, given the degree of her hearing loss.

The subtest scatter in the verbal section suggests that Erin has strong skills in the area of abstract thinking. This indicates that she possesses more verbal ability than is reflected in her other subtest scores. Information and comprehension subtests are lowest, in keeping with the effects of hearing loss. Slightly higher scores are those of arithmetic and vocabulary, more dependent upon, and reflective of knowledge obtained in structured learning experiences and language intervention. These scores are impressive for a child who was pre-lingually affected with hearing loss like hers.

Both the performance IQ score and the Bender Visual Motor Gestalt suggest intact visual motor organization and memory. Erin appears to be more adept in dealing with details within a structured framework than with few organizational guides. The slightly depressed arithmetic and coding scores may indicate that attention and concentration are variable.

The Slingerland Test for Specific Language Disability indicates that all modes of information processing are intact and that they are strongest when used in combination. No evidence of learning disability is present. In the classroom, Erin will benefit from use of visual cues such as outlines on the blackboard or on paper that summarize the main ideas of the lessons presented. Checking to see that Erin has understood material presented in class would be beneficial. Problem areas can be addressed in the resource room.

Achievement testing indicates that Erin's reading comprehension level is slightly below her grade placement. Given her vocabulary scores on the WISC-R and in the speech and language evaluation, this is a consistent finding. The receptive vocabulary delays appear to be hindering her reading progress. Although she is only two months below her grade placement and at the 50th percentile for her educational group, she has the potential to do better. Because the use of inference is integral to more difficult reading material, it will be important to monitor this area more closely in the coming year in her resource room work. Mathematics computation is well above her grade placement and consistent with her ability. Although this score is inconsistent with that of the WISC-R, the task and its presentation (oral vs. pencil and paper) may account for the difference in the scores. These tests were not timed.

Adaptive behavior domains were assessed by using the Vineland Adaptive Behavior Scale, with Erin's mother as the informant. Development of communication skills, including reading and writing as well as spoken communication, is at age level. Socialization skills are consistent with her age level. Erin's knowledge of social skills is more pronounced than her actual practice of them. Frustration and loss of control erupt when she is feeling most vulnerable and have been related to communication and social difficulties. Daily living skills are below age expectancy largely because Erin is not required to help with household chores. However, in other tasks of daily living she is age-appropriately independent.

The projective tests and interview suggest an active inner life and a strong ego. Erin turns within to find resources to cope with the world at large. Erin senses her difference from others and feels isolation and anger especially associated with social needs. Her self esteem needs to be enhanced and she should be taught communication strategies to help her relate to her peers.

Comments A top priority in building Erin's confidence was to help her understand that, although she was not at the head of her class, her accomplishments, given her hearing loss, were quite remarkable. Erin needed to know that her efforts were commendable. The recommendations for Erin were to continue resource room support one hour per day, with emphasis on vocabulary and concept development relative to material presented in her regular classes. Erin appeared to have the cognitive and language skills to make more progress in reading if vocabulary was strengthened.

Erin was making good progress in all academic areas, yet feeling increasing pressure in social areas as peer relationships became more group oriented. Strategies for use by the school staff and social strategies for Erin herself to use to facilitate social participation were needed. Skills such as asking for repetitions or clarifications that would allow her to function more effectively in social situations would be useful. Her teacher of the hearing impaired in the resource room and her speech-language pathologist were enlisted to teach and encourage her to use these skills.

In addition, it was felt that Erin would have more to share with her peers if she had access to a television decoder. Reading the captions might also help her reading skills. It was recommended that Erin meet other hearing-impaired children with whom she could share her experiences and find common ground. Suggestions were given to help the parents encourage skills for independence.

With better communication strategies for interacting with others, it was expected that Erin's stress would be reduced and that there would be more energy for concentrating and for attention in school.

Psycho-Educational Evaluation: Morris

Background Morris is a nine-year-old fourth grade student who has a moderate-to-severe congenital sensorineural hearing loss for which he uses binaural postauricular hearing aids and an FM system. For part of his school day, Morris has been in a self-contained learning disabilities classroom and he has received the services of a teacher of the hearing impaired, speech and language services, occupational therapy, and adaptive physical education. He was mainstreamed for reading with the third grade and with the fourth grade for non-academic subjects.

Morris's early development was remarkable for fetal distress resulting in seizures. His hearing loss was diagnosed early and early intervention was obtained for motor difficulties and for speech and language delays. His family was very involved and supportive. Morris was referred for evaluation to obtain a differential diagnosis relative to learning disabilities and the hearing loss and to plan for a unified school program that would meet his diverse needs.

General Observations   Morris impressed the examiner as a congenial, relaxed, soft spoken youngster who clearly enjoys the company of others and responds eagerly to new situations and tasks. He was diligent in his work throughout the sessions although some impulsivity was noted in his written work. Problem solving was generally unsystematic, signaling difficulties in organizing tasks. Nevertheless, he persevered for as long as he was asked. Morris's poor motor control in writing was troublesome.

Amplification was checked at the outset and determined to be in good working order. Morris's speech was intelligible to the unclued listener. Repetitions by the examiner were needed on occasion.

Test Results and Interpretation
Wechsler Intelligence Scale for Children-Revised:

Information	8	Picture Completion	6
Similarities	6	Picture Arrangement	11
Arithmetic	6	Block Design	6
Vocabulary	5	Object Assembly	5
Comprehension	7	Coding	5
Verbal IQ score	78		
Performance IQ score	75		

Bender Visual Motor Gestalt—age equivalent: 6–6½ years
Bender Recall: 3 designs.

Draw A Person—Koppitz Developmental Scoring: low average.
Stanford Achievement Test:

Primary 2 Form F

	Grade Equivalent
Word Reading	2.0
Reading Comprehension	2.4
Mathematics Computation	2.7

Primary 2 Form E (presented orally)

	Grade Equivalent
Word Reading	3.7
Reading Comprehension	2.6

Slingerland Test for Specific Language Disability:

Strengths:	auditory modality
Weaknesses:	visual discrimination
	visual/motor
	visual/auditory
	visual memory

Vineland Adaptive Behavior Scale:

Communication Domain	9 years, 10 months
Daily Living Skills Domain	10 years, 5 months
Socialization	9 years, 8 months

House-Tree-Person Drawings

Diagnostic Component	Weak	Strong
VIQ		*
PIQ	*	
Reading	*	
Arithmetic	*	
Visual Motor Skills	*	
Visual Memory	*	
Auditory Memory		*
Multimodality Integration	*	
Writing	*	
Speech Reception		*
Comprehension	Vocabulary	Syntax
Expression		*
Speech Intelligibility		*
Attention		*
Social-Emotional		*
Problem Solving		*
Use of Amplification	FM	HA

On the Wechsler Intelligence Scale for Children-Revised, Morris obtained a Verbal IQ score of 78, and a Performance IQ of 75. Given Morris's hearing loss and multisensory involvements, these scores represent function and not potential as all modalities of information processing are affected. Because he shows adaptive strength at age level or above for other areas of his life, as indicators of potential these scores should be viewed cautiously. Nevertheless, diagnostically, these results demonstrate where difficulties and strengths lie.

The subtest scatter in the verbal section, though not remarkable, suggests that Morris learns incidental information with greater ease than information that is dependent on school experience. The low similarities score suggests that abstract thinking skills are relatively weak, but this might be related to the effects of his hearing loss.

The subtest scatter in the performance section is remarkable for the high score in picture arrangement. Because this subtest requires finding a "story line," an underlying verbal/social component may be helpful to him. The other subtests are quite low and consistent with the results seen in the Bender, suggesting severe deficits in visual/motor perception. Morris's weakest modes of input/output appear to be visual/motor, with auditory information input/output the most reliable avenue of information processing, *despite his hearing loss.* Verbal skills, in direct spoken language and incidental learning, appear to offer his best access to information.

The Stanford Achievement Test was given twice in different formats. First, it was given as the directions require except for the extended time. Morris obtained grade equivalents for Word Reading and Reading Comprehension, 2.0 and 2.4 respectively. Mathematics was slightly higher (2.7). In a second testing session Morris was given another form of the same test orally and achieved a 3.7 and 2.6 in Word Reading and Reading Comprehension. These scores suggest that he understands more than his reading skills indicate and learns information more efficiently when he receives it auditorily only. Many of the errors that Morris made were in the use of the inference, consistent with the similarities score on the WISC-R. He made few errors on questions that did not require inferences.

The Slingerland Test of Specific Language Disability was given to explore Morris's use of the various modalities alone and in combination. Testing revealed that his use of visual and motor modalities was far weaker than his use of auditory alone, supporting the comments above. Visual discrimination was highly unreliable and variable; this was especially evident when Morris was asked to look at words or letters, remember, and then identify them in a group of similar letters or words. Morris could recognize a word and then not know it in another context. His writing contained reversals and transpositions. A learning disability that Johnson and Myklebust (1967) describe as *visual dyslexia* is indicated. It appears that Morris' preferable mode for learning is auditory alone, which will have a significant effect on how he is taught.

The Vineland Adaptive Behavior Scale suggests that all areas of adaptive behavior are at or above age level. Moreover, his social and emotional adjustment has been far superior to his success in academic areas in school. Morris appears to have the social wherewithall and emotional strength to make adaptations and derive satisfaction from the accomplishments he has made. He tends to see the positive rather than the negative. The projective drawings, which may be questionable emotional indicators given his visual motor difficulties, do suggest that Morris feels some confusion about himself in relation to his environment but has a positive self image.

Table II. Questions to Use in the Assessment Process for Mainstreaming Children with Hearing Loss

1. What do I need to know about this child, and which test instruments will give the widest, truest picture of his or her capabilities?
2. When verbal measures of intellectual ability are given, how should they be interpreted relative to the hearing loss?
3. What strengths and weaknesses does this child possess, and how will they affect the school experience?
4. What does the integrated assessment (audiological, speech and language, and psycho-educational) tell us?
5. What preschool/academic skills has this child developed for mainstream readiness (language, attention, socialization, concepts, vocabulary, reading, math, abstract reasoning, etc.)? How does he or she compare with hearing/hearing-impaired peers?
6. How do these skills compare with those of the children in his or her educational setting?
7. What material does the curriculum cover? How does this compare with the needs addressed in the Individualized Education Program?
8. How much progress is being made each year? What are long range predictions based on this?
9. Does this child possess the independence skills necessary for the mainstream?
10. Will present socialization skills development allow the child to "fit in" with his or her class?
11. Is the child motivated to make mainstream adjustment (X factor)?
12. Is there support from parents for mainstream adjustment (too much, too little)?
13. What support services will be needed for this child to succeed in the mainstream placement?
14. Is there support from school staff to allow for special needs of this student and make adjustments?
15. How will school staff collaborate on a frequent basis to monitor progress and focus their efforts?

Comments   Because it was determined that Morris was a stronger auditory learner than visual, it was recommended that he make more frequent use of his FM system in instructional situations. Teaching strategies that emphasize auditory input were suggested, such as use of tapes, tape recorders, records, oral tests, and computer-aided instruction to reduce the motor component. With his instruction emphasizing intervention for the learning disability, a curriculum could be developed that would not fragment services. It was felt that Morris's learning disability was his primary handicap and that the hearing loss was secondary to it. It was recommended that speech and language services continue to build his receptive vocabulary, inference skills, and articulation.

DISCUSSION

The questions listed in table II provide a guide for the psycho-educational assessment paradigm (see figure 1). In drawing up recommendations for a child, after all evaluations are complete, a multidisciplinary conference should be held to integrate all the data available and answer the questions listed in table II. This guide can help to identify needs and chart goals to be accomplished. The group input should result in recommendations that will address the child's needs in a holistic manner and utilize the resources available in a coordinated fashion toward unified goals.

GLOSSARY

Cognition—process of understanding information. Cognition occurs through the five senses to the brain for organization and retention.
Criterion-reference—tests based on mastery of a hierarchy of skills.
Inference—a conclusion or interpretation from partial information—meaning supplied by drawing on person's understanding.
Metacognition—awareness of one's own thinking, reflecting on one's activities and knowledge such as problem solving or planning.
Nonverbal—activities that are non-language based.
Norm-reference—measure based on comparison of the skills of many other students.
Projective testing—a test that allows a person's personality characteristics or feelings to be reflected in his or her response.
Verbal—knowledge related to language based activities.

REFERENCES

Brigance, A. H. 1977. *Brigance Diagnostic Inventory of Basic Skills*. North Billerica, MA: Curriculum Associates.
Garguilo, R. M. 1985. *Working with Parents of Exceptional Children*. Boston: Houghton-Mifflin Co.
Gould, S. J. 1981. *The Mismeasure of Man*. New York: W. W. Norton Co., Inc.
Johnson, D. J., and Myklebust, H. R. 1967. *Learning Disabilities: Educational Principles and Practices*. Orlando: Grune & Stratton, Inc.
Koppitz, E. M. 1963. *The Bender Gestalt Test for Young Children*. New York: Grune and Stratton.
Pflaster, G. 1981. A second analysis of factors related to the academic performance of hearing impaired children in the mainstream. *The Volta Review* Feb–March: 71–81.
Sattler, J. M. 1982. *Assessment of Children's Intelligence and Special Abilities* 2nd Edition: Allyn & Bacon, Inc.
Seligman, M. 1983. (ed). Parenting moderately handicapped persons. In *Family with a Handicapped Child Understanding and Treatment*. Orlando: Grune & Stratton, Inc.

Slingerland, B. H. 1984. *Slingerland Screening Tests for Identifying Children with Specific Language Disability.* Cambridge: Educators Publishing Service.

Sparrow, S., Balla, D., Cicchetti, D. 1984. *Vineland Adaptive Behavior Scale.* Circle Pines, MN: American Guidance Service.

Wechsler, D. 1967. *The Wechsler Preschool and Primary Scale of Intelligence–Revised.* Cleveland: The Psychological Corporation.

Wechsler, D. 1974. *The Manual for the Wechsler Intelligence Scale for Children–Revised.* Orlando: The Psychological Corporation.

Wechsler, D. 1981. *The Manual for the Wechsler Adult Intelligence Scale–Revised.* Orlando: The Psychological Corporation.

Ying, E., and Brackett, D. 1984. Communication evaluation: Academic and social considerations. *Seminars in Hearing* 5(4)4:367–84.

Chapter • 5

Developing an Individualized Education Program for the Mainstreamed Hearing-Impaired Student

Diane Brackett

The concept of an Individualized Education Program (IEP) was developed to ensure that students receive a quality public education despite handicapping conditions. Since its inclusion in Public Law 94-142, the IEP has evolved into a useful document for establishing, in writing, the extent of each child's program.

The law establishes the parents' role in designing and approving the special education plan for each child and provides the legal vehicle through which they can appeal if they are dissatisfied with the outcome. The parents' responsibilities do not end with the development of the initial IEP, because the plan should be reexamined at least yearly to document progress and review the required services.

The IEP has standard components that are required regardless of the exact format that the particular school system chooses. Of particular relevance for the mainstream hearing-impaired student are the following components:

1. Classification of handicapping condition: deaf or hard-of-hearing
2. Extent of participation in regular education: full mainstreaming or part-time mainstreaming for specific subjects

3. Related services: frequency; length of session; individual or group; group size
4. Service providers: name; title; and goal responsibility
5. Special equipment: FM unit
6. Management needs: preferential seating; use pattern for FM unit; extended time for standardized tests; individually administered standardized tests; coordination time for special and regular education staff; daily amplification monitoring program; interpreter; acoustically adapted environment
7. Level of performance
8. Annual goals
9. Short term objectives: instructional materials; evaluation timetable
10. Participants in the planning conference: parents and multidisciplinary team.

MODEL

The model described in Table I delineates the process by which an IEP can be developed by professionals and parents for a mainstreamed hearing-impaired student following a comprehensive multidisciplinary evaluation. *Process* is the key word, since it describes the approach by which deficit areas shape and focus the remedial program and classroom management. This approach requires that professionals discuss their evaluation results, determine common elements, generate a comprehensive profile of the student's needs, and jointly determine appropriate management. Each heading will be described in detail in the remainder of the chapter.

Profile of Strengths and Weaknesses

Through multidisciplinary evaluations and the resulting statement of level of performance, a profile of the student's strengths and weaknesses emerges from which goals for the student can be written on the IEP. These evaluations (see related chapters) also provide the raw material for building a management plan that reflects the unique needs of each hearing-impaired child. The audiological evaluation describes the student's ability to hear and perceive auditory information under controlled conditions. The communication evaluation documents how the student receives, understands, expresses, and produces speech. The education evaluation assesses the impact of the communication deficit on the child's academic performance. The psychological evaluation characterizes the student's learning potential and provides a baseline

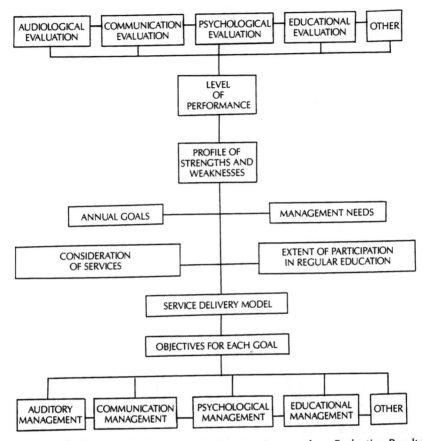

Table I. Developing an Individualized Education Program from Evaluation Results

against which the student's communication and academic performance can be compared. While each evaluation provides specific information, together they reflect the overall deficit pattern imposed by hearing loss.

There are different approaches to "synthesis" that can help portray the multidisciplinary nature of each of the child's problems. The traditional way of organizing the evaluation results is according to the expertise of the professional administering the test. Even though the underlying problems may be the same, each discipline presents a profile of the student's performance that reflects the professional's specific expertise. For example, the special educator may document a delay in reading that needs to be addressed in the academic support program; the speech-language pathologist may determine that the student has deficient speech production and expressive language skills that necessitate enrollment in speech-language therapy. Yet both of these profiles reflect one common problem, a vocabulary deficit. If each discipline is going to address the same identified weakness, then close coordination between the disciplines is essential in order to avoid professional conflicts.

Another way of organizing the data is according to the parameter being assessed, as shown in table II. By looking at the title of tests or subtests, it is possible to identify similar skills being tapped via different modalities or test formats. There is a vocabulary subtest included in achievement tests, speech/language tests, and on the verbal portion of the intelligence test. An analysis of the student's performance on these vocabulary subtests provides a view of how the child handles word meaning across modalities, whether spoken, written, or read. The remedial program evolving out of this analysis will address spoken, written, and read vocabulary. Similar cross-disciplinary analyses can be performed for speech reception, grammar/syntax, and paragraph understanding.

Annual Goals

A logical progression from multidisciplinary evaluation through interpretation to goal development allows all the deficits to be addressed in the written goals. Unlike many children with communication disorders, the hearing-impaired child experiences weaknesses in all aspects of communication, which in turn have an impact on social and academic skill development. Therefore, joint goals generated by the speech/language pathologist, audiologist, special education personnel, and the regular educator should address general deficits identified during the evaluation process. Goals are written to reflect behaviors that can be accomplished realistically in one year.

Management Needs

Management needs are adaptations required to make the learning environment accessible to the mainstreamed hearing-impaired student so that annual goals can be achieved. These needs, which are listed in

Table II. Categorization According to the Parameter Assessed

Parameter	Discipline	Evaluation
Vocabulary	Communication	Comprehension (spoken) Production (spoken) Production (written)
	Education	Vocabulary (read)
	Psychology	Vocabulary (spoken)

the IEP, are derived from the student's performance on multidisciplinary evaluations. Hearing-impaired students have two kinds of special learning requirements: those that circumvent hearing loss by enhancing visual reception of speech and those that deal with hearing loss by optimizing auditory reception of speech. It is imperative that these requirements be written into the IEP so legal recourse is available if the program does not proceed according to plan.

The first step in visually enhancing speech reception is accomplished by adapting visual aspects of the environment. Ensuring that the classroom is well-lighted and that the teacher's face is illuminated without backlighting from a window allows the student to make use of speechreading cues. Consideration should be given to using an interpreter (oral, cued speech, or sign language) to ensure that the teacher's utterances are received by the child. A notetaker should be provided for those students responsible for the material discussed during classroom presentations. The grade at which a notetaker becomes necessary depends upon the educational philosophy of the school and the specific teacher.

It is possible to optimize auditory reception of speech by modifying acoustic characteristics of the listening environment. The addition of any sound absorbing materials can dramatically reduce the amount of classroom noise that might interfere with what is being said. Preferential seating frequently is recommended in order to keep the distance between teacher and student minimal; this provides optimal intensity of the teacher's voice as long as he or she remains in the chosen spot. To further offset negative listening conditions that exist in mainstream classrooms, classroom listening devices should be recommended for students with even the mildest of hearing losses, and their use should be described in detail in the IEP. There is a section on the IEP form to list specialized equipment, but it does not have a place for indicating the use pattern of the equipment. Too often children are instructed to use their FM units only in one-to-one therapy situations or in the resource room. This application is contrary to the intended purpose of an FM system, which is most useful in noisy situations or where there is a large distance between speaker and listener. To avoid misunderstandings it is important to designate on the IEP the subject areas in which the device must be used as well as those times for which a choice is possible. For the sensitive junior high or high school student, specifying that the device need not be worn in the hallway between classes could defuse a potentially explosive situation.

Modifications in the administration of standardized testing are listed under management needs or, in some cases, in a special section of the IEP. In addition to designating the testing category, i.e., the ex-

Table III. Examples of *Objectives* that Logically Evolve from the *Level of Performance* Demonstrated during the Evaluations

AUDITORY MANAGEMENT

Annual Goal

To improve the use of aided residual hearing.

Level of Performance

Is aware when amplification is turned off, but not when severe distortion is present.

Is unaware when /t/ and /d/ are added to words to indicate past tense, except when stressed.

Lacks confidence in his or her ability to functionally use his or her hearing for speech reception for sentence and paragraph material.

Short Term Objective

Will correctly indicate the quality of the amplified sound when asked during daily troubleshooting at 60% accuracy.

Will recognize /t/ and /d/ used to denote past tense when the sentence stimuli are presented listen alone at 75% level.

Will paraphrase the content of a three sentence paragraph presented without visual clues at 90% level.

COMMUNICATION MANAGEMENT

Annual Goal

To improve reception of spoken language.

Level of Performance

Instead of indicating when he or she has not understood, the student either nods head or has a blank expression.

Has deficient word knowledge that affects the student's ability to understand lecture material.

Lacks flexibility in word use as evidenced by limited use of idiomatic expressions, multiple meanings, antonyms, and synonyms.

Short Term Objectives

Given an unintelligible/ambiguous utterance, child will indicate his or her confusion by requesting clarification specifically indicating that part of the utterance misunderstood at 70% level.

Will demonstrate understanding of 150 new words based on school-related topics at 80% level.

Will provide a minimum of two meanings for each of 25 common words and use them appropriately in sentences at 75% level.

PSYCHO-SOCIAL MANAGEMENT

Annual Goal

To demonstrate age-appropriate social behavior.

Level of Performance

Enjoys the company of other children but seems to be led astray or leads the others into unacceptable behavior.

Uses aggressive means of interacting with his or her peers in situations where negotiation is the socially-acceptable alternative.

Short Term Objectives

Given peer/peer interaction, child will demonstrate or suggest socially acceptable behavioral alternatives at 75% level.

Will demonstrate his or her verbal negotiation skills during role playing activities which mirror potential situations in the classroom at 85% level.

EDUCATIONAL MANAGEMENT

Annual Goal

To achieve age-level reading and writing skills.

Level of Performance

Reading is at age level for concrete material with breakdown occurring when inference is required.

Has difficulty interpreting the information being requested in essay questions.

Short Term Objectives

Will demonstrate understanding of inference in grade level paragraphs at 85% level.

When presented with essay questions that require the student to *describe, compare* and *contrast,* or *list,* he or she will provide a well-organized answer that accurately addresses the question at 60% level.

tent to which the student participates in city and statewide testing, this section stipulates if extended time and one-to-one administration are required.

Extent of Participation in Regular Education

Each year the degree of each student's participation in mainstreamed education must be reassessed in order to determine how well the regular classroom can accommodate the student's academic needs. A level of participation that is appropriate in the early elementary years may no longer meet his or her needs in middle school or high school. Conversely, a student who has been in a self-contained class during the early grades may show sufficient progress to warrant more involvement in regular education for some subject areas.

Each potential placement has its own set of communicative demands and educational requirements. Self-contained classes are small, maintaining student-to-teacher ratios of 8 to 1 instead of the typical 20 to 1, and are acoustically adapted to the needs of hearing-impaired students. Because the curriculum is geared to the language skills of students, the content is, in most cases, below that to which same-aged normal-hearing students are exposed, and the communicative requirements are reduced. As more mainstreaming is included in the student's program, he or she must be able to converse easily with peers and adults, and learn in an environment that has minimal accommodations for hearing-impaired students. Decisions regarding the most appropriate placement should be based upon the student's performance during the multidisciplinary evaluation and the educational and communicative demands of the setting.

The role of the regular classroom teacher should be delineated in detail in the IEP. This should be done whether participation in regular education is to be fairly minimal, limited to social experiences only, or whether academic subjects will be learned in the regular classroom. If the student participates fully in all aspects of the learning experience, then the classroom teacher is responsible for planning and implementing the curriculum. The student should have the entry skills necessary to learn from the lesson as it is presented to all the students in the class. As a class participant, the hearing-impaired student works under the same grading scheme and class requirements as the other students. Any confusion on the teacher's part regarding the grading of tests, homework, and expected performance should be resolved before the mainstream placement begins. Often if the student has been in a more protected environment, the teacher and parent will agree to a short transition period between the smaller supportive setting and the pressured regular classroom environment. If transition is the purpose of the placement, then the teacher should be informed so that he or she can set appropriate expectations and act accordingly.

Consideration of Services

Because of the heterogeneity of the hearing-impaired population in auditory, communicative, academic, and social skills, it is not possible to prescribe specific services based on age or degree of hearing loss. Instead, the following is a comprehensive list of services that might be needed by a student with a hearing loss. It is a summary of the information appearing in other chapters of this book. Whether a service is appropriate for a particular child can only be determined by a thorough evaluation of the child's skills in and out of the classroom. These services should be considered for inclusion on the IEPs of all hearing-impaired children and omitted for a specific child only when his or her performance has ruled out the need.

POTENTIAL SERVICES FOR
MAINSTREAMED HEARING-IMPAIRED STUDENTS

   I. Comprehensive audiological and amplification evaluation (minimum, once per year)
       A. Unaided testing: to include pure-tone air and bone conduction; speech detection and recognition
       B. Assessment of middle ear function (as needed)
       C. Aided testing (aids and FM): to include sound field warble tone thresholds; speech detection and recognition measures, in quiet and noise
       D. Electroacoustic analysis of hearing aids and FM system
   II. Comprehensive communication evaluation (minimum, once per year)
       A. Assessment of preferred receptive mode: to include word, sentence, and paragraph material presented auditorily only, visually only, auditorily-visually combined, in quiet and noise and at varying speaker/listener distances.
       B. Assessment of comprehension of spoken language: to include single word, sentence, and paragraph level material.
       C. Assessment of production of spoken language: to include single word, sentence, and paragraph level material.
       D. Assessment of speech intelligibility
       E. Assessment of written language

III. Educational evaluation (annual)
    A. Assessment of reading: to include word knowledge, sentence comprehension, and paragraph understanding
    B. Assessment of math: to include calculation and word problems

IV. Psycho-social evaluation (triennial)
    A. Assessment of intellectual status (performance subtests)
    B. Assessment of social skills and adjustment

V. Evaluation of classroom learning environment (minimum, once per year)
    A. Child/teacher communicative interactions
    B. Child/child communicative and social interactions
    C. Child participation in classroom activities
    D. Classroom modifications used by the teacher to ensure understanding
    E. Strategies employed by the child to facilitate learning
    F. Use of FM systems by the child and teacher
    G. Analysis of noise sources in the classroom that can interfere with speech reception
    H. Analysis of visual distractions in the classroom that can interfere with speech reception
    I. Use of classroom aide/interpreter to facilitate communication in the classroom

VI. Classroom audiological management
    A. Improving classroom acoustics
    B. Recommending and using FM systems
    C. Daily troubleshooting of personal aids and FM system
    D. Assessing use of FM system in various settings
    E. Monitoring of middle ear problems with appropriate referrals

VII. Speech-language management
    A. Remedial program: focus on deficit areas that have an impact on academic performance and social interaction
    B. Classroom communication management: coordinate with support personnel and classroom teacher; improve classroom presentation by paraphrasing, directing classroom discussion, and using visual aids

VIII. Educational management
    A. Academic support: preview/review tutoring of academic vocabulary and academic concepts
    B. Classroom support through suggestions to increase the student's access to the content material: locate favorable seating that is close to the primary sound source; assign a

"buddy" to keep the student abreast of changes in class-room routines; provide a peer notetaker during lecture classes; provide classroom amplification to reduce inter-ference from background noise and large speaker/listener distances; coordinate the vital exchange of information from the classroom teacher to the academic support per-sonnel; provide an interpreter to ensure optimal reception of classroom lecture and discussion

IX. Psycho-social management
   A. Individual support: to include adolescent support group, career counseling, parent support group, participation in extracurricular social activities
   B. Classroom adjustment through teacher-facilitated group interaction

X. In-service training
   A. Staff: to include all school personnel once per year and di-rect-service personnel twice per year
   B. Peers: once per year

The kind and frequency of each evaluation by the multidisciplin-ary team should be specified in the IEP because evaluation information is critical to the planning process, permitting a longitudinal view of the child's status. Without an accurate indication of progress in each area, it is not possible to adapt the existing program to meet changing skills.

With respect to the mainstreamed hearing-impaired student, any form of intervention, whether audiological, communicative, or educa-tional, has an impact on both individual and classroom management. Because the regular school environment lacks the special modifications present in the special education setting and regular educators have little experience with hearing-impaired students, a major focus of the intervention program must deal with ramifications of placing students in this setting, i.e., assisting those educators in enhancing the environ-ment. Support from the audiologist is required for the teacher to en-sure optimal use of classroom amplification; the speech-language pa-thologist can suggest ways of enhancing classroom communication to utilize the child's strengths and the special educator can suggest learn-ing strategies for the teacher to employ when difficulties in under-standing arise. The individual remedial program, in addition to addressing typical deficit areas, must include an academic support program coordinated with the classroom curriculum through frequent meetings between special and regular educators. This particular aspect of the remedial program is essential for the mainstreamed student whose primary educational program occurs in the regular classroom.

Careful and complete selection of services is critical. If the foregoing outline is employed for all hearing-impaired students in mainstreamed settings, there will be fewer children receiving services they do not need or not receiving the most salient services because their need was not obvious.

Service Delivery Alternatives

Once the services have been selected, the IEP team must determine how the designated services will be delivered, taking into consideration student motivation, school finances, and availability of resources.

Child Factors It is crucial to determine the student's motivation to learn and his or her learning style. A student who is challenged by tough competition is best suited to the stimulating environment of the mainstream classroom. The availability of home reinforcement to supplement school work is important. The absence of home support will be apparent. When home support is present, the professionals involved must use it effectively. The "parent" factor can not be ignored.

School Factors Factors such as the availability of support personnel play a role in deciding which service delivery model will be best for the student and the school system. Some school districts, especially those in rural communities, do not have staff specifically trained or with appropriate credentials for working with hearing-impaired students. With no teacher of the hearing impaired to provide academic support, and with only one itinerant speech-language pathologist to cover a 150 mile area and visit schools twice weekly for the most severe cases, the question arises, "Is it possible to provide a quality program with the personnel who are available?" The answer may be "no" if caseloads are heavy and coordination time is difficult to arrange. Or the answer may be a resounding "yes." Many highly individualized programs have been implemented by support personnel who, with some in-service consultation, provide exactly what a child needs even though they do not possess the "correct" professional credentials.

The school district's attitude toward mainstreaming can affect the service delivery model selected. A district may not want the bother of generating a local program, preferring instead to send the student to an already existing out-of-district program. Conversely, a small district may be able to hire that special teacher who can effectively design a suitable program for a specific child. Economics also affect the choice of a model for a particular child. It may be less expensive to initiate a program locally, rather than pay a large tuition to centralized special education services. However, it is difficult to effectively implement a quality program without sufficient resources.

These child and school factors must be considered as the decision regarding the service delivery model is made. No single approach is right for each student or each school district. Finding the approach that best matches the student's motivation level and the school's economic needs and attitude is the challenge.

Objectives

Once the service delivery model has been selected, the service providers write objectives for each identified deficit area and designate the timetable for evaluating the student's performance. Multiple objectives typically are needed for each annual goal to ensure that all deficits described in the evaluation section are addressed in the IEP. Table III displays objectives designed to meet the needs of a hypothetical hearing-impaired student whose communicative, academic, and social functioning are described under the section labeled *Level of Performance*. Table III should not be considered all inclusive or even applicable to another student, but represents the objective-writing process that logically evolves from the deficits described under the *Level of Performance* and addressed by the *Annual Goal*.

Once the objectives have been generated, the teacher selects instructional materials that will facilitate learning. Although it is impossible to anticipate all potentially useful remedial activities, written descriptors give parents an opportunity to confirm methods that have been useful in the past or negate others that are contraindicated based upon the child's previously demonstrated learning style.

The final section of the IEP specifies evaluation tools that have been selected to assess the child's progress in learning targeted skills. The timetable for completing re-evaluations may vary, depending on the anticipated rate of skill acquisition and the specificity of the objectives. In general, progress is assessed at least annually so that changes can be made in the IEP that reflect this new level of performance. Parental signature indicates agreement with the services, goals, objectives, and timetable stated in the IEP.

SUMMARY

Thus the IEP process is complete, from evaluation and interpretation, to service selection and implementation. Each step is intricately interwoven with the other; none can effectively stand alone.

The IEP stands as a detailed written description of services to be rendered, goals and objectives to be met, and a time frame in which the skills are to be learned. It represents an agreement among the educators and parents regarding the "appropriate" environment to facilitate learning and provides a written document as legal evidence. Care in its preparation and design is critical if the unique needs of the mainstreamed hearing-impaired student are to be met.

RECOMMENDED READINGS

Dublinske, S. 1978. P.L. 94-142: Developing the individualized educational program. *ASHA* 20(5):393–97.

Nober, L. W. 1978. Developing effective IEPs for the hearing-impaired: Considerations and issues. In *Periscope: Views of the Individualized Education Program*, ed. B. B. Weiner. Reston, VA: The Council for Exceptional Children.

Nober, L. W. 1981. Developing IEPs for hard of hearing children. In *Special Education in Transition: Educating Hard of Hearing Children*, eds. L. Nober and M. Ross. Washington, DC: A. G. Bell Association for the Deaf.

Ross, M., Brackett, D., and Maxon, A. 1982. *Hard of Hearing Children in Regular Schools*. Englewood Cliffs, NJ: Prentice-Hall Inc.

Chapter • 6

Managing Classroom
Amplification

Jane R. Madell

Under the best of situations, almost every classroom offers a poor acoustic environment. The rooms are large, the ceilings are high, there are hard wall surfaces for sounds to bounce off of, and the windows may face a busy street or a playground. In addition, there is unwanted noise within the rooms. Children are, by their very nature, not quiet. They whisper to their neighbors, shuffle their feet, and move papers and books around. To complicate matters even further, the teacher is, at best, several feet away from the child who is listening. He or she may be facing away from the child toward the blackboard or another child, eliminating the possibility that the child can use speechreading clues. In addition, the person from whom the child must receive information is not always the teacher in the front of the room. Other children in the room may take turns speaking. It will probably be difficult for the hearing-impaired child to identify who is speaking so that he or she can look at the speaker. This all adds up to a difficult listening condition that requires special assistance. Fortunately, technology and classroom management can help.

SPEECH ACOUSTICS

It is important to have some basic information about speech acoustics in order to understand some of the factors that affect classroom listening. Figure 1 presents a basic overview of the frequency and intensity com-

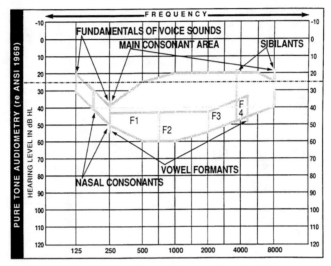

Figure 1.   General description of speech acoustics plotted on an audiogram.
Reprinted with permission from Ross, Brackett, and Maxon (in press).

position of speech. Vowels have most of their energy in the low frequencies (60–500 Hz). They account for 60% of the power of speech
information but account for only 5% of the intelligibility of speech.
Consonants have their energy in mid and high frequencies (1000–8000
Hz). They carry only 5% of the power or energy of speech but are responsible for 60% of the intelligibility (Levitt 1978; Gerber 1974). There
is a 30 dB range from the softest speech sounds to the most powerful
throughout the frequency range. Low frequency information provides
us with suprasegmental information (rhythm and inflection) as well as
perception of some vowels and low frequency consonants. High frequencies convey most of the information for perceiving the majority of
consonants. They are also critical for recognizing verb tense ("walks"
vs. "walked"), pluralization ("book" vs. "books"), possession
("yours," "John's"), and contractions ("it's," "he's," "what's").

The perception of the higher frequencies is therefore obviously
critical for language learning. Detecting higher frequencies, however,
is difficult because they contain less energy than the lower frequencies
and they can be easily masked by noise. To complicate things even further, most hearing-impaired children have poorer hearing in the
higher frequencies, making reception of high frequency components
even more difficult. Our goal is to provide these children with amplification that permits them to hear speech sounds over a wide range of
frequencies and intensities. This provision is the critical prerequisite
for maximizing the auditory contribution to the development and comprehension of speech and language.

CLASSROOM ACOUSTICS

Noise and Reverberation

When speech and noise are equally intense they are said to have a signal-to-noise ratio of 0 (0 S/N). If speech is 15 dB louder than noise, the S/N ratio is +15. If the noise is 15 dB louder than the speech the S/N ratio is −15. The higher the S/N ratio, the easier it is to understand speech. A hearing-impaired person needs a S/N ratio of +20 to +25 in order to maximize speech perception. Work by Finitzo-Hieber and Tillman (1978), Tillman, Carhart, and Olsen (1970), Bess and McConnell (1981) and others have demonstrated the effect that different S/N ratios have on the perception of speech.

Reverberation also has a negative effect on the perception of speech. Reverberation time is the length of time it takes for a sound to decrease 60 dB after the source has ceased. If a speech sound reverberates for a long time it will become combined with other speech sounds that arrive later and will interfere with the ability to understand speech. For normal-hearing people the ideal reverberation time is about 0.6 to 0.8 seconds for larger rooms and 0.4 for smaller rooms (Bess and McConnell 1981; Ross 1978). Reverberation begins to degrade word recognition significantly for hearing-impaired children when it exceeds 0.4 to 0.5 seconds (Bess 1981). Table I, from the work of Finitzo-Hieber and Tillman (1978) demonstrates the effect of different levels of

Table I. Speech Intelligibility Scores for Normal Hearing, Unaided Hard-of-Hearing, and Aided Hard-of-Hearing Children Under Different Reverberation Times and Signal-to-Noise Ratios (Used with permission from Finitzo-Hieber and Tillman 1978.)

Reverberation Time (sec)	Signal-to-Noise Ratio (dB)	Normal Hearing	Unaided Hard-of-Hearing	Aided Hard-of-Hearing
0.0	Quiet	95	88	83
	+12	89	78	70
	+6	78	66	60
	0	60	42	39
0.4	Quiet	93	79	74
	+12	83	69	60
	+6	71	55	52
	0	48	29	28
1.2	Quiet	77	62	45
	+12	69	50	41
	+6	54	40	27
	0	30	15	11

competing noise and reverberation times on speech perception for normal-hearing and hearing-impaired children. Figure 2, from the work of Finitzo-Hieber and Tillman (1978) displays the same kind of information for four reverberation levels. These data demonstrate the significant negative effect that noise and reverberation can have on the functioning of hearing-impaired children in classrooms.

Effect of Distance

Distance between the listener and the speaker has a significant impact on how speech is received. Figure 3, from Ross, Brackett, and Maxon (1982), clearly demonstrates this effect. If a child is standing three feet from the person speaking (the best one could expect in a classroom), speech will arrive at his or her ear at about 46 dBHL. If the child is six feet from the person speaking, the signal at the ear will be 40 dBHL. If the child is 12 feet away, the signal will only be 34 dBHL. On the other hand, if the child is 4½ inches from the person speaking, the speech will be 84 dBHL at the child's ear. It is not likely that a teacher would be able to arrange to have his or her mouth 4½ inches from the child's ear throughout the day, but an FM microphone 4½ inches away from the teacher's mouth would have the same effect.

Classroom Noise

The noise levels in a standard classroom should not exceed 30 to 35 dB (on the "A" scale of a sound level meter) if optimal learning is to take

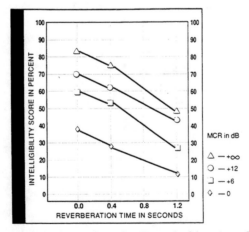

Figure 2. Speech intelligibility scores for 12 normal-hearing children as a function of four reverberation times and four signal-to-noise levels. (Reprinted with permission from Finitzo-Hieber and Tillman 1978).

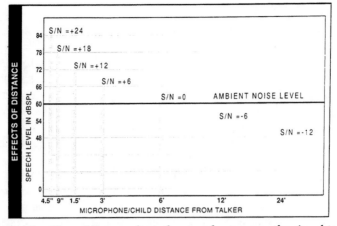

Figure 3. The effect of distance from the speech source on the signal-to-noise ratio with an ambient noise level of 60 dB assumed to be present in the room. (Reprinted with permission from Ross, Brackett, and Maxon 1982).

place (Bess and McConnell 1981; Gengel 1971; Olsen 1988; Finitzo-Hieber 1981). A number of authors have investigated the problem of classroom noise and their reports are significant. Sanders (1965), Ross and Giolas (1971, 1978), and others have demonstrated that in average kindergarten rooms, when students are present, the mean noise level is about 69 dB (on the "C" or linear scale). Noise levels in elementary school classrooms are appoximately 59 dB and in high school classrooms are approximately 62 dB. When one considers the effects on speech recognition of competing noise and reverberation, it is clear that there is a need to provide alternative listening devices (FM systems).

FM SYSTEMS

What Is An FM System?

An FM (frequency modulated) system is a wireless amplification system in which a speech signal is transmitted from a microphone via FM radio signals to an FM receiver. The microphone is worn by the teacher or parent, and the receiver is worn by the student. The FM signals can be transmitted on a number of different radio frequencies. The frequencies used for FM systems are designated by the Federal Communications Commission (FCC) and compete with several other systems (some paging devices and garage door openers).

Advantages of FM Systems

A hearing-impaired child in the regular classroom is at a disadvantage in the ability to receive information. First, the child probably will have some language delay that interferes with his or her ability to comprehend the speech that is heard. In addition, the hearing loss itself will preclude the perception of some speech signals. Distance from the speaker, noise in the classroom, and reverberation will all significantly decrease the acoustic information available. These factors make it critical that every attempt be made to improve the classroom listening situation. The teacher of the hearing-impaired, the speech-language pathologist, the resource room teacher and the parents will focus on the language delay. Managing the acoustical conditions in the classroom is the responsibility of the audiologist. Some of the problems can be reduced by modifications of the classroom itself. (This will be discussed later in this chapter.) Fortunately, FM systems will significantly reduce the negative effects of poor classroom acoustics. With the FM transmitter placed appropriately 4–6 inches from the teacher's mouth, the problem of distance will be eliminated (see figure 3). Although noise and reverberation in the classroom cannot be eliminated completely, their impact upon speech intelligibility will be reduced because the speech signal reaching the child from the FM transmitter will be louder than the classroom noise. The FM system should provide a signal that is 15–20 dB more intense than that arriving directly at the child's ear through his or her hearing aid.

Figure 4 demonstrates the advantage of an FM system over standard hearing aids for a child with severe to profound hearing loss. The most gain one can hope to obtain with a hearing aid is about 60 dB. The astericks (*) represent the expected aided thresholds. This figure clearly demonstrates that although the hearing aid is providing a significantly louder signal, there are still many speech sounds that are not being perceived. Simply by using an FM transmitter, one can improve the audibility of the signal. Because an FM transmitter is only 4–6 inches from the mouth of the person who is speaking, the signal at the FM microphone will be 15–20 dB more intense than would occur with a hearing aid. The triangles on the audiogram represent the advantage that the FM system provides in this example. Although the child is still not receiving *all* the acoustic components necessary to obtain *optimal* speech perception (see Chapter 2), there is significantly more auditory information available with the FM system than without it.

Figure 5 shows the same relationship for a child with a severe hearing loss and figure 6 for a child with a moderate hearing loss. Even for a moderate hearing loss, when a gain of about 40 dB is appropriate, the advantage of the FM system is still clear.

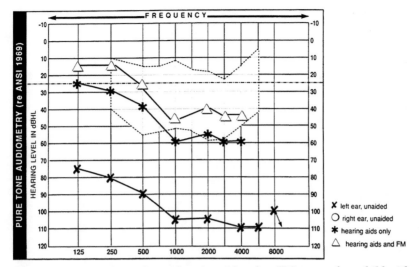

Figure 4. Expected gain from a hearing aid and an FM system for a child with a profound hearing loss.

Figures 7 and 8 demonstrate the FM advantage for children with moderately-severe and profound hearing losses. Of specific interest in figure 7 is the word recognition information in quiet at soft conversational levels (35 dB) and in the presence of competing noise. Although the FM advantage at normal conversational levels (50 dB) in a quiet test

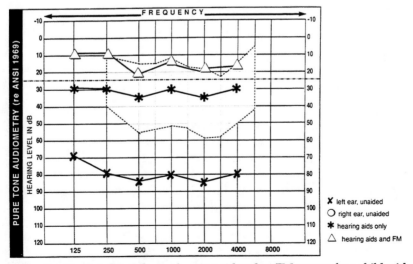

Figure 5. Expected gain from a hearing aid and an FM system for a child with a severe hearing loss.

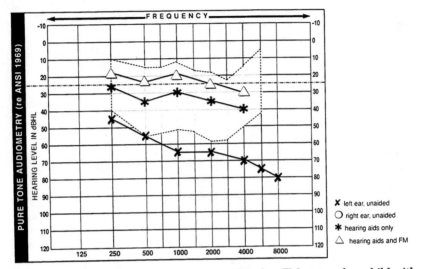

Figure 6. Expected gain from a hearing aid and an FM system for a child with a moderate hearing loss.

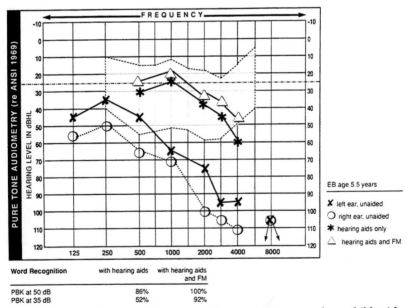

Word Recognition	with hearing aids	with hearing aids and FM
PBK at 50 dB	86%	100%
PBK at 35 dB	52%	92%

Figure 7. Speech recognition and warble tone responses for a child with a moderately-severe hearing loss comparing hearing aid and FM responses.

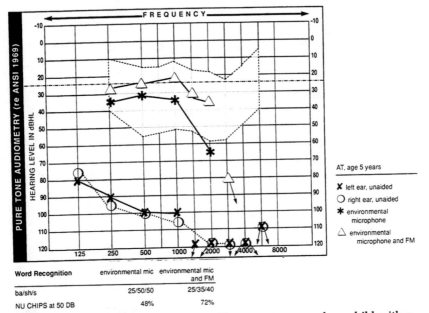

Word Recognition	environmental mic	environmental mic and FM
ba/sh/s	25/50/50	25/35/40
NU CHIPS at 50 DB	48%	72%

Figure 8.   Speech recognition and warble tone responses for a child with a profound hearing loss comparing hearing aid and FM responses.

room is limited, the advantage of reducing microphone distance is very clearly apparent at the 35 dB level. Figure 8 demonstrates the advantage of an FM system for a child with a profound hearing loss. With this degree of hearing loss the FM advantage is apparent at the 50 dB speech input level.

Who Needs an FM System?

An FM system will benefit anyone who functions under adverse listening conditions. Every hearing-impaired child, simply because of the hearing loss, functions under adverse listening conditions. Although children with mild or moderate hearing losses may not appear to have any listening difficulty at close range in the quiet of a test room, this will not be true in noise, or when the speech source is far from them. Even if they appear to do fairly well at soft speech levels, the listening effort may make it difficult for them to concentrate for long periods of time.

To demonstrate the difficulty of listening at soft sound levels one can turn the television to a level where speech can barely be understood. After a few minutes, it will be difficult to concentrate. Now turn on a radio set to a "talk" station. Set it at a sufficiently soft level so that the television can still be understood. Try again to concentrate on what is happening on TV; after a few minutes, concentration will be difficult. Imagine being a young child in a classroom where it is important to comprehend speech all day long. It would not be reasonable to expect a child to attend to soft speech under these conditions for any length of time. Without additional assistance, the child will lose interest, cease to pay attention, and fall behind in school work. Every hearing-impaired child, regardless of the degree of hearing loss, needs an improved signal in the classroom. The FM signal, simply by increasing the loudness of the teacher's voice, will reduce listening fatigue and improve speech comprehension.

FM System Options

The audiologist must select the type of microphone transmitter to be used by the classroom teacher, the receiver to be worn by the child, and the method of coupling the receiver to the child's ear.

Transmitters. FM microphone/transmitters come in three varieties. The lavalier microphone (figure 9) hangs from the neck by a cord worn around the neck. Because of its position on the neck, the microphone is always at an appropriate distance from the speaker's mouth.

The clip-on microphone (figure 10) is attached to the speaker's shirt or jacket and connected by a wire (which serves as the antenna) to a transmitter pack worn in the pocket or on a belt. If the clothing to which the microphone is attached is loose, its position may change with movement. As a result, it will not necessarily be in the correct position at all times.

A miniature boom microphone (figure 11) is also available with some systems. It is worn on a headband with the microphone near the mouth. This provides the most ideal signal but is viewed by some as awkward and uncomfortable to wear. Its location near the face may also interfere with speechreading.

Receivers. FM receivers come with a variety of options. Some are designed to be coupled with hearing aids, and others contain environmental microphones so that they also can function as body-worn hearing aids. They may be monaural or binaural. The binaural self-contained receiver allows the audiologist to adjust electroacoustic settings separately for each ear. (Some units are adaptable for use as either monaural or binaural systems, with or without environmental microphones.) It is important that the FM system include environmental microphones, located either in the FM receiver or in a personal hearing aid, so that the child can hear his or her own voice and that of children

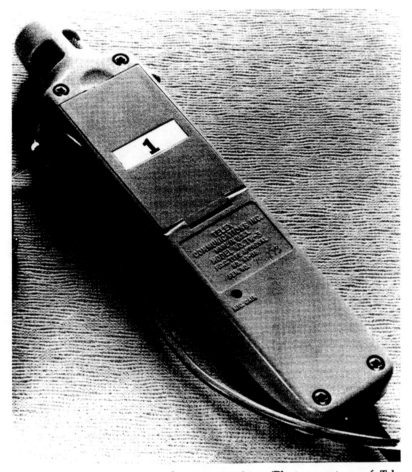

Figure 9. FM lavalier microphone transmitter (Photo courtesy of Telex Corporation).

seated close by. If environmental signals are being detected through hearing aids or behind-the-ear (BTE) transducers (explained below, see figure 13), the FM receiver can be worn attached to a belt, or in a pocket under or over the clothing.

Coupling Systems.   A number of different methods are available to transmit the signal from the FM receiver to the child's ear.

1. *Button transducers.* These attach by wires to the FM receiver and snap directly into standard earmolds (figure 12). In this case, the self-contained FM system is also functioning as a body hearing aid. It therefore must include environmental microphones and have the capability to modify the amplification pattern in both

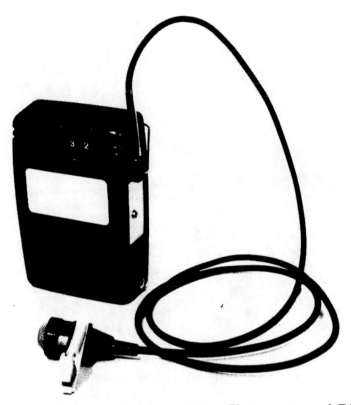

Figure 10. FM lapel microphone transmitter (Photo courtesy of Telex Corporation).

ears. The environmental microphones should be placed high up on the chest so that the child can receive a clear signal from his or her own voice.

2. *Behind-the-ear transducers*. These look like BTE (behind-the-ear) hearing aids, except that they contain only a microphone and a miniature loudspeaker (figure 13). The other components are located in the FM receiver. A wire attaches the BTE transducer to the FM receiver. This system has the advantage of placing the microphones at ear level and permits certain earmold acoustic changes (see Chapter 2). The amplified signal frequently contains less low frequency and more high frequency information than occurs with button transducers and a body location for the environmental microphones. Because the environmental microphones are located at ear level with BTE transducers, the FM receiver can be worn under the clothing or at the waist.

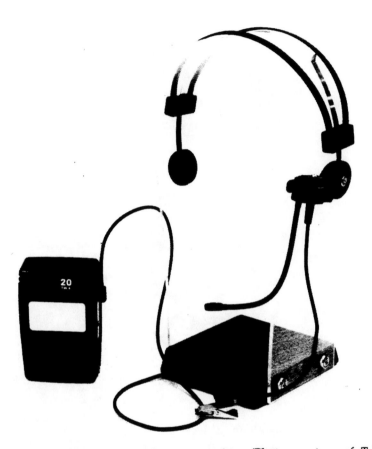

Figure 11. FM boom microphone transmitter (Photo courtesy of Telex Corporation).

3. *Direct audio input.* In a direct audio input connection, the child's own hearing aid is coupled to the FM receiver by a "shoe" or "boot" via a wire cord (figure 14). This coupling mode requires a hearing aid that includes a special electrical connection to accept the FM signal from the FM receiver. Because the environmental microphones on the FM system will not be used, it is possible to wear the receiver under the clothing. The wires to the hearing aids, however, still will be visible. Different types of audio boots are available. Some cut off the environmental microphone and others do not. Except in very special circumstances, a boot should be chosen that will not deactivate the environmental microphone on the child's hearing aid.

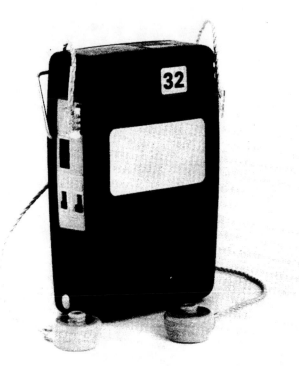

Figure 12. FM receiver with button transducers (Photo courtesy of Telex Corporation).

4. *Neck loop.* This is a loop of wire worn around the neck and connected to the FM receiver (figure 15). When the child's hearing aid is turned to the telephone switch (the "T" setting), a small coil is activated in the hearing aid. The FM signal is transmitted to the wire loop. This creates a magnetic field around the loop. This magnetic energy is picked up by the telephone coil in the hearing aid, amplified, and converted to sound. If the hearing aid has an "MT" (microphone-telephone) switch, the child will be able to use the hearing aid microphones for environmental signals. If not, the child will not be able to hear his or her own voice or hear people who are speaking at a distance from the FM transmitter. The advantage of the neck loop is that it can be worn under clothing. However the magnetic signal is subject to interference from other signals in the environment. The strength of the signal depends on the strength of the telephone coil of the hearing aid and upon the distance of the hearing aid from the neck loop. Very small increases in distance can significantly reduce the signal the telecoil picks up from the teleloop.

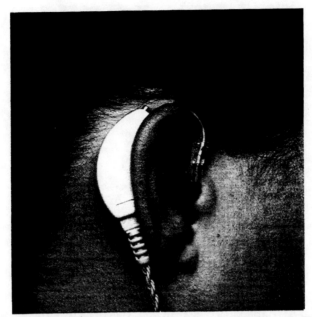

Figure 13.   Behind-the-ear microphone transducer for use with FM system (Photo courtesy of Phonic Ear Corporation).

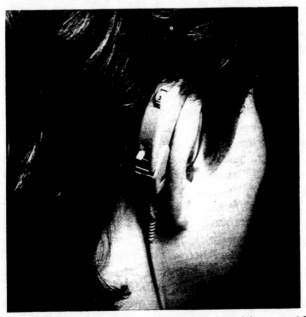

Figure 14.   Hearing aid with audio-input boot and cord for use with FM system (Photo courtesy of Phonic Ear Corporation).

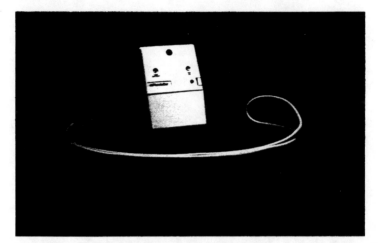

Figure 15. FM receiver with neck loop (Photo courtesy of Phonic Ear Corporation).

5. *Silhouette inductor.* This device is a loop incorporated in a thin piece of plastic shaped like a hearing aid. It is placed alongside the hearing aid, which is switched to the "T" or "MT" position. The closeness of the inductor to the aid creates a stronger signal in the telecoil than that produced with a neck loop. The inductor is connected to the FM receiver by a wire cord. This system is useful when a standard neck loop is not strong enough and the hearing aid does not have audio-input capabilities.

FM System Specifications

Electroacoustic characteristics vary from system to system and between different coupling systems (Hawkins and Van Tassell 1982; Hawkins and Schum 1985). Figure 16 displays the response of an FM system coupled to a hearing aid through a neck loop and with audio-input. Figure 17 demonstrates the response resulting from a different hearing aid/FM system, also coupled to a neck loop and an audio-input boot. With the system used in figure 16, the neck loop reduces the response in the low frequencies. The system used in figure 17 does not cut the low frequencies with the neck loop, but does increase the low frequency amplification when audio-input is used. Figure 18 shows the difference in response when button transducers, a BTE transducer, and audio-input are used on the same FM system. In figure 19 the effects of different button transducers are displayed. For the most part, the results are not predictable from information about the individual components. To be certain that a particular system is functioning as

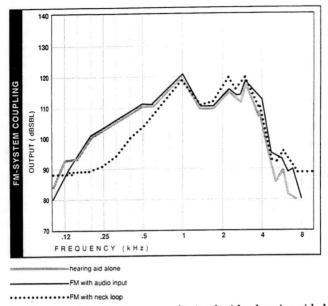

Figure 16.   Frequency response curves obtained with a hearing aid alone and with the hearing aid connected via a neck loop and an audio-input boot to an FM receiver; output was matched at 1000 Hz.

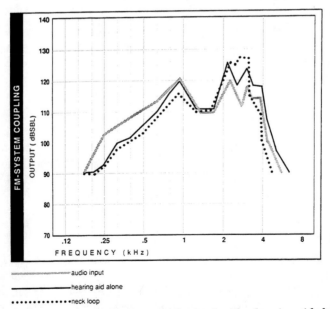

Figure 17.   Frequency response curves obtained with a hearing aid alone and with a hearing aid connected via a neck loop and an audio-input boot to an FM receiver; output was matched at 1000 Hz.

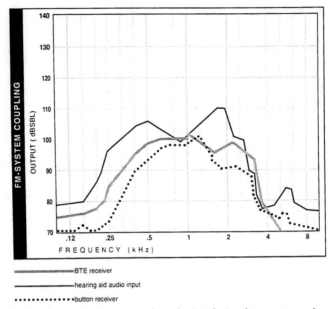

Figure 18. Frequency response curves obtained via a button transducer, a behind-the-ear transducer and a hearing aid with audio-input connected to an FM system; output was matched at 1000 Hz.

desired, the entire system must be evaluated electroacoustically and behaviorally. Without such an evaluation, it is not possible to ensure that the system is functioning as desired.

THE FM EVALUATION

An FM evaluation has two main purposes. First, it is necessary to demonstrate to the child, parents, and school personnel that an FM system will be beneficial. Second, evaluation of different systems will permit the selection of one that will best suit the child's needs.

Test Room Setup

The child should be seated three feet from the loudspeaker and facing it in the same way that he or she would be seated for a hearing aid evaluation. The FM transmitter should be hung 4–6 inches in front of the loudspeaker, simulating its typical placement 4–6 inches from the speaker's mouth (see figure 20). A 50 dBHL signal from the audiometer is calibrated to reach the child's ear three feet away from the loud-

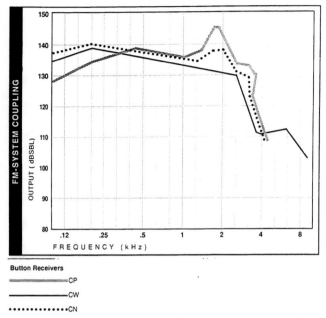

Figure 19.   Frequency response curves obtained with three different button receivers coupled to an FM system.

speaker at 50 dBHL. It will reach the FM transmitter at about 65 dBHL because the FM transmitter is located closer to the loudspeaker than is the child's ear. This simulates the normal listening situations with and without an FM system. To test with competing noise it is necessary to introduce the noise through a loudspeaker placed three feet behind the child (180 azimuth) or directly above the child's head.

Test Conditions

To demonstrate the FM contribution, aided sound-field thresholds should be measured, first in the hearing aid/environmental micro- phone only condition, and then combined with an open FM micro- phone. This will demonstrate the increased sound available through the FM system. If the child is ever in a situation in which he or she uses the FM system without the hearing aid or environmental microphone, then the FM only condition should be tested as well. (We do not rou- tinely evaluate this condition because we believe that a child only rarely should be in a situation in which he or she cannot hear his or her own voice.)

Following aided thresholds, it is necessary to measure word rec- ognition scores with hearing aids alone and with hearing aids and FM

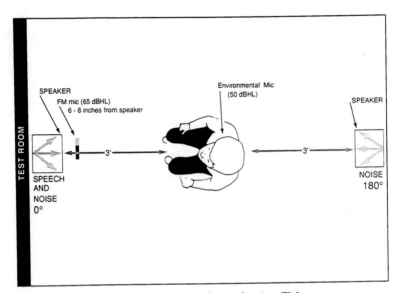

Figure 20.   Test-room arrangement for evaluating FM systems.

system together. Testing should be performed at normal conversational levels (50 dBHL), soft conversational levels (35 dBHL), and in the presence of competing noise at 0 S/N or +6 S/N. (For information about selection of word recognition tests and competing noise see Chapter 2.)

By looking at scores under the different test conditions it is possible to delineate the FM advantage. The improvement in warble tone and speech test results with the FM system should be clearly evident, especially at soft conversational levels and in the presence of competing noise (see figure 7). Note particularly that with the FM system, speech recognition scores are significantly improved in all test conditions. In addition, it is often helpful to demonstrate the FM advantage by having the child turn the FM system on and off while listening to speech in a noisy location. These evaluations should convince virtually every child, parent, and teacher that it is much easier to hear with the FM system than without it.

Acceptance of Use of the FM System

The younger the child, the easier it is to get him or her, the parents, and school personnel to accept the need for an FM system. Young children almost never resist. They are not yet at a stage where vanity is a concern and they usually follow directions from parents and teachers. As children grow older, social concerns become a factor. Still, children who rely on audition for communication purposes will not easily give up the FM advantage. If a child becomes resistant, the audiologist should consider modifying the type of coupling system to make it less visible. It is frequently beneficial to demonstrate to other students and school personnel how much an FM system helps. This can be done by demonstrating what it sounds like to listen through a hearing aid with and without an FM system (through audio or videotapes). If the hearing-impaired child wants to participate he or she can, for example, demonstrate how well speech can be understood from the back of the room or in the presence of competing noise.

MAINTAINING THE AMPLIFICATION SYSTEM

Personal amplification is the responsibility of the parents and the child. Classroom amplification is the responsibility of the school system and the child. Even very young children can be taught to trouble-shoot their amplification devices and to report equipment failure. We strongly recommend that children be given this responsibility as soon as possible. In the school, however, an adult must be responsible for monitoring the equipment. This includes a daily listening check of the system each morning before the student puts it on to be certain that it is working well, that the signal is strong and free from distortion, and that there is no interference. Most systems have rechargable batteries that must be charged each night. Otherwise, spare batteries need to be available at all times. The school must also have a supply of spare parts because cords, audio boots, and neck loops can break. There should also be a spare FM system to replace an inoperable receiver or transmitter. When a malfunction occurs it can take two to three weeks to get the appropriate parts from the manufacturer. If replacements are not available at the school, the child will be deprived of optimal auditory functioning in the classroom. Once a child has learned to rely on an FM system this can be very distressing. It is not unusual for a child to refuse to go to school when the FM system is not available, and from our point of view, this is perfectly reasonable behavior.

MONITORING THE CLASSROOM

The work of Finitzo-Heiber and Tillman (1978), Crum (1974), Nabelek and Nabelek (1985), and others have shown that noise and reverberation degrade speech intelligibility for all people, but more so for people who are hearing impaired. As a result, it is critical that every effort be made to monitor noise, especially in rooms in which hearing-impaired children spend the day. Although it is useful to come into the room with a sound level meter and measure the intensity of the noise, a great deal can be learned by simply surveying the room and analyzing the sources of sound. Are there open windows facing a playground or other heavy traffic area? Is the door to the classroom kept open so that hallway noise inteferes? Is the hearing-impaired child sitting next to a noisy air conditioner? Are noisy activities such as block building and hammering going on where the child is trying to listen to the teacher?

Classrooms can be modified to improve the acoustical environment (Ross 1978). If possible, carpets and draperies should be installed. Dropped ceilings and acoustic tiles on the ceilings and walls will reduce noise and reverberation. Windows should be closed as much as possible because even the quietest street has noise. If air conditioners are used, they should be quiet ones that are well maintained to reduce noise. Only solid doors should be used to attenuate the amount of noise that comes into the room. The door should be sealed with weather stripping and kept closed to eliminate hallway noises. The classroom with the hearing-impaired child should be located on the side of the school away from the playground, traffic noise and trains, and be far from the gym, cafeteria, and bathrooms. Finally, the classroom must be acoustically separate from adjacent rooms. A classroom with a sliding wall, or one in which several classes meet in the same room, will present a very difficult listening situation for any child. It will be impossible for a hearing-impaired child.

Modifications in Teaching Style

By making minor changes in teaching style, a classroom teacher can greatly improve the hearing-impaired child's ability to function. The child needs to be seated so that he or she can see the teacher in order to employ speechreading. If the teacher gives some lessons from the front of the room and some from the rear, the child should be allowed to move his or her seat. The appropriate use of the FM system is critical. Because the child will be receiving information only from the person wearing the transmitter, he or she will miss comments from other children in the classroom. It is important, for both academic and social reasons, to hear classmates' comments. This problem can be partially resolved if the teacher repeats the other students' comments. For some classes it may be possible for the students to pass the FM transmitter to whomever is speaking.

As important as it is for a child to hear everything he or she is intended to hear, it is equally important that the child not overhear conversation not intended for him or her. When the teacher is assisting another student individually, or talking with another teacher in the hall, the FM system should be turned off. In this instance, the child will be able to hear the speech of those close by through the hearing aids or the environmental microphone of the FM system. As a basic principle, the FM system should be "on" when the child should be hearing the teacher, either individually or as a member of a group, and "off" when it is not relevant for the child to hear the teacher. Other suggestions for assisting the hearing-impaired child in the classroom are found elsewhere in this text.

SUMMARY

Although the acoustical conditions of mainstream classrooms can be deplorable, this situation can be ameliorated with the use of an FM system and with appropriate classroom modifications. These are prerequisite considerations to ensure that a hearing-impaired child can reach his or her performance potential in a classroom. It is incumbent upon parents, classroom teachers, audiologists, speech-language pathologists, and teachers of the hearing-impaired—all of whom are involved in a child's education—to make sure that audiological management in classrooms becomes an educational priority. The results are worth the effort.

REFERENCES

Bess, F., and McConnell, F. 1981. *Audiology, Education and the Hearing Impaired Child*. St. Louis: C. V. Mosby.

Crum, M. A. 1974. Effects of speaker to listener distance upon speech intelligibility in reverberation and noise. Ph.D. diss., Northwestern University, Evanston, IL.

Finitzo-Hieber, T., and Tillman, T. 1978. Room acoustics effects on monosyllabic word discrimination ability for normal and hearing-impaired children. *Journal of Speech and Hearing Research* 21:440–58.

Finitzo-Hieber, T. 1981. Classroom acoustics. In *Auditory Disorders In School Children*, eds. R. Roeser and M. Downs. New York: Thieme-Stratton.

Gengel, R. W. 1971. Acceptable speech-to-noise ratios for aided speech discrimination by the hearing impaired. *Journal of Auditory Research* 11:219–22.

Gerber, S. 1974. *Introductory Hearing Science*. Philadelphia: W. B. Saunders.

Hawkins, D., and Van Tasell, D. 1982. Electroacoustic characteristics of personal FM systems. *Journal of Speech and Hearing Disorders* 47:355–62.

Hawkins, D., and Schum, D. 1985. Some effects of FM-system coupling on hearing aid characteristics. *Journal of Speech and Hearing Disorders* 50:32–141.

Levitt, H. 1978. The acoustics of speech production. In *Auditory Management of Hearing-Impaired Children: Principles and Prerequisites for Intervention*, eds. M. Ross and T. G. Giolas. Baltimore: University Park Press.

Nabelek, A. K., and Nabelek, I. V. 1985. Room acoustics and speech perception. In *Handbook of Clinical Audiology*, ed. J. Katz. Baltimore: Williams and Wilkins Co.

Olsen, W. 1988. Classroom acoustics for hearing-impaired children. In *Hearing Impairment In Children*, ed. F. Bess. Parkton, MD: York Press.

Ross, M. 1978. Classroom acoustics and speech intelligibility. In *Handbook of Clinical Audiology*, Second edition. ed. J. Katz. Baltimore: Williams and Wilkins Co.

Ross, M., and Giolas, T. G. 1971. Effects of three classroom listening conditions on speech intelligibility. *American Annals of the Deaf* 116:580–84.

Ross, M., and Giolas, T. G. 1978. Issues and exposition. In *Auditory Management of Hearing-Impaired Children: Principles and Prerequisites for Intervention*, eds. M. Ross and T. G. Giolas. Baltimore: University Park Press.

Ross, M., Brackett, D., and Maxon, A. 1982. *Hard of Hearing Children in Regular Schools*. Englewood Cliffs: Prentice Hall.

Ross, M., Brackett, D., and Maxon, A. (In press). *Evaluating and Managing Mainstreamed Hearing Impaired Children*. Austin, TX: Pro-Ed.

Sanders, D. 1965. Noise conditions in normal school classrooms. *Exceptional Children* 31:344–53.

Tillman, T. W., Carhart, R., and Olsen, W. O. 1970. Hearing aid efficiency in a competing speech situation. *Journal of Speech and Hearing Research* 13:789–811.

Chapter • 7

Communication Management of the Mainstreamed Hearing-Impaired Student

Diane Brackett

A communication management program is an outgrowth of a comprehensive evaluation. Each of a child's observed strengths can be employed to teach new skills and deficit areas can be addressed with specific goals and objectives. Intervention must include helping the child receive speech optimally, understand the speech that has been received, generate messages that express the intended idea, and produce speech that is intelligible to others. Rather than attack each isolated communication skill, it is best to look at the overall effect of communication on social interaction and academic performance and address those skills that have the greatest impact on both of these areas. An effective management program addresses the requirements for both social/interactive and academic communication. Addressing either one of these in isolation results in a child ill prepared to benefit from the mainstream experience where learning occurs during structured sessions as well as during spontaneous interactions with peers.

The need to emphasize either social or academic communication changes somewhat with chronological age (see table I). In preschool years, social aspects of communication predominate, since the goal of

Table I.   Changing Communication Focus Across Chronological Age

Preschool Child = Social/interactive is primary

School-aged Child = Academic and social/interactive language are equal

Young Adult = Social/interactive is again primary

early childhood education is to prepare the child for social interactions within a group. Each contact that hearing-impaired children have with normal-hearing peers brings with it the potential to learn some aspect of social language that will assist them in future similar situations. Language as simple as "Move over," or "Don't touch it. It's mine," is best learned in realistic situations where motivation is high and the context clear. During the preschool years, children are exposed to beginning-level concepts in preparation for kindergarten, with the intent being to familiarize students with the material rather than demand mastery. For example, numbers, name reading, letter names, and shapes are introduced through play and routine activities but are not expected to be mastered until kindergarten. With academics playing this ancillary role, it is not surprising that hearing-impaired students with the best social language excel in this preschool environment, whereas students displaying strong academic readiness skills but limited social language are limited to showing their expertise for only a short period of each day.

Once the hearing-impaired child becomes school-aged, there is a more equal balance between social requirements and academic necessities. While academic demands in a mainstream educational setting seem obvious, it is unrealistic to assume that the child is merely an academic being. There are many situations, in the educational environment, in which children are called on to interact with each other in large or small groups during class activities or non-academic classes or routines. These other aspects of life have to be considered.

As students mature into young adults and begin to consider their employment possibilities, academic communication decreases in importance as social interaction rises in prominence. Concerns relating to job interviews, communication with co-workers, and development of outside interests and relationships become paramount and require different communicative abilities than those that were useful in the academic setting.

Communication management must therefore be viewed within the framework of the educational and social environment. Each deficit area revealed in the evaluation must be viewed as it effects the student's functioning in these contexts.

SOCIAL CONVERSATION

Social contact is established by initiating an interaction through verbal or nonverbal means. There are certain communicative prerequisites that are necessary if social interaction is going to be effectively initiated and maintained. If speech is used as the vehicle for establishing social contact, then the intelligibility of that speech becomes critical. The intended message must be understood, i.e., be intelligible, if the partner is going to react as intended.

Although intelligible speech is a reasonable goal given most degrees of hearing loss, "normal" speech is highly unlikely. While the student's speech must be intelligible, it does not have to be "normal" to be understood. Regular educators must understand this distinction. If they react first to the "different" aspects of the student's speech, i.e., different vocal quality, distortions, and cadences characteristic of hearing-impaired speech, without delving below the surface to examine what the child knows, they may erroneously decide that the student cannot be accommodated in a regular school. Yet as long as a high degree of intelligibility is present, social interaction with peers and adults can be effective, positive, and productive.

Conversational competence develops gradually during preschool years, as children become aware of how conversation is structured. Hearing-impaired children may miss some of this indirect instruction, or shaping, since they are still in the early stages of acquiring spoken language when this modelling occurs. For example, while normal-hearing four- and five-year olds are chastised for interrupting adults, hearing-impaired children of the same age are encouraged to talk whenever and to whomever they choose in an effort to increase the quality of their spoken language. By the time they have acquired a sufficient degree of language competence to benefit from this informal instruction, they are no longer captive audiences for the speech models of their parents, but have moved into a larger sphere of influence—school.

Hearing-impaired students, like their normal-hearing counterparts, have to learn to adapt to their listener, and be able to understand the rules that govern conversation. It is difficult for these children to learn the rules that govern conversational interaction—how to enter conversations without interrupting, how to terminate conversations, and how to initiate conversations on a variety of topics. The social appropriateness of a topic—those peer-to-peer topics that are inappropriate to discuss with parents and teachers—must be learned and used selectively during social communication.

In social interactive conversation, students have the opportunity to select the topic discussed thus increasing the likelihood that they will know something about it. This element of control is missing in academic settings where the teacher picks the topic and obligates the student to converse or give answers relative to the teacher-chosen topic.

Social context—gesture, the person, the face, the situation—provides support for the words said during social interactions. Often hearing-impaired students look better in a social situation where they can nod their heads, appearing to understand the topic, rather than in an academic situation where they are held accountable for information that is given. It is important to help students acquire strategies for providing feedback to the speaker regarding how completely they have understood the information.

The pattern of conversational-turn exchanges is different in social situations from those in academic settings. During social interaction, turns are usually fairly short and equal among the conversational partners. Conversely, in an educational setting the teacher takes a long turn while lecturing and teaching the materials, with the student answering briefly in response to a question. Students must realize that this difference is part of the social contract of school life, which is different from the social obligation of interpersonal interactions.

ACADEMIC CONVERSATION

Being aware of the social interactive components of communication is only part of the skill "package" that must be learned if the student is going to be successful in the mainstream educational setting. It is within the demands of the academic environment that hearing-impaired students demonstrate the inadequacies of their language. They may have difficulty interpreting aspects of "teacher talk," such as indirect requests like "Don't everyone jump in so fast." In this example, the hearing-impaired student may take the comment literally even though the teacher is actually asking for an answer to a question or comment. To avoid misunderstandings in the classroom, the hearing-impaired student needs to be exposed to these unique forms of academic conversation prior to experiencing them in the classroom.

Hearing-impaired students approach classroom learning with significantly reduced vocabulary skills. To participate effectively, they will require strategies for understanding when they have identified unfamiliar words. Using linguistic context or applying prefixes, suffixes, or roots can be effective approaches. In addition to the difficulty these students have in learning content vocabulary, they require specific instruction on words, phrases, and syntax contained in test or lesson directions. Typically these students "eyeball" the page and try to figure out from the pattern on the page what they are supposed to do, instead of reading and comprehending the instructions.

Written language competence also has an impact on students' performance in the classroom. These children are often penalized on essay questions because they are unable to express a logical progression of ideas on paper. If they had had the opportunity to respond orally, they can often explain their answer acceptably at a more sophisticated level. They must be taught to prepare a narrative answer that *discusses*, *compares*, or *contrasts*; this skill is critical for full participation in the upper grades.

Together the social and academic communication demands of the educational environment should tailor the focus of the communication management program. This huge task faces speech/language pathologists as they design effective intervention for hearing-impaired students in mainstreamed settings.

MANAGEMENT MODEL

The management model in figure 1 synthesizes information gathered from the communication evaluation and classroom observation into individualized speech/language therapy and classroom communication management. Using this two-pronged management program—one component to remediate communication deficits and the second component to facilitate communication needs in the classroom—it is possible to address all the areas assessed in the comprehensive evaluation, i.e., reception, comprehension, production, and speech intelligibility. See Chapter 5 for a full description of the communication evaluation.

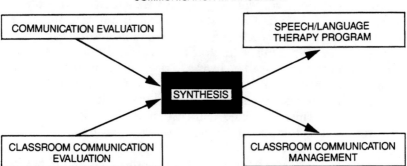

COMMUNICATION MANAGEMENT

COMMUNICATION EVALUATION

SPEECH/LANGUAGE THERAPY PROGRAM

SYNTHESIS

CLASSROOM COMMUNICATION EVALUATION

CLASSROOM COMMUNICATION MANAGEMENT

Figure 1. A realistic communication management program is developed by synthesizing the evaluation results derived from the detailed communication evaluations and classroom observation.

It is difficult to describe the components of a communication management program for mainstreamed hearing-impaired students in a general way because of the high degree of heterogeneity that exists in this population. The extent of a student's communication problems depends on the degree of hearing loss, configuration of loss, age of identification, amplification history, parent involvement, innate potential, learning style, and kind and extent of early involvement. While there are children with mild hearing losses who exhibit communication deficits, their needs are very different from children with severe to profound hearing losses who are mainstreamed. Nevertheless, both groups require a comprehensive communication management program, the focus of which is determined by the child's performance during the communication evaluation. The heterogeneity of this population is also manifest in the degree to which two children with identical hearing losses exhibit surprisingly different levels of communicative competence. An example of this is the exceptional severely or profoundly hearing-impaired student who is fully mainstreamed, doing outstanding work, in the top reading class, communicating effectively, while another student with an identical hearing loss and supportive family does not have the skill level to be able to progress in a mainstreamed environment. It is this unpredictability that makes programming for the hearing-impaired student in the mainstream such a challenge.

MANAGEMENT

Speech Reception

Since the communication problems exhibited by hearing-impaired children in social and academic interactions are a direct result of hearing loss, it is logical to first address the issue of optimizing speech reception. In planning speech reception programs for mainstreamed hearing-impaired students, educators often ignore listening-related issues and concentrate instead on trying to circumvent the problem with visual enhancements. It is more effective to adopt an approach for improving speech perception that incorporates the full use of a child's residual hearing. This, combined with use of available speechreading cues, results in better speech recognition scores than would be obtained if the modalities were employed singly.

To utilize an approach that emphasizes audition, the amplification system worn by the student must provide an optimal auditory signal, i.e., affording the fullest possible accessibility to speech for the particular degree and configuration of the hearing loss. (If questions exist regarding the student's amplification, consult the audiologist). Given appropriate amplification, the first step in an auditory management program is to design a system for monitoring personal and classroom amplification. *Daily* troubleshooting of equipment is required if students are to utilize their aided hearing to its maximum extent. Starting in the early elementary grades, the student needs to join the professional in the monitoring process by noting when amplification is malfunctioning and reporting it to the personnel responsible for maintenance. This level of sophistication requires that children be made responsible for handling their personal amplification equipment during the preschool years. When they reach school age, they should feel comfortable in putting it on and recognizing when it is not working.

In-service programs (see Maxon, Chapter 15) should be scheduled for the classroom teacher to teach the appropriate use of classroom amplification (FM units) and personal hearing aids and to ensure that interfering factors such as background noise and distance from the primary speaker are considered. Classroom observation makes it possible to document the actual use pattern within the room and to suggest modifications when necessary. To "de-mystify" FM units or hearing aids, the hearing impairment specialist needs to provide an informational and hands-on workshop for normal-hearing students in the classroom. Often, when classmates understand how these amplification systems function they ignore their presence on the hearing-impaired child.

In addition to these general auditory management considerations, which are specified on the Individualized Education Program (IEP), specific speech reception goals and objectives pertaining to the child's functioning in the remedial program and classroom need to be addressed (table II). Suggestions unique to the mainstreamed hearing-impaired student are highlighted in this section.

Speech Production

Speech production needs of hearing-impaired students in mainstreamed settings do not differ dramatically from those of other speech-impaired children, i.e., the need for stimulation, reinforcement, and practice of targeted phonemes at the syllable, word, phrase, or sentence level (see table III). The biggest difference lies in the reason for the speech errors. Errors are related directly to the child's inability to perceive phonemes correctly either at the present time or during the developmental period in which sounds were emerging. If changes in the child's speech production are expected, then the therapy regime must stress auditory self-monitoring.

Table II. Description of Remedial and Classroom Objectives for Speech Reception Improvement

Speech Reception	
Speech/Language Therapy (Objectives for child)	Classroom Communication Management (Objectives for teacher)
Resolve perceptual errors through minimal pair contrasts	Gain student's attention
	Repeat answers to questions
Introduce or reinforce new sounds, words, or grammar, listen-only	Direct classroom discussion by naming participants
	Use visual demonstration
Increase dependence on audition for speech reception	Write key words on board
	Avoid turning back to student
Monitor own speech skills	Alternate speaking and demonstrating
Practice under negative listening conditions (background noise, distance, no context)	Ensure that teacher's face is fully visible, well-lit, away from glare
Increase knowledge of maintenance and repair of amplification	Seat student away from obvious noise sources

Vocabulary

The single most obvious delay in communication skills of mainstreamed hearing-impaired students is in lexical development. Their inability to hear words repeatedly used in a variety of contexts results in vocabulary delays of six months to four years or more. Children with mild hearing loss exhibit deficient vocabulary acquisition, which has a dramatic impact on academic learning. Due to the all-encompassing

Table III. Description of Remedial and Classroom Objectives for Speech Production Improvement

Speech Production	
Speech/Language Therapy (Objectives for child)	Classroom Communication Management (Objectives for teacher)
Practice recognizing own errors	Ask student to write unintelligible answer
Accept responsibility for making oneself understood	Ask for repetition of a misunderstood word
Give back more precise speech following request for clarification	Give student a limited number of choices from which to pick answer
Refine phoneme production; facilitate carry-over into spontaneous speech	Repeat that part of student's statement that is understood
Gradually reduce external feedback	

nature of the vocabulary deficit, it is often difficult to designate words or category of words to be learned. Further indicators of deficient word knowledge are evident when the student over-uses nonspecific designators (it, this, that, these, there) in place of specific words or is unfamiliar with multiple meanings, antonyms, or synonyms. To address this relentless problem, an active vocabulary development plan (table IV) must be instituted in the remedial program with the cooperation of the classroom teacher.

Form

While errors exhibited by hearing-impaired students are similar to those of language-impaired children, the reason the deficits exist is different. Ambiguous auditory signals received by the hearing-impaired student are insufficient to convey all acoustical information necessary to develop the structural aspects of the language. Many important morphological markers in English are carried by high frequency phonemes and/or unstressed syllables, both of which are difficult for most hearing-impaired students to perceive. Syntactic errors occur due to lack of repeated audible exposure to the more sophisticated elements of English in meaningful contexts. Therefore, any communication management program must include a concentrated period of simultaneous exposure to and use of the linguistic forms (see table

Table IV. Description of Remedial and Classroom Objectives for Vocabulary Improvement

Vocabulary	
Speech/Language Therapy (Objectives for child)	Classroom Communication Management (Objectives for teacher)
Learn vocabulary from content material in classroom	Write important words on board
Review old words at regular intervals	Define words by using in a sentence
Must know "sound" of new words, not just look	Give list of vocabulary to support staff
Enlist parent support and reinforcement	Select vocabulary from academic material in the lessons
Expand language with multiple meanings, synonyms, idioms, and antonyms	Ensure that directions are understood
Use high interest words from board games, sports, or hobbies	Encourage child to give specific answers
Use old words to learn new "instruction" words	

V). Self-monitoring of word endings should emerge when listening and speaking are combined.

Use

Problems in using language appropriately are evident as mainstreamed hearing-impaired students attempt to interact with their peers socially and academically. Although the deficits seem similar to those of the pragmatically impaired, normal-hearing students, remediation must again reflect the causative factor, i.e., lack of audible exposure in meaningful contexts. Therefore, an approach that repeatedly exposes students to the appropriate social language models is necessary in order to improve pragmatically inappropriate behavior (table VI).

General Principles of Communication Management

Regardless of the deficit areas to be addressed in remedial sessions and classroom management programs, there are general principles that apply in both areas.

Selecting Targets By selecting targets that are within the developmental grasp of the student, it is possible to advance rather effortlessly from one stage to the next. When correction of inappropriate phonemes, vocabulary, or syntactic forms are targeted, progress may be minimal until such time as the student is developmentally ready or has acquired the prerequisite skills to move to a more advanced level.

Teaching Techniques The same techniques that are applied to hearing students with speech-language deficits can be utilized with

Table V. Description of Remedial and Classroom Objectives for Morphological/ Syntactic Improvement

Form	
Speech/Language Therapy (Objectives for child)	Classroom Communication Management (Objectives for teacher)
Expand simple forms	Check comprehension of lecture and instruction
Self-monitor morphological endings	Paraphrase into simpler form
Recognize obligatory context and respond accordingly	Write assignments on board
Produce audible morphological endings	Give different grade for content and grammar
Increase flexible use of grammatical forms	

Table VI. Description of Remedial and Classroom Objectives for Pragmatic Improvement

Use	
Speech/Language Therapy (Objectives for child)	Classroom Communication Management (Objectives for teacher)
Learn rules of conversational appropriateness	Explain "teacher talk" style at the beginning of the year
Adapt speech to the listener	Insist that the student maintain topic
Learn a variety of ways to ask, state, and direct	Require child to assume responsibility for making himself or herself understood
Learn colloquialisms and slang	Insist on adherence to non-interruption rules
Adhere to obligatory contexts	

mainstreamed students, as long as the audibility of the stimuli is taken into account. Targets that appear frequently in everyday speech can be practiced often without having to contrive the situation. Phrases such as "I don't want to," "Is it time for _____?", or "Can I have _____?" are useful vehicles for practicing particular phonemes or grammatical elements. Recognizing and identifying these routine utterances is the challenge facing the speech-language pathologist.

Relevance of the target to more than one area of function may determine how quickly the skill is learned, generalized, and automatized. For example, carry-over occurs more quickly if the /s/ phoneme can be trained and reinforced simultaneously as the marker for plurality, possession, and verb tense, as well as in various positions in words. Further, using old, familiar information to assist in learning new words, sounds, or phrases provides an associative context. For example, if /t/ is the target, then using the *place* information of the familiar /d/ or /l/ can speed up the initial learning process; if *astronaut* is the vocabulary item, then assisting the student in recalling other words with the "astro" root (astronomy, astrology, astronomical), and applying the root to the new word, is a useful teaching and reinforcement strategy.

Diagnostic Teaching Careful diagnostic evaluations lead to effective management. The process does not stop with formal evaluation; rather, it continues during therapy. As stimuli are introduced, the child's responses must be analyzed in order to correct observed errors. For example, an incorrect response to the word "cats" may occur if the child does not know that the /s/ denotes plurality or because the /s/ was not heard due to its high frequency characteristics.

Practice To accelerate the rate at which new skills are acquired, practice must occur not only in the therapy setting where they are introduced, but also in the less structured environment of the classroom and home. Although this is ideal, it is the most difficult goal to implement because the therapist's control is reduced. Enlisting the assistance of the parent in providing practice is effective as long as parameters for evaluating the accuracy of responses are explicit. Each social/interactive encounter where the child has an opportunity to practice the targets correctly means more rapid acquisition of the skill and knowledge of when to use it. Although having the classroom teacher assist in monitoring correct productions would be ideal, it is difficult to arrange due to the large number of children that he or she manages. The teacher's support may be obtained in specific contexts, e.g., requiring correct speech during oral reading or encouraging longer utterances when answering content questions in small reading groups.

Generalization Generalization or carry-over occurs when the student begins to monitor his or her own productions or use of targeted forms. Assimilating newly learned forms into automatic use is the most time-consuming aspect of the hearing-impaired student's remedial program. Often this process is prolonged due to misguided efforts of professionals and parents who continue to provide external feedback about the accuracy of the student's production long after it is necessary. Until external reminders, in the form of corrected repetitions, questions ("What?"), or quizzical looks, are reduced or eliminated, the student will not have to rely on his or her own monitoring ability.

CONCLUSION

Evidence of disruption in communication skills and academic achievement of even mildly hearing-impaired students corroborates the debilitating effect of hearing loss. A communication management program that concentrates exclusively on one isolated aspect of communication leads to a student who is unprepared to handle the demands of the mainstreamed environment. An aggressive, effective communication management program must address deficits in speech reception, comprehension, production, and intelligibility as they are manifest in the social and academic domains of the challenging regular classroom.

Chapter • 8

Issues Relating to Classroom Management

Laraine C. Conway

INTRODUCTION

With the trend to place handicapped students in their home schools, more hearing-impaired students are being programmed into mainstreamed settings. Seventy-five percent of the hearing-impaired student population is partially to totally mainstreamed (Ninth Annual Report to Congress on the Implementation of the Education of the Handicapped Act 1987). These students are mainstreamed as early as preschool and sometimes remain in this setting throughout their education. Therefore, regular classroom and resource teachers, by necessity, have become involved in the education of hearing-impaired students. These teachers are well-prepared to fulfill the role of teacher for hearing students but may feel ill-prepared to meet the needs of hearing-impaired children. In an effort to support regular classroom and resource teachers, this chapter focuses on educational, environmental, and instructional issues to provide them with ideas for creating quality education for mainstreamed hearing-impaired students.

Two issues relating to the management of hearing-impaired students in the mainstream setting are addressed in this chapter. Aspects relating to classroom communication interactions and management

---

*The author would like to extend her thanks to Diane Schmidt, graphic artist, for the illustrations contained in this chapter.

suggestions are discussed in the first portion. Language and cognitive issues that relate to curriculum and instructional procedures, along with suggested adaptations, are emphasized in the second section. Not every consideration raised or instructional adaptation discussed in this chapter will apply to all hearing-impaired students. The purpose of these discussions is to provide regular classroom and resource teachers with insights into the effects hearing impairment has on academic achievement as well as to suggest approaches for managing the classroom and educational programming of mainstreamed hearing-impaired students.

CLASSROOM INTERACTION CONSIDERATIONS

When hearing-impaired students are placed in regular classes, hearing students, as well as teachers, often are concerned about how they will communicate with these youngsters. Will they be able to understand the students' speech? Will these youngsters understand what they are saying? What can be done to facilitate positive communication interactions? Although the answers to these questions may vary depending on the type of communication system used by the hearing-impaired students, the main issue remains the same. How can an atmosphere be created that will allow for open exchanges between students and teachers and among the students as a group?

Classroom Interactions Adaptions

One significant factor that contributes to learning is the classroom environment. This is especially true for hearing-impaired students because background noise, lighting, mannerisms of speech, and context of the communicative interaction can influence greatly the quality of information the students are able to obtain. Hearing-impaired students generally are attuned visually to their environment. Because of this tendency, they can be distracted if there is an excess of visual information present in the classroom. Consideration needs to be given to the auditory, as well as visual environment. Even in the most optimal situation, hearing-impaired students do not receive the same acoustic information as their hearing peers.

Acoustic Environment An optimal acoustic environment contributes significantly to hearing-impaired students' reception of classroom instructions. Issues relating to classroom acoustics and to the care and use of audiological devices have been discussed in the chapter of this book entitled *Managing Classroom Amplification*. Regular classroom teachers need to be knowledgeable about these issues in order to plan carefully for and to implement classroom modifications that will enhance hearing-impaired students' acoustic environment.

Speechreading Some hearing-impaired students use speechreading to obtain information from a speaker's lips to supplement their limited auditory input. This task is difficult because many factors affect speechreading. Similarity of words on a person's lips, such as the words *mat* and *bat*, can make these words hard to distinguish. A hearing-impaired person can have difficulty speechreading linguistically complex sentences because of the language demands of the task. Distracting physical features, such as a moustache or a beard, or mannerisms of a speaker like moving around the room while instructing, tend to draw the speechreader's attention away from the speaker's lips. Environmental factors, such as poor lighting, distance of speaker from student, or objects that cover a speakers lips can interfere with the quality of information hearing-impaired persons are able to perceive visually.

Effects of Lighting When speaking to hearing-impaired students, it is important to ensure that light is on the speaker's face and not in the youngsters' eyes. It is extremely difficult to speechread when a person is standing in a bright light, such as in front of a window. In such a setting, the speaker's face is shadowed, and the student may be looking into a glare.

It is also difficult to speechread in a darkened room. If the teacher lectures while showing a film or slide presentation, even if the hearing-impaired student is using an FM unit or has an interpreter, the speaker's face or the interpreter's signs will be difficult to see. Additionally, this student must attend to two visual inputs simultaneously—the media and the speaker/interpreter. Suggested adaptations for this situation include: (1) giving the student information in advance, (2) providing the student with a manuscript of the film that can be used to prepare the student to view the film and/or used as a review, (3) using a captioned film, and (4) saving instructional comments to the end of the film.

Preferential Seating Traditionally, preferential seating has been recommended because of hearing-impaired students' reliance on visual input to support the auditory. Concerns about the limitations of personal hearing aids, the amount of background noise present in the classroom, and the distance of the speaker from the student resulted in a stationary preferential seat for most students, namely a seat at the front or side of the classroom. Two factors that have altered this rigid notion of preferential seating are use of the FM units and the dynamic nature of classroom interactions today. These changes permit more flexible seating arrangements. Factors to be considered in deciding upon seating arrangement should include: (1) the auditory and visual reception needs of the child, (2) the type of communication system used, particularly one requiring an interpreter, (3) the type of amplification used by the student, and (4) the communicative interactions demanded by the learning activities. A well-planned mobile seating arrangement enables the mainstreamed hearing-impaired student to have optimal auditory input regardless of the communicative interactions that transpire during the school day.

Speaker's Mannerisms   When communicating with hearing-impaired persons, speakers should use natural speech at a moderate pace and with a normal speaking voice. Use of exaggerated mouth movements, extremely slow or quick rates of speaking, or overly loud speech destroys the natural rhythm and intonation of speech. A full view of the speaker's face at all times facilitates the speechreading task. Even with amplification, youngsters with moderate and severe hearing losses require the additional support of speechreading to perceive correctly the spoken message. When the teacher is not facing hearing-impaired students directly, the students miss information because of their significant difficulty in understanding auditory input alone.

Other Factors   Even with optimal amplification and ideal speechreading conditions, hearing-impaired listeners are not able to receive the total spoken message. Therefore, they often rely on other visual information, such as situational clues, facial expressions, body language and gestures, and/or shared knowledge to make conjectures about incomplete information. Sometimes, a mismatch between the visual setting and the speechread message can confuse the student or result in a misconception. For example, during a social studies class about the signing of the Declaration of Independence, interjecting information about a current event relating to the drafting of a new bill might confuse the student because the context no longer supports the message. Care should be taken that the student makes these transitions with the rest of the class. When students do not speechread the message correctly, the speaker should first repeat it. If the student still experiences difficulty comprehending the spoken message, other factors besides speechreading abilities may be the underlying cause of the problem. Hearing-impaired students' correct reception of spoken utterances does not guarantee comprehension of the message. Other factors, such as their language abilities, can affect their interpretation of the information.

Communication Adaptations of Classroom Interactions

Several factors affect the hearing-impaired students' participation in classroom communication interactions. In addition to physical considerations, the students' present level of language and knowledge can have an impact on the extent of their involvement. Additionally, some communication aspects can influence classroom communication exchanges.

Communication Exchanges   Communication exchanges that take place within the classroom can be extremely demanding for hearing-impaired students, who often encounter difficulties hearing and locating the speaker. By the time the speaker is located, these students often have missed relevant information or may need to locate the next speaker. It assists hearing-impaired students if the teacher reiterates other students' questions and comments, if the FM microphone is passed to the speakers, or if student speakers clearly identify themselves before speaking.

At times, hearing-impaired students may have difficulty understanding classroom instructions or exchanges yet be unaware of these comprehension difficulties. Therefore, they do not seek or request the additional information or clarification. Some students develop ineffective coping mechanisms for dealing with misunderstood or insufficient auditory or linguistic information. Two counter-productive strategies hearing-impaired students often use are nodding when they do not understand, or looking around the classroom for visual clues that will assist them to understand the instructions. Some of these students make cognitive assumptions based on limited or incomplete linguistic information and use their experiential and acquired knowledge base to decipher the meaning of the message. Although these strategies can be successful, their use can result in inaccurate assumptions, misinterpretations, and/or inappropriate responses. In such cases, the students need to be made aware of their comprehension difficulties, as well as to learn expressions for appropriately requesting clarification.

Questions   Questions are an essential tool teachers use for instruction and evaluation. Yet, questioning tasks can prove to be difficult for hearing-impaired students. Similar to all students, they may not know the answer. Yet, even if these students know the answer to the question, they may not understand the question form or may have difficulty correctly interpreting the question. A hearing-impaired student could interpret a regulatory question, such as "Would you like to read that paragraph?", as a true question and respond accordingly. When hearing-impaired students give an incorrect or inappropriate response, it can assist them to analyze the error for themselves. Sometimes, allowing extra response time for students to formulate their answers or simply restating the question using a different question form can result in a correct response. Questions requiring the use of complex language and cognitive skills can be difficult for these students.

Such questions might require students to analyze information, to make inferences or predictions, to determine causes or solutions to problems, or to compare and contrast information. Because of an underlying language or learning difficulty, students may require individual assistance from a speech/language pathologist and/or a resource teacher to enable them to comprehend questions and statements that increase in complexity and abstraction.

Inattention In spite of their best efforts, hearing-impaired youngsters sometimes have difficulty attending in school. Inattentive behaviors may be related to frustration and/or fatigue. Sometimes the language demands, the level of difficulty of tasks, an insufficient knowledge base, and/or a lack of visual information to support spoken information result in inattentive behavior. In such cases the students simply may not have sufficient information to comprehend the instructions or directions. Inattention, especially toward the end of the day, may be the result of fatigue. It takes tremendous effort for these students to speechread or watch an interpreter for an entire school day. Additionally, they are often attempting to attend to the variety of visual information in an effort to understand communicated information.

When a hearing-impaired student demonstrates inattentive behaviors, it is necessary to determine the underlying cause of the problem. Suggested strategies for assisting hearing-impaired students to increase their attention include: (1) daily schedule adjustments, like scheduling demanding language-based subjects earlier and less difficult ones later in the school day; (2) providing additional visual context or instructional support; or (3) presenting information at a language level closer to the students' present abilities.

Use of Interpreters Educational interpreters provide a vital communication support service to mainstreamed hearing-impaired students. Because of the requirements of this position, they should be trained professionals and, when possible, certified. During class instruction, it is the interpreter's responsibility to translate or transliterate the teacher's spoken communication to hearing-impaired youngsters and to verbalize the students' signed utterances to the teacher and/or class. Because there are different sign systems and sign languages (such as American Sign Language, Signing Exact English, Pidgin Sign English) it is essential to identify the one used by the student. When choosing an interpreter, it is important to select one proficient in the same sign system used by the student. Similarly, students who use Cued Speech, which supplements the visual cues of speechreading with hand positions to eliminate ambiguity, need an interpreter skilled in this system (Henegar and Cornett 1971). Oral interpreters, trained to translate verbatim with only occasional substitutions or rewording of the speaker's message, are beneficial to aural/oral students. Interpreters who lack certification should be evaluated by a professional skilled in that sign language/system. Using an interpreter who has had a few sign classes is inappropriate and could result in poor academic achievement by the student.

Educational interpreters are often assigned additional classroom duties. These assignments can include: (1) assisting hearing-impaired students to understand class routines or instructions by clarifying or explaining concepts, (2) supporting these students in their completion of independent tasks, (3) providing tutoring and follow-up instructions, and/or (4) serving as a liaison between the special education and regular classroom teacher (Irwin and Morgan 1985). When defining responsibilities for the educational interpreter, it is important to emphasize that, although they are well-trained persons qualified to facilitate communication between deaf and hearing people, they are not trained teachers. Therefore, they require direction and supervision from a certified teacher in order to perform the educational tasks required of them in the regular classroom.

Classroom Cuing Mechanisms   Classroom interactions are general, as well as idiosyncratic, systems for conducting communication exchanges—verbal and nonverbal. The organization of the general system evolves from the daily classroom schedule, the demands of a particular subject, and the teacher's instructional style. During interactions that take place the first few days of school, stated and subtle rules governing these classroom communication interactions are established (Kretschmer 1990). Hearing-impaired students are often knowledgeable about the organizational aspects, such as the daily schedule. They often are observant of visual cues that contribute to classroom management, such as watching other students in order to determine which page to open to in the text book. Yet, they can be unaware of the subtle nonverbal and indirect verbal cues that are used by the teacher to manage the class routine and students. Lack of awareness of these verbal conventions can result in inappropriate or potentially troublesome classroom behaviors.

Knowledge of cuing mechanisms used in the regular classroom to govern routines and behavior patterns can facilitate hearing-impaired students adjustments to the mainstream setting. It is advantageous to the hearing-impaired student for a professional to analyze these conventions and to assist students to understand and learn strategies for responding appropriately to verbal nuances, such as "Does anyone else have anything to share?", as a signal to the end of a lesson. This information can be obtained by observing or videotaping lessons in different classes. Spoken and unspoken cuing mechanisms used by teachers and students can be analyzed and explained to the hearing-impaired student. Their awareness of different classroom cuing mechanisms enables them to function more effectively in the mainstream setting (Johnson and Griffith 1985).

Incidental Classroom Information   Hearing-impaired students often do not hear incidental information from teachers or other students. This can happen because the information is given over the loudspeaker or during transition times when direct instruction is not taking place. Independent work time and less formal classroom routines such as lining up for lunch are examples of times hearing-impaired students will miss incidental information. If information, such as the lunch menu or a change in schedule, is given to students, then the teacher, interpreter, or "buddy" should ensure that the hearing-impaired students are informed.

Peer Interactions   Attempts at communication between a hearing and hearing-impaired student require patience and understanding on both parts. Talking with a hearing-impaired youngster can be frustrating to the hearing person because of the need to make sense out of partially articulated words and incorrectly sequenced sentence structures. An oral hearing-impaired youngster can have difficulty speechreading an unfamiliar person. In addition, the hearing-impaired person may not have sufficient vocabulary knowledge nor adequate ability to understand the complex language structures used. For students using total communication, the hearing person's limited ability to use signs can present significant communication problems. Hearing and hearing-impaired persons need to take the time and make the effort to work through this communication challenge. In a mainstream setting, professionals can devise opportunities for hearing and hearing-impaired students to communicate with each other.

LANGUAGE/COGNITIVE CONSIDERATIONS

Educational Development Considerations

The linguistic abilities and knowledge base that students bring to their learning tasks greatly influence their rate of academic progress. For hearing-impaired students in the mainstream setting, it is essential that consideration be given to the match between linguistic and cognitive demands of learning tasks and the students' present language abilities and general knowledge base. A mismatch can affect the students' academic achievement negatively, often resulting in frustration and a sense of failure for both student and teacher.

Hearing-impaired students demonstrate varying degrees of difficulty keeping pace with growing linguistic and cognitive demands of the curriculum. As they progress through their educational years, their abilities increase, but so do the demands of academic tasks and teachers' expectations of students. The degree of difficulty of language/ cognitive demands of learning activities in comparison to hearing-impaired students' present abilities needs to be continually monitored so that appropriate adaptations can be implemented. If extensive instructional adjustments are required, the collaborative team should consider whether additional support services or an alternative educational program would be in the students' best interest.

Primary Level During the beginning school years, teachers tend to employ teaching approaches that are especially beneficial for hearing-impaired youngsters. Concrete hands-on activities, like growing plants while learning about plant life or consistently linking personal experience with academic demands (such as a language experience approach in reading) are strategies that allow students to associate their real life experiences with the cognitive and linguistic demands of the task. Extensive use of visual materials, such as pictures in reading books, also supports linguistic information. Many instructional procedures in preschool through primary grades encourage tangible language/learning experiences that promote active student involvement. Such educational experiences greatly facilitate hearing-impaired students' learning.

Intermediate Level The transition from a primary, skills-oriented approach, to an intermediate language-based content curriculum, results in many hearing-impaired students encountering increasing difficulties. It is assumed that all students at the intermediate level possess sufficient cognitive, language, and academic skills to support the demands of the curriculum. Students are expected to be competent users of previously taught information and skills, so they are provided with less contextual/visual support. Previously successful hearing-impaired students may begin to demonstrate signs of frustration or increased difficulty with schoolwork due to increased lecture time, the introduction of more complex, abstract cognitive and linguistic information, and/or higher level academic tasks that require students to operate on a metalinguistic level.

Advanced Level The educational environment at the junior high and high school levels becomes more complex and difficult for hearing-impaired students because of the nature of linguistic and cognitive demands of the learning task. The assumption is that students are on their way to becoming independent learners who are capable of using printed information as a tool for learning. Students are expected to use their knowledge base and linguistic abilities to generate new ideas. Therefore, the emphasis of teaching is on discussion of new principles and concepts and the usual mode of instruction is lecture. Visual support and active-learning experiences are minimal in classes other than science and vocational courses. Because of the strong linguistic mode of instruction, language-based problems, subtle as they may be, can have an impact on hearing-impaired students' progress in one or more areas of the curriculum. This appears to be true for students with significant residual hearing, as well as those with minimal residual hearing.

Recent research indicates that even students with unilateral hearing experience "a variety of auditory, linguistic, and cognitive difficulties that appear to be compromising educational progress" (Bess 1986). Although these students can converse easily on a social level, their communication abilities often conceal language-based problems that have the potential to effect their academic performance negatively. Therefore, hearing-impaired students, even with minimal hearing-losses, require additional support services and/or special instructional adaptations.

Curriculum Considerations

Reading   Reading is a complex process that demands more than isolated knowledge of phonetics, grammar, and comprehension skills. The goal of reading is to construct meaning from printed text. Thus, the process of reading requires interactions of the reader's experiential, linguistic, and cognitive knowledge bases (Smith 1977). Similar to their hearing peers, students with a hearing loss approach reading tasks with different experiential backgrounds, as well as different levels of cognitive, linguistic, and reading abilities. Their levels of proficiency in relation to the demands of the reading task affect their ability to read and comprehend printed information. Some hearing-impaired students approach reading tasks with insufficient background knowledge, and/or a limited understanding of the linguistic structures and decoding skills needed to process the information successfully (LaSasso 1990). Yet, consideration is not always given to the effect this can have on their reading performance.

Hearing-impaired students do not have access to the same phonological information as do their hearing peers. However, they can acquire a knowledge of phonology in certain linguistic situations (Hanson and Wilkenfeld 1985). Hearing-impaired students with minimal hearing losses can be expected to learn phonetic skills with minimal instructional adaptations. Students with severe-to-profound losses, who are able to make use of their residual hearing, may require special instructional adaptations to develop phonetic skills. These students may rely on kinesthetic cues, that is, how a speech sound feels when it is produced, and visual clues, such as letter patterns, rather than auditory input. For hearing-impaired students to be able to "sound out" an unfamiliar word, they need to associate their auditory input, speech knowledge, and learned phonetic rules. Students versed in cued speech sometimes use this system to assist them in decoding a word. Others may use fingerspelling. Similar to their hearing peers, hearing-impaired students profit from knowledge of a variety of strategies, such as whole word configuration or word analysis, to apply to decoding tasks.

For hearing-impaired students, correct decoding and pronunciation of words does not always indicate word comprehension. Rather, it is possible that students may not understand or may only have superficial comprehension of the meaning of words and concepts. Many hearing-impaired students have limited and/or delayed receptive and expressive vocabulary, which has an impact on their comprehension (Yoshinaga-Itano and Downey 1986). Vocabulary knowledge or word concept entails more than the simple definition of a word. A person's unique experiences with a word, as they hear or see it in a variety of contexts, results in the formation of his or her meaning of a word (Johnson, Toms-Bronowski, and Pittelman 1982). In comparison to their hearing peers, hearing-impaired students may have limited exposures to a given word. When these students have insufficient knowledge of a word, they tend to have literal or inflexible understanding of the word's meaning. Inadequate and/or superficial knowledge of vocabulary can result in their comprehending only one meaning of multimeaning words or can prevent them from deciphering subtle inferences or deductions. Often, these students can be unaware of their limited comprehension of vocabulary and its negative effect on reading comprehension.

The type of syntactic structures used in reading material can influence hearing-impaired students' comprehension. Even at a simple sentence level, some hearing-impaired students can experience comprehension difficulties. For example, a simple sentence containing an active verb would be easier for them to understand than one containing a passive verb (Robbins and Hatcher 1981). Given the sentences, "John pushed Mary" and "Mary was pushed by John," a hearing-impaired student would probably interpret the first sentence correctly, but conclude that Mary pushed John in the second. Hearing-impaired students often have difficulty understanding complex sentences, especially those containing relative clauses, conjunctions, pronouns, and indirect objects (Robbins and Hatcher 1981). For example, a hearing-impaired student may interpret the sentence, "The *boy*, *who* lives next door to my neighbor, is coming over to play with me," as the neighbor being the one who is coming over to play. Compared to their hearing peers, hearing-impaired students may experience more difficulties comprehending negative forms, determining the antecedent for pronouns, using morphology to determine a time or sequence, or filling in implicit information, such as "John is taller than I (am tall)" (Quigley et al. 1976). The greater the gap between the students' syntactic knowledge and the complexity of syntactic structures contained in the text, the more difficulty the student will have comprehending the text. If it appears that the student's comprehension problem is related to his or her knowledge of syntax or the syntactical structures encountered in texts, it would be worthwhile for the classroom teacher to consult with a teacher trained for hearing impaired students. Together they could determine strategies or devise materials that would build from the student's syntax base.

Hearing-impaired students often have difficulties interpreting figurative language, such as idiomatic expressions or metaphorical language. These difficulties can be related to their exposure to figurative language and/or their language abilities. Thus, a simple idiomatic expression, such as, "Stop pulling my leg!", could be interpreted literally. Additionally, comprehension of figurative language can be compounded by the level of vocabulary and complexity of syntax used in these expressions. Some hearing-impaired students may require special instruction and repeated exposure to figurative language before they demonstrate comprehension.

Teachers require students to read for a variety of purposes. Comprehension demands of the task can range from locating specific information contained in a sentence to making evaluative judgments about ideas presented in an extended text. As demands of the comprehension task increase, students need to rely on their ability to make connections between the text and their knowledge base. Because different reading tasks require different levels of comprehension, the ability of students to demonstrate comprehension is related to the type and kind of information they are able to obtain from the text.

Hearing-impaired students tend to have greater difficulty making inferences than their hearing peers (Wilson 1979 as cited in Quigley and Kretschmer 1982). Often insufficient background experience and knowledge of vocabulary and syntax, coupled with ineffective reading strategies, result in hearing-impaired students experiencing comprehension difficulty with reading tasks requiring them to make inferences, predictions, conjectures, and judgments, as well as to draw conclusions or form evaluations. These tasks are difficult because they require the student to go beyond the content contained in the text and to supply additional information from their knowledge base. Ways of assisting these students to increase their knowledge base are: (1) providing them with opportunities to read a variety of materials, (2) engaging students in a discussion about vocabulary and concepts contained in a story prior to the reading experience, (3) increasing their awareness of organization of different reading materials, and (4) teaching them cognitive and/or language strategies that will assist them in comprehending text.

Hearing-impaired students can benefit from knowledge of comprehension strategies, such as contextual analysis or semantic mapping, because application of these techniques require readers to focus on the meaning of the text and to utilize their knowledge base. Some hearing-impaired students demonstrate ineffective comprehension strategies that result in superficial or incorrect understanding of the text. They tend to attain only a general sense of the text without fully understanding it (King and Quigley 1985), or to employ some type of a visual matching strategy to attain requested information without necessarily understanding their response. For example, their response may contain key words stated in the comprehension question with some words preceding or following those words in the text (LaSasso 1985). Students' use of such strategies can indicate comprehension difficulty that may relate to their inability to understand the question form itself and/or the information contained in the text.

Knowledge of discourse organization, that is the structure of stories and texts, can enable students to comprehend text, as well as to locate and organize information. Students usually are instructed in the general organization of texts so they will be able to locate information. For example, they are taught how chapters are organized and how to use a table of contents. Although these reading/study skills assist all students, hearing-impaired students can benefit from additional knowledge of the underlying structure of stories and texts, such as the organization of information presented in a detective story as opposed to a romance novel or a science text as opposed to a social studies textbook. Such knowledge provides the student with a conceptual framework for organizing and associating information contained in various reading materials.

Given the complex nature of the reading task, it is not surprising that the reading performance of many hearing-impaired students is below that of their hearing peers. Although hearing-impaired students can encounter difficulties developing their reading abilities, it is encouraging to note that given a combination of favorable factors, it is possible for hearing-impaired students with profound losses to achieve reading skills commensurate with those of their hearing peers (Geers and Moog 1989; Moeller and Johnson 1988).

Written Language As most educators would agree, the emphasis in written language instruction for years has been on the mechanics of writing (e.g., spelling, grammar, punctuation, and capitalization.) Today, the process of writing is being emphasized. Rather than requiring students to practice isolated skills, they are engaging in creative written language activities. These endeavors provide students with the opportunity to work through various stages of writing, specifically, rehearsing, drafting, revising, and editing to achieve the final product (Calkins 1986). This does not mean that mechanics are disregarded. Rather, the students' products can be used to target goals that will assist them in improving the quality of their written language expression, in addition to assisting children to grow as writers. Because many hearing-impaired students have difficulty developing written language competence, a process-oriented writing approach, coupled with meaningful instructions based on students developing writing mechanics, grammar, and discourse needs, should assist them to improve their written language abilities. Such an approach should benefit hearing-impaired students, who may be developing written language abilities more slowly than their hearing peers, because it capitalizes on their interest and provides them with meaningful writing experiences based on their instructional level and personal needs.

Acquisition of spelling skills can present a challenge to hearing-impaired students. Yet, many of these students learn to spell. As in the case of phonics, they may apply their knowledge of letter patterns and word structure to spell words. Associating their speech knowledge with spelling tasks or teaching phonics and spelling as a unit can assist these students to integrate their knowledge of word structure.

Hearing-impaired students with a limited vocabulary often use generic terms in their writing. Frequently, they use basic content words, such as nouns, verbs, and some adjectives. Other word forms such as articles, auxiliaries, prepositions, and conjunctions (Quigley and Kretschmer 1982) are regularly omitted or used incorrectly in their written products. These factors can depreciate the quality of their written work.

Hearing-impaired students, like their hearing peers, may have a variety of topics they like to write about, but their topic choices may be substantially different. During their early attempts at writing, hearing-impaired students often choose to write about topics that are similar to those of their hearing peers (Conway 1985). However by the middle grades, differences in the quality and quantity of hearing-impaired students' topic selection may become evident. This discrepancy is the result of a quantitative difference between hearing and hearing-impaired students' knowledge and linguistic base, and can affect the quality of the students' written product.

Written language produced by hearing-impaired students may differ in length from that of their hearing peers. Written products may be shorter because hearing-impaired students tend to write simple sentences. Limited knowledge about the topic also can result in a short text. Brainstorming for ideas relating to the topic, as well as writing ideas on the board, can provide students with a means of increasing the length of their written product.

Hearing-impaired students' knowledge of syntax also influences the quality of their writing. Frequently, morphological endings are omitted from words. Incorrect word order or verb tense errors often are observed in their written text. They may have a tendency to express their ideas in simple declarative sentences. The conjunction "and" may be overused, as in connecting a series of run-on sentences. Complex sentence structures may seldom be observed in their writings. When a student's work manifests several of these features, the result is a rigid written language product that is qualitatively different from that of his or her hearing peers (Quigley and Kretschmer 1982).

Mechanical aspects of written language are just as essential for hearing-impaired students as they are for their hearing peers. Students with language-based problems frequently encounter difficulties learning and applying capitalization, punctuation, and grammatical rules. They may not understand that a sentence is a unit of thought; therefore, the concept of the beginning and end of a sentence may not make sense to them. Additionally, they may not understand, and thus be unable to distinguish between, different types of sentences.

Giving instructions accompanied by modeling of and exposures to different sentence forms, as well as providing students with the opportunity to use these forms in a variety of writing activities, may assist them to acquire these skills. If the linguistic errors noted on students' written language product consistently prevent them from communicating their ideas to others, a language-based problem, not simply their written language abilities, may be the underlying cause of the students' difficulties. Additionally, these students may need assistance from a speech/language pathologist to develop their language competencies.

To attain a quality written language product, it is necessary to express one's thoughts in a well-organized, cohesive style. This is not an easy task. Not only do students need to have sufficient knowledge about the topic, they must also be able to use correct syntactic, mechanic, and discourse structures to express their ideas so that others will comprehend their written expression. Working through the various stages of the writing process can result in quality written language products. Hearing-impaired students have demonstrated the ability to increase both the length and level of complexity of their written product when provided with the opportunity to engage in the writing process (Truax and Edwards 1984).

Content Area   The difficulties, noted in the section on reading comprehension, apply to hearing-impaired students' accomplishments in the content areas of curriculum, such as social studies, science, and health. As concepts and vocabulary become more abstract and language structures become more complex, hearing-impaired students tend to demonstrate increasing difficulty and frustration in their attempts to comprehend the teacher's instruction and concepts presented in various content areas of the curriculum.

The student's inability to process information and interpret classroom instructions can result in misconceptions, lack of comprehension, difficulties organizing, storing, and/or retrieving information. Their ability to use verbal reasoning skills and to be flexible thinkers affects the quantity and quality of information they are able to acquire in these areas. Due to language-based problems, these students sometimes have not achieved the prerequisite language and cognitive skills needed to sequence events, to make inferences, predictions, and generalizations, to perceive cause and effect relationships, and/or to formulate comparisons, contrasts, or explanations based on the available facts. Yet, these abilities are vital to obtaining information in the content area.

Other difficulties encountered by hearing-impaired students in content areas relate to notetaking, class discussions, and independent assignment issues. Notetaking requires students to write and listen simultaneously. Hearing-impaired students' reliance on visual information, such as speechreading, sign language, and visual clues, makes it extremely difficult, if not impossible, to take adequate notes. Because they are unable to watch the teacher and write notes simultaneously, attention to one task results in missed relevant information in the other.

The difficulties hearing-impaired students have participating in class discussions are related not only to identifying the speaker but also to comprehending the expressed information. The concepts discussed may be within the hearing-impaired students' cognitive capabilities but not their language capabilities. In such situations, it can be difficult for the teacher to decide whether to emphasize the content or to assist the student in understanding the unfamiliar vocabulary or complex language structure. If the student consistently experiences difficulties understanding context, for either reason, then the teacher should meet with the team to determine whether the student is in need of additional assistance from a resource teacher.

The variety of independent reading and writing assignments given in the content area can be quite challenging to hearing-impaired students. Depending on their present language, reading, and writing abilities, they may need assistance to accomplish independent reading and writing projects, reports, and research papers required of students in content areas. Hearing-impaired students have the ability to make academic progress in content areas of the curriculum, but they may require specific directions or additional support in order to complete these learning tasks successfully.

Mathematics   Mathematics calculation can be an area of relative strength for many hearing-impaired youngsters. Because these youngsters can keep pace with their hearing peers on calculation tasks, the language-based demands of the math curriculum are sometimes not considered to be a problem.

Applied math problems, involving word problems, measurement, money, time, geometry, estimation, or probability, are difficult for hearing-impaired students because of the vocabulary, linguistic, verbal reasoning, and problem-solving demands of the task. These students may not comprehend the meaning of specific math vocabulary terms, such as *least, ruler, quadrilateral,* or *quarter-to-nine.* In such cases, they require specific vocabulary instruction in math vocabulary and/or basic concept words in conjunction with the math lessons. Hands-on activities and use of real objects, even at an advanced level, can enhance their comprehension of these math tasks.

When solving word problems, some hearing-impaired students may be able to read the problems correctly, but are unskilled at identifying the key facts or at interpreting the question stated in the word problems. Teaching them the meaning of specific terms and language structures used in word problems can increase their skills in solving word problems, but may not assist them to understand the problem itself. Acting out the problem or making the problem visually clear to the students can assist them in understanding how math relates and applies to life's experiences.

Instructional Adaptations

Academic achievement, even for normally hearing students, can be challenging at times. This is especially true for hearing-impaired students, whose language, cognitive, and/or academic achievement may not be commensurate with their hearing grade peers. These students can require one or more instructional and/or special adaptation to be implemented in order for them to succeed in a mainstream educational program.

Concrete/Experiential Context   When introducing a new concept, it is beneficial to provide hearing-impaired students with concrete learning activities, relate the new concepts to their previous experiences, or give them background knowledge. These activities can provide the student with a foundation for new information. These learning activities can be an actual experience, a role-playing activity, or a class discussion about background information relating to new concepts. The main goal of these activities should be to establish the students' language and knowledge bases for new information. Once conceptual background has been established, instruction can focus on new concepts.

Visual Organizational Frameworks Hearing-impaired students benefit from instruction that is supported by visual context and tangible materials. Manipulative material and visual representations provide them with the link between their experiential knowledge and symbolic or abstract linguistic and cognitive information. Functional charts and graphs can be developed as new skills and concepts are taught. Initially, real objects, pictures, and/or printed words can be used as visual aids, until the students can interpret the information independently. Charts containing learned skills or concepts can be hung in the classroom or made into individual charts. Students then can use these as references during independent learning assignments. Learning how to use and apply visual organizational approaches such as networking, semantic mapping, or outlining can provide students with a method of identifying relevant facts and an understanding of how these facts are related. Initially, these cognitive/linguistic strategies will need to be taught to the students, but gradually they should develop independent use of these methods. Students can learn to use these methods across the curriculum, in reading, written language, content areas, and even math activities. Visual organizational approaches can provide the hearing-impaired student with the means of becoming an independent learner.

The methods and techniques presented below can be effective strategies for hearing, as well as hearing-impaired, students. The ideas are meant to stimulate the teacher's thinking. Proposed techniques and adaptations should be tailored to the specific needs of the individual student.

Charts A few examples are given below:

Phonics/Spelling: The teacher can develop charts containing the primary and secondary letter patterns for sound/symbol relationships, or charts with learned word structure rules (see figure 1). Relevant examples should be given for each sound or rule.

Science: A chart could be constructed around a specific unit, such as dinosaurs. As different dinosaurs are presented in class, specific information relating to different distinctive characteristics can be

VOWEL CHART

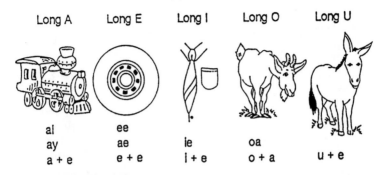

Long A	Long E	Long I	Long O	Long U
ai	ee		oa	
ay	ae	ie		
a + e	e + e	i + e	o + a	u + e

Figure 1. A phonics chart.

added to the chart (see figure 2). Such information can be used to teach categorization or definitions.

Networking: A method that teaches the student to identify and visually represent six different types of relationships often represented in instructional content developed for deaf students at National Technical Institute for the Deaf (Long et al. 1980). The six types of relationships are definition, characteristic, example, sequence, result, and compare/contrast. A few examples are shown in figures 3, 4, and 5.

Once the six basic structures of networking are mastered they can be combined and used to depict ideas contained in paragraphs, chapters, and stories visually.

Semantic Mapping: Semantic mapping is a categorical structuring of information in graphic form (see figure 6). This technique is not new, but has been referred to in a variety of ways, such as semantic webbing, semantic networking, or plot mapping. Semantic mapping has been mostly used for general vocabulary development, for pre- and post-reading activities, and as a study skill technique

DINOSAURS

TYPE	SPECIAL NAME	FOOD	SPECIAL FEATURES
Brontosaurus	Thunder Lizard	Plants	Big As 10 Elephants
Stegosaurus	Armored Lizard	Plant	Hard Plate Of Bones
Triceratops	Three-Horned Face	Plant	Fought With Horns
Tyrannosaurus	Tyrant King	Meat	Big Jaw/Sharp Teeth

Figure 2. A science chart.

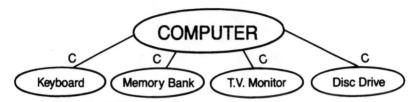

Figure 3.   Characteristics—A computer has a keyboard, memory bank, t.v. monitor, and disc drive.

(Heimlich and Pittelman 1986). It can be used to expand hearing-impaired students comprehension of specific vocabulary words and concepts (Johnson, Toms-Bronowski, and Pittelman 1982). When the vocabulary word or concept is discussed, the students and teachers share information they know about the topic. Then ideas are organized according to different categories and used to formulate the semantic map.

Pre-/Post-Teaching   Prior to being taught new material, students need to have both a list of vocabulary words and an outline of the content to be taught during the lesson. This information can be written on the board or presented in a handout. If students are working with re-source teachers, providing a copy of the handout helps to integrate the students' lessons. Pre-teaching activities, conducted either in the class or resource room, should assist the students in establishing the knowledge base needed to understand new information as well as exposing them to new terms and concepts. Post-teaching sessions can be used to review key concepts, clarify misconceptions, organize information, and expand the students' knowledge of content or skills emphasized during the lesson.

The semantic mapping technique can be used in pre- and post-teaching situations. After new vocabulary words and concepts have been presented during instruction or reading activities, the initial map can be altered to allow for new or more specific facts. Information contained in the semantic map can be a guide for independent reading and

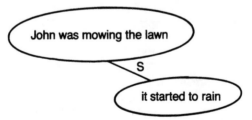

Figure 4.   Sequence—It started to rain before John finished mowing the lawn.

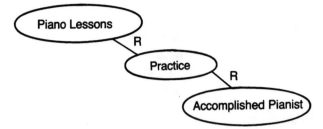

Figure 5. Reason/Result—If you take piano lessons, and practice daily, you can become an accomplished pianist.

writing activities related to the topic. The semantic map is also a useful study tool because it provides the student with relevant information to review for tests.

Monitoring of Linguistic Information   Because one cannot assume that students with hearing losses possess the same language and conceptual bases as their hearing peers, it is beneficial to hearing-impaired students if teachers frequently monitor these students' comprehension of key vocabulary words and concepts presented during instruction and independent reading assignments. Sometimes students are unaware of comprehension difficulties and lack of strategies for requesting clarification or additional information. If the student has consistent difficulties comprehending relevant information, tutoring or resource assistance should be considered.

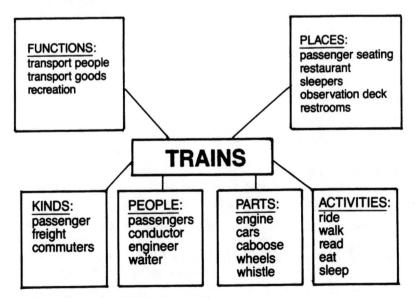

Figure 6.   Example of semantic mapping.

Restating Information When hearing-impaired students demonstrate difficulty in understanding a specific concept or process, it can be helpful to restate information. Some strategies for clarifying information are: (1) rephrasing sentences using familiar vocabulary and less complex sentences, (2) reducing the complexity of the tasks, (3) providing an experiential frame of reference, (4) providing response choices, or (5) establishing the students' knowledge base, and/or analyzing the students' difficulty, then reteaching information based on this knowledge.

Adapting Materials Adapting material contained in texts to the students' level of ability can help them to understand the content more fully. Aspects to consider in adapting materials are: (1) Using presentation formats that complement the students' proficiency level, such as providing hearing-impaired students with visual context to support instruction, such as tables or graphs; (2) establishing the students' knowledge base prior to introducing new information, such as relating information to previous experience or discussing background knowledge; (3) reducing the amount of extraneous information present by highlighting main points contained in the text, such as providing an outline or diagram; (4) controlling the amount and complexity of new vocabulary words being introduced; (5) simplifying grammar by using simple sentence structures and reducing the use of complex sentences, especially when introducing new information; and (6) constructing paragraphs so that the main topic is clearly presented and the supporting details are correctly sequenced (Short 1989). Implementing these adaptations enables students with language-based difficulties to understand concepts and to expand their knowledge base until they develop the higher level language/cognitive skills to gain knowledge from independent reading of the text.

Special Adaptations

Special adaptations refer to additional support services that can assist hearing-impaired students to function successfully in the mainstream setting. These adaptations may include resource assistance from other professionals or help from another student. Suggestions for special adaptations are presented in the following sections.

Supplementary Assistance If hearing-impaired students are experiencing consistent difficulty with any area of the curriculum, or their language and academic abilities are falling behind their hearing grade peers, additional support service may be required for them to make academic progress.

Peer Support/Buddy System   The buddy system is a support service that can assist both the classroom teacher and the hearing-impaired student. As previously noted, a hearing-impaired student can often miss relevant information. Given the student-teacher ratio, it can be an impossible situation for the teacher to keep the hearing-impaired student totally informed about changes in routine, announcements made over the intercom, unexpected events like visitors, or incidental occurrences such as students' reactions to a loud outburst of noise in the adjoining classroom. Repetition of directions can also interrupt class procedures. In such situations, a designated student—a buddy—would provide the hearing-impaired student with the required information. Additionally, providing hearing-impaired students with opportunities for being buddies to other students in the class allows them to be contributing members of the class. Such a system can foster class spirit, while encouraging sensitivity for others.

Peer Notetaker   Because the hearing-impaired student has to attend to the teacher or interpreter visually, taking notes can become a frustrating and futile experience. A hearing student who is capable of taking complete, well-organized, legible notes, can be a notetaker for the student with a hearing loss. Prior to initiating this support service, the notetaker should be provided with guidelines and materials for accomplishing the task (Osguthorpe 1980). Furthermore, the notetaker should be instructed about the procedures that produce quality class notes. Quality peer notetakers provide the mainstreamed hearing-impaired student with an important service that enables him or her to obtain more information from class instruction.

Peer Tutoring   The practice of having a student assist another student to learn is commonly referred to as peer tutoring. A classmate who shares a similar conceptual and experiential base by explaining the new information contributes to the success of this program. Peer tutors should demonstrate sensitivity and knowledge to work with hearing-impaired students in a positive manner. Hearing-impaired students also need to be given the opportunity of being a peer tutor. Guidelines and appropriate procedures should be established and clearly understood by the students. This approach can become a powerful means for promoting learning and creating a positive interpersonal climate in the classroom.

Cooperative Learning   Cooperative learning is a technique in which students jointly work on learning activities and are rewarded based on the group's performance. This technique has three essential components: a task structure, a reward structure, and an authority structure (Slavin 1980). Teachers are required to be trained in this tech-

nique so that they learn the logistics needed to set up the structure and
to assist students to learn the process. The cooperative learning approach can facilitate constructive interactions among the students, promote growth in learning, and foster positive interaction between hearing and hearing-impaired students in a learning activity that can be
rewarding to the whole class.

Use of Technology

For the past 20 years, technology increasingly has influenced education. Technological devices have become useful tools for learning and
instruction. Some of these devices are especially beneficial to hearing-
impaired students.

Captioning   Filmstrips and slides are used to supplement and
enhance information presented in many areas of the curriculum. Because films are a great source of knowledge, as well as entertainment,
captioning of films is a service provided for hearing-impaired people.
There are over 60 libraries in the United States that distribute captioned
films. Many of these films have accompanying study guides. Filmstrips, slides, transparencies, and other visual materials are also available to teachers working with hearing-impaired students.

Closed captioning is a process in which the dialogue portion of a
television program is translated into captions (subtitles), converted to
electronic codes, and inserted in the regular broadcast television signal
in a portion of the picture that normally is not seen. In order to see the
captions, viewers must have televisions equipped with special decoding devices called "decoders" (Caldwell 1981). A decoder is the device
attached to the television that decodes the portion of the broadcast signal containing the captions. Decoders can be used effectively in the
school setting to show captioned educational television programs used
to supplement instruction. Many scientific programs, such as *NOVA*,
are captioned. Look for the logo, CC, next to a program listing in the
television guide; this means that a show is closed captioned.

Real Time   Real time is a system for transliteration of speech into
print. A court stenographer attends class and enters the classroom instruction verbatim using speech sounds in phonetic shorthand into a
minicomputer that generates English. The script is displayed on the
classroom television set seconds after the spoken utterances. The hearing-impaired student reads the script as it appears on the screen
(Stuckless 1983). A hard copy of a lecture can be transcribed and given
to the student immediately after class. The cost of implementing such a
system is a major consideration for school districts.

Overhead Projectors   The overhead projector is helpful to use for instruction because it allows the teacher to face the students and stay in one place while teaching. These factors make speechreading accessible to the students. New vocabulary words and key points can be written easily by the teacher and seen by the class.

Computers   Computers are another tool for assisting instruction and can be used as a reinforcer. Computer programs are available for use in all areas of the curriculum. The combination of visual information and immediate feedback about the accuracy of a student's responses are advantageous features for hearing-impaired students. These programs, coupled with supervision, can be used as effective supplementary instructional tools.

Instructing hearing-impaired students in a word-processing program provides them with a potent tool for written expression. The computer can be used for written language assignments, such as paragraphs, stories, letters, or reports. Additionally, the word-processing program allows the student to make corrections easily, add information, and correct spelling errors, especially with the use of the spell check. Enabling these students to become proficient computer users provides them with a useful skill.

CONCLUSION

One of the greatest challenges for a classroom teacher is to manage the learning environment in such a way that all students are provided with educational opportunities needed to develop them to their fullest potential. Given the unique composition of students in a regular education class, successful management of a hearing-impaired student in this setting may be perceived as herculean in nature. Although the student's designated team collaborates to design the general educational program, the regular classroom teacher often becomes the person primarily responsible for making necessary adaptations needed for its effective implementation. Due to the changing dynamics of classroom interactions and the balancing of linguistic and cognitive demands of academic tasks, the teacher often is required to make decisions about interactive or instructional adaptations needed to facilitate the student's acquisition of knowledge. At times, a student may need additional support from other professionals in order to make academic progress. In such cases, the teacher can work jointly with other team members to implement needed changes. The challenge of enabling hearing-impaired students to be mainstreamed in their neighborhood school, with their families and friends, is a formidable goal, both for the student and the regular classroom teacher. Yet, for over a decade, many regular education and resource teachers have met this challenge head-on. These teachers have worked diligently to provide handicapped students with the abilities needed to achieve successfully in the mainstream educational setting. Their arduous efforts are to be commended and supported.

REFERENCES

Bess, F. 1986. The unilaterally hearing-impaired child: A final comment. *Ear and Hearing* 7 (1):52–54.

Caldwell, D. 1981. Closed-captioned television and the hearing impaired. *The Volta Review* 83 (5):285–90. [Annual Monograph].

Calkins, L. 1986. *The Art of Teaching Writing.* Portsmouth, NH: Heinemann.

Conway, D. 1985. Children (re)creating writing: A preliminary look at the purposes of free-choice writing of hearing-impaired kindergartners. *The Volta Review* 87 (5):91–107. [Annual Monograph].

Geers, A., and Moog, J. 1989. Factors predictive of the development of literacy in profoundly hearing-impaired adolescents. *The Volta Review* 91 (2):69–85.

Hanson, V., and Wilkenfeld, D. 1985. Morphophonology and lexical organization in deaf children. *Language and Speech* 28 (3):269–80.

Heimlich, J., and Pittelman, S. 1986. *Semantic Mapping: Classroom Applications.* Newark, Delaware: International Reading Association.

Heneger, M. E., and Cornett, R. O. 1971. *Cued Speech Handbook for Parents.* HEW Contract #OEC-O-8-001937-4348(019). Washington, D.C.: Gallaudet College.

Irwin, C., and Morgan, S. 1985, April. Educational interpreters—A new breed. Paper presented at the Annual Convention of the Council for Exceptional Children (63rd). Anaheim, CA. (ERIC Documentation Service No. ED 257 301).

Johnson, H., and Griffith P. 1985. The behavioral structure of an eighth-grade science class: A mainstreaming preparation strategy. *The Volta Review* 87 (6):291–301.

Johnson, D., Toms-Bronowski, S., and Pittleman, S. 1982. Vocabulary Development. *The Volta Review* 84 (5):11–24. [Annual Monograph].

King, C., and Quigley, S. 1985. *Reading and Deafness.* California: College-Hill Press.

Kolzak, J. 1983. The impact of child language studies on mainstreaming decisions. *The Volta Review* 85 (5):129–37.

Kretschmer, R., Jr. 1990, March. The hearing impaired child in the mainstream interpersonal, print and school discourse issues. Paper presented at the meeting of the Nebraska Education of the Hearing Impaired 9th Annual Spring Conference, Lincoln, NE.

LaSasso, C. 1985. Visual matching test-taking strategies used by deaf readers. *Journal of Speech and Hearing Research* 28:2–7.

LaSasso, C. 1990, March. Impacting on reading achievement of hearing-impaired students. Paper presented at the meeting of the Nebraska Education of the Hearing Impaired 9th Annual Spring Conference, Lincoln, NE.

Long, G., Hein, R. Coggiola, D., and Pizzente, M. 1980. *Networking: A Technique for Understanding and Remembering Instructional Material* (2nd ed.). New York: National Technical Institute for the Deaf and Rochester Institute of Technology.

Moeller, M. P., and Johnson, D. L. 1988, November. Longitudinal evaluation of deaf students learning signing exact English. Paper presented at ASHA Convention, Boston, MA.

Ninth Annual Report to Congress on the Implementation of the Educational of the Handicapped Art. 1987. Washington, DC: Department of Education.

Osguthorpe, R. T. 1980. *The Tutor/Notetaker: Providing Academic Support to Mainstreamed Deaf Students.* Washington, DC: Alexander Graham Bell Association.

Quigley, S., and Kretschmer, R. 1982. *The Education of Deaf Children: Issues, Theory and Practice.* Baltimore, MD: University Park Press.

Quigley, S., Wilbur, R., Power, D., Montanelli, D., and Steinkamp, M. 1976. *Syntatic Structures in the Language of Deaf Children.* Urbana, IL: University of Illinois, Institute for Child Behavior and Development.

Robbins, N., and Hatcher, C. 1981. The effects of syntax on the reading comprehension of hearing-impaired children. *The Volta Review* 83:105–115.

Short, D. 1989. *Adapting Materials for Content-Based Language Instruction.* Washington, DC: ERIC/CLL News Bulletin 13 (1), 1–8.

Slavin, R. 1980. Cooperative Learning. *Review of Educational Research* 50 (2):315–41.

Smith, F. 1977. Making sense of reading—and of reading instruction. *Harvard Educational Review* 47:386–95.

Stuckless, E. 1983. Real-time transliteration of speech into print for hearing-impaired students in regular classes. *American Annals of the Deaf* 128 (5):619–24.

Truax, R., and Edwards, B. 1984. Creating Stories as a means of communication. Short course presentation at the International Convention of the Alexander Graham Bell Association, Portland, OR.

Wilson, K. 1979. Inference and language processing in hearing and deaf children. Unpublished doctoral dissertation, Boston University.

Yoshinaga-Itano, C., and Downey, D. 1986. A hearing-impaired child's acquisition of schemata: Something's missing. *Topics in Language Disorders* 7 (1):45–57.

Chapter • 9

Psycho-Social Aspects of Mainstreaming

Sue Schwartz

Mainstreaming is not a new concept. In the early 1800s, J. P. Arrowsmith wrote about the education his younger deaf brother received in "ordinary" schools (Markides 1989). Arrowsmith advocated early education and strongly recommended parent support to supplement the school education. Similarly, in 1900, Alexander Graham Bell wrote that deaf children should be in "constant personal contact with their friends and relatives." Further, Bell wrote that "it would be better to send the teachers to these children, rather than send the children to the teachers. . . ." Bell goes on, in agreement with Arrowsmith, that the teachers should instruct the children as well as "their parents, relatives, and friends" (Blatt 1985).

Seventy-five years after Bell's letter was written, Public Law 94-142, which has come to be known as the "mainstreaming law," was signed by President Ford. Education for the hearing impaired has come to be what was envisioned by Arrowsmith and Bell, as well as others. The majority of hearing-impaired students are educated in "ordinary schools," and often teachers are sent to the students rather than vice versa. Today, nearly fifteen years after this signing, we can examine and question the impact of P.L. 94-142 on the psycho-social development of hearing-impaired students. With relatively little having been written on this topic, a brief review of the pertinent literature will bring us up to date on the issues that face us heading into the twenty-first century.

Garrettson (1977) discusses an "unwritten curriculum," which he describes as a variety of informal interactions that routinely occur between students in schools. He cites, for example: conversations on the bus and in the halls; participation in extra-curricular activities; attendance at social functions; interactions with a variety of students and teachers. These encounters provide much of the substance of the social interactions that can occur in school settings.

Foster (1987) expands this concept further by saying that one of the primary functions of the schools is the socialization of youth into the values and culture of adult society. She explains that the deaf learn in this mainstream environment what it means to be deaf in a hearing world, i.e., how to adapt and how to cope.

Gresham (1982) tells us that mainstreaming has been built on three faulty assumptions relative to the psycho-social domains. These are:

1. that the physical placement of handicapped children in regular classes will result in an increase in social interactions;
2. that placement of handicapped children in regular classes will result in increased social acceptance of the handicapped child by non-handicapped peers;
3. that mainstreamed handicapped children will model or imitate the behavior of non-handicapped peers as a result of increased exposure to them.

Gresham (1982) goes on to say that handicapped children placed in a mainstreamed environment without the requisite social skills that are crucial for peer acceptance are more likely to find increased social isolation and more restrictive social environments than might otherwise occur. In fact, the studies reviewed by Gresham found that the handicapped were not well-liked, not chosen as friends, nor accepted by others; that interest in them as individuals was low; and that the handicapped children did not model the behavior of the non-handicapped.

These studies and others (Antia 1982; Farrugia 1980; Ladd, Munson, and Miller 1984; Mertens 1989; Ross 1978; Salend 1984) show us that merely putting the students in "constant personal contact," as suggested by Dr. Bell, is not sufficient to insure interaction if we do not also add the needed social skills training.

Studies in this area of the psycho-social domain, as well as two informal surveys conducted for this report, show that there are clear factors that contribute to the success students feel on a psycho-social level in their educational environments.

CLEAR COMMUNICATION

Clear communication is any communication system that works for the student. The key is understanding between speaker and receiver. Deaf students in research studies have spoken highly of environments where educators and hearing students use effective total communication with the hearing-impaired (Foster 1987; Green 1976; Mertens 1986). Students in these learning situations feel very comfortable with both educators and hearing peers. It is not necessarily true that students with spoken communication fare better than those who choose not to use speech. It is possible, though, that their speech production may not be clear enough for hearing peers to understand and that their receptive skills may not be sharp enough for them to understand all that is said to them. Today there are many academically and socially successful hearing-impaired people who use available communication methods. There are choices and we must make them match the abilities of our students and their families (Schwartz 1987). The end result must be clear communication between sender and receiver.

In preparation for this paper, an informal questionnaire was mailed to twenty-seven students who are mainstreamed in the Montgomery County Public School Auditory Program in Maryland. Eighteen of the students responded. They represent varying levels of mainstreaming, with the majority being mainstreamed for all of their classes. These students also represent each of the communication methods used in this program: oral, total communication, and cued speech. They all have access to an interpreter for their classes; however, half reported that they did not use this service. It should be noted that the students have hearing losses that range from moderate to profound. All of the students responded that they use their own voices to answer in class. Additionally, some of the students said that they use the interpreter to respond for them some of the time.

In response to the questions, "How do you interact with hearing people?" and "What causes problems for you?", many of the students answered that communication was often the difficulty. They had varying strategies for dealing with this problem. Some wrote things down, others felt confident to ask the hearing person to slow down, others moved from a noisy environment to a quieter one, which enabled them to hear and speech-read better.

Helping students develop varying strategies is a key ingredient to providing communicative success. In our communication classes, auditory communication specialists use a variety of techniques to develop confidence in communicating. In addition to specific speech target sound practice, students are given real life situations in which to practice their communication skills. At the senior high level, for example, students are offered opportunities to practice in situations such as going to restaurants, to the post office, for a medical visit, and returning or exchanging merchandise at a store. The vocabulary of each experience is developed first, the speech production of the vocabulary is practiced, and each student is able to use his or her own communication system at this point. The students use role playing with their peers and are videotaped at various points in the process. A final culminating activity is an actual visit to the real-life place for which they have been practicing. A recent group visited a restaurant. They were driven by the communication specialist who sat at a distant table observing the communicative environment. The students were on their own to order, eat, and pay the bill. Their skills were evaluated, and after the experience each student met individually with the specialist to discuss his or her performance (Fernandez 1989). Practicing these skills with their own hearing-impaired peers provides them with the confidence to go out with hearing friends and to understand better the social environment.

Providing adequate communication support systems is critical to the success of students. The interpreter staff is central to our program, providing interpretation in all three methodologies. It is available for mainstreamed students on a needs basis from kindergarten through high school in our five center schools. The supervisor and interpreter coordinators are careful with the role of the interpreter in the classroom, so that she or he is the ears and/or voice of the student and not an aide helping the student with school work (Doctors 1989; Lee 1989; Gregory 1989). It is important that interpreters be facilitators of communication and not barriers. The interpreter coordinators offer students several sessions through the year in which they are trained in how to make the best use of an interpreter; the purpose of these sessions is to try to forestall some of the dependencies we have seen develop in the past (Lee 1989; Gregory 1989). The interpreter will often facilitate discussions between hearing and hearing-impaired students, again acting as ears and/or voice but not becoming personally involved in the discussion. By the time our students reach adolescence, most are comfortable with using an interpreter both for receiving information and, if necessary, giving it back.

Interpreters serve an educational as well as social role in our program, but an additional boon for our students has been a geographical one. Several years ago, school system administrators determined that it was important to consolidate our center schools into one county administrative area. Therefore, our three center elementary schools feed into one junior high and one senior high school. This often has allowed our students to attend school with the same hearing students for all of their educational years. This arrangement has developed a core of students who are comfortable around hearing-impaired students, who have learned a communication system, and who have learned to appreciate the social qualities of an individual who happens to be hearing impaired, thereby expanding the social opportunities for our students.

The junior and senior high schools have offered sign language as an elective course taught by members of the auditory staff (Gershowitz 1989; Lee 1989). These classes have helped some hearing students develop skills in the use of sign language to a level where they are the interpreters for high school plays that may include hearing-impaired students in key roles.

At our elementary school that uses total communication, the music teacher has become a fluent signer. She teaches signs to the words in the music so that every class learns signs in this way. Each performance has a nice balance of songs that are sung and signed by all of the performing students. Additionally, she has a volunteer chorus composed of approximately sixty hearing students with three or four hearing-impaired students, which meets at recess to learn songs in sign. This group, the Fabulous Flying Fingers, was invited to perform at the White House when Nancy Reagan was there. Through the medium of music, these hearing students learn sign language and begin to feel comfortable using it with their hearing-impaired schoolmates (Burdette 1989).

At the elementary school that houses the oral/aural program, a regular education teacher established a group of young children who sing and perform and has included hearing-impaired students in this group (Johnson 1989).

Whatever the system, clear communication is a key ingredient to successful integration of hearing-impaired students with hearing students. Many resources need to be drawn upon to ensure success in this area.

PARENTAL SUPPORT

Green (1976), in looking at the psycho-social aspects of mainstreaming, suggests that the child's acceptance of himself or herself as a hearing-impaired individual is dependent on the parents' attitude and degree of acceptance. She goes on to say that if parents become overprotective, their child may translate this into "I am not able." Hearing parents faced with the diagnosis of their child's deafness face confusion, anxiety, guilt, and perhaps disappointment, which may lead to rejection. Programs must provide support for parents in dealing with these feelings.

For many years, we have focused on academic and communication issues with our students, so that parents have taken a back seat. Parents' needs must be attended to so that they can be free psychologically and available to their children. They must learn to understand the unique role that they play in their child's education and personal life.

This can only happen with support for their emotional needs and for the psychological as well as social issues that will arise for their hearing-impaired children.

An informal survey was sent to teachers of the hearing impaired and teachers in the mainstream who have had hearing-impaired students in their classroom. Two questions were asked: (1) What skills do students need to succeed in the mainstream? and (2) What can parents do to support these skills? A full list of responses to both of these questions can be found in Appendix A, but see table I for a summary of the parent skills.

Many hearing parents are not prepared for the demanding job of raising hearing children and certainly are not prepared for the large amount of new information they must absorb about their hearing-impaired child. We often program this parent support for the infant–toddler years; but we fail to recognize that this need goes on into the adolescent and young adult years, when children face many psycho-

Table I.   Parent Skills

Summary of Parent Skills	Behaviors
Parental relationship with child	Learn communication system of child
	Include child in all family discussions
	Be realistic about the child's strengths and weaknesses
	Have consistent consequences for behaviors
	Have positive attitude toward child's hearing impairment
Parental relationship with school	Achieve mutual trust and support
	Attend conferences
	Learn school expectations for all students
Encouraging school-related behaviors	Provide a rich variety of supplemental language experiences
	Provide assistive devices such as TDD and captioner to help child broaden general experiences
Supporting academic growth	Read and discuss widely with child
	Continually build and expand language and vocabulary
	Provide space and opportunity for child to do homework under supervision
Encouraging socialization	Provide before and after school transportation for clubs and sports
	Encourage participation in activities such as church, synagogue, and Girl and Boy Scouts with hearing peers

social problems. What special skills and support this group of parents requires at these times as well as in the early years! Education is indeed a three-legged stool. We must have the educators, students, and parents all working together to make the entire educational program succeed.

Meadow-Orlans (1986) discusses three tasks of adolescence: to develop autonomy, achieve independence, and master self-determination. These skills are best encouraged and enhanced in the home. She strongly states that parents need to learn and use the child's communication system because this is critical to establishing the opportunities for free and accessible discussions with the child. She suggests that opportunities for independence be provided in the preschool years with increasing levels of self-reliance as the child matures, while maintaining a balance by establishing limits. Because the hearing-impaired child lacks many avenues of access to the hearing world, it is best to provide every possible opportunity for independence by acquiring assistive devices such as vibrating or flashing alarm clocks, TDDs, and captioners, so that the hearing-impaired child can be as independent as today's technology allows.

In her book, *Deafness and Child Development* (1980), Meadow talks about parental attitudes and child-rearing practices that slow the development of social maturity in deaf children. She feels that over-protectiveness is a major contributor and cautions against allowing this to develop. Once again, she stresses the vital importance of successful communication, stating that social development and language acquisition are intertwined. Additionally, she feels that social development and self-concept go hand-in-hand and that self-concept is enhanced by family climate, school achievement, and of course, clear communication.

Parents of adolescents often are concerned about feelings of social isolation that their children experience. As a possible solution, parents need to feel comfortable opening their home to teen activities, sponsoring a movie and soda party, being the chaperone on the class trip to facilitate communication, and organizing after-school activities that focus on needs of hearing-impaired children but include other students as well. Often it is the parents' own needs that are keeping the child socially isolated.

Parental involvement is an important element in the socialization process. Parents who support their children are essential to the success of the social and psychological domains of mainstreaming.

Today, of course, we have many working parents and the reality is not as simple as the expectation. Coupled with this increasing phenomenon, however, is the increased involvement of fathers in our programs and in our parent groups. In many cases, there are two parents who can help drive carpools, participate in field trips, and otherwise contribute to the social life of the hearing-impaired child.

The students mentioned earlier in the informal survey were asked, "If you were talking with parents of a young deaf child, what would you suggest to them to help them integrate their child with hearing people?" Several verbatim responses of these students are quoted in table II. These students' responses provide provocative insights into the life experiences of these young people.

EXTRACURRICULAR ACTIVITIES

Almost every article discussing the psycho-social factors in mainstreaming points out that participation in extracurricular activities is a key ingredient in the successful total integration of the student. Where

Table II.   Verbatim Responses

Student	Response
Male (PTA 90 dB)	Don't push their children too hard or they will fall; and don't spoil their children or they will become dependent. Give their children the loving and caring support they need to stimulate their minds.
Male (PTA 75 dB)	Constant determination. The experience will be as painful for the parents as for the child. Don't give in. The pain now will be far less than that of an isolated deaf person (adult) in society. Get involved with your kids' school. My teachers were involved in my life not because of my deafness, but simply because my parents and I showed an interest in school and learning. Emphasize strength of friendships/relationships rather than quantity.
Male (PTA 95 dB)	Give constant positive encouragement. Very often it's the deaf child who has to make the first contact and it's scary. Continue to give communication a high priority— the child will hopefully transfer the communication skills he/she learns to his/her social surroundings.
Male (PTA 55 dB)	I would suggest them taking their child to an older deaf person and explain to them what to expect and try to make the child give a better understanding of life. Being deaf is hard to live with; but after accepting their loss, and trying to get the best out of life despite of many failures and successes one would be enjoying life.
Male (PTA no responses)	Suggest the following ideas: educate yourself on hearing impairment, enroll in auditory service, combination of programs for both hearing and deaf children. Let child get used to hearing aids right away, and finally be prepared for *years* of *hard* work which will result in a rewarding future!

non-mainstreamed environments were preferred by students, the reasons stated were the availability of extracurricular participation with ease of communication. Where mainstreamed environments were preferred for other reasons, the lack of participation in extracurricular activities was cited as a drawback.

Opportunities for participation are often available, but barriers can preclude involvement. The primary barrier, of course, is communication. Making interpreters available to students for participation in extracurricular activities is vital. Providing opportunities for hearing students to learn sign language or cued speech is important for training a new personal resource. Parental support for the inevitable car pooling is a major issue. Building confidence in the students to venture into these social groups is also critical.

Several years ago, in Montgomery County, an innovative program was started by the Superintendent's Advisory Committee on the Rights of Handicapped Individuals to promote acceptance of children with handicaps. This program, called the "Montgomery County Exceptional Leaders," involves high school students with a variety of handicapping conditions. Since its inception, approximately thirty students with different handicapping conditions have been selected to participate. The training for these students has two phases. In the first phase the students spend a weekend together in the early autumn for the purpose of developing friendships within the group, sharing educational experiences (the difficulties as well as the successes), gaining comfort in making presentations, building teams from the members for school visitations, and planning programs for the coming year. After this initial planning, the teams meet periodically to discuss and practice their classroom presentations. The actual presentations are made in regular education classrooms in the elementary schools. The benefits of such a program are obvious: the students giving the presentations have to be prepared to answer difficult questions from their young listeners, they have to gain confidence to present themselves as achieving teens in spite of their handicapping condition, and they must have problem-solving skills to field situations as they occur. The students who are listening and responding to these speakers have a first-hand experience with a young person who is handling a handicapping condition in an effective way (Fagen 1989; Moore 1989).

Interacting through this program as well as in sports, clubs, and other fun activities, will provide a hearing-impaired student with the opportunities for social skills development that sitting alongside a hearing student in an academic classroom is not going to provide. Clubs and varsity sports are vehicles for access to hearing students. Sport stars, leading actors and actresses, and class officers are respected by peers and are roles hearing-impaired students should strive to attain. We have focused, and rightly so, on the academic and communication needs of our students and have not stressed the vehicles available for effective participation in extracurricular activities; but these vehicles represent an area that is vitally important to our students, one that enables them to feel a part of their school community.

TEACHING SOCIAL SKILLS

The structured teaching of social skills is the most critical and least implemented facet of mainstreaming. It is the essence of what will add to the psycho-social success of hearing-impaired students in mainstream environments. Two excellent resources have emerged from the regular education domain. These are *MegaSkills* by Rich (1988) and the *Skillstreaming Series* by Goldstein et al. (1980).

Rich states that megaskills are the values, attitudes, and behaviors that determine success in and out of school. She goes on to say that "you know in your bones that they are important but you may not know how to teach them. This book shows you how." Dr. Rich uses materials found easily around the home to help develop these skills (see table III).

There are special activities for each of these megaskills, which are geared for children ages four through twelve. The activities seem simplistic at first glance, but they do reach out to show children how to maximize each of these skills. The activities are for parents and children to do together, which helps remind us to shift our time priorities back to our children.

While *MegaSkills* focuses on parents and children at home, it certainly also can be used in schools. *Skillstreaming the Adolescent* (Goldstein et al. 1980) and *Skillstreaming the Elementary School Child: A Guide*

Table III.   Megaskills

Megaskill	Definition
Confidence	Feeling able to do it
Motivation	Wanting to do it
Effort	Being willing to work hard
Responsibility	Doing what's right
Initiative	Moving into action
Perseverance	Completing what you start
Caring	Showing concern for others
Teamwork	Working with others
Common sense	Using good judgment
Problem solving	Putting what you know and what you can do into action

for Teaching Prosocial Skills (McGinnis et al. 1984) are geared for a school environment. The authors of this series state in their introduction that educators are more and more frequently frustrated by the problematic behaviors that children show in school. The authors realize that educators' time could be better spent in preventing the problem-behavior than in punishing the student or trying to find the ultimate culprit in the dispute. While educators may succeed in reducing the unwanted behaviors, they often find that the children simply do not know an appropriate way to behave in a given situation. The skills identified by these authors are those with which hearing-impaired students often have difficulty, perhaps because they do not know the appropriate language or have never been in a similar situation before. The skills are taught through a structured sequence with role playing to facilitate learning. Follow-up sessions are held to review skills periodically. There are sixty skills that are covered in the elementary guide and fifty in the secondary level guide. A few of these skills are described (see table IV).

Tables V and VI give an example of one of the skills that is in both the elementary and adolescent guide and shows how it is taught.

It is apparent that these as well as the other skills covered in these two guides are useful skills for the hearing-impaired student to practice to help in successful social interactions. In communication and resource sessions in Montgomery County, several of our staff members are beginning to use these materials to teach the pragmatics of language. These social situations provide a way to practice vocabulary and speech drills.

Table IV. School Skills

Skill	Description
Asking for help	Does the student decide when he or she needs assistance and ask for help in a pleasant manner?
Saying "thank-you"	Does the student tell others that he or she appreciates help given, favors, etc?
Deciding on something to do	Does the student find something to do when he or she has free time?
Introducing yourself	Does the student introduce himself or herself in an appropriate way to people he or she doesn't know?
Beginning and ending a conversation	Does the student know how and when to begin and end a conversation with another person?
Joining in	Does the student know and practice acceptable ways of joining an ongoing activity or group?
Playing a game	Does the student play games with classmates fairly?
Giving a compliment	Does the student tell others that he or she likes something about them or something they have done?

Table V. Skill 51: Dealing with Being Left Out (at the elementary level)

Steps	Notes for Discussion
1. Decide what has happened to cause you to feel left out.	Discuss possible reactions as to why a student may be ignored by peers.
2. Think about your choices. a. Ask to join in.	 Students should be taught the skill, "joining in" (skill 17).
b. Choose someone else to play with.	
c. Do an activity you enjoy.	Students should generate and discuss personal lists of acceptable activities.
3. Act out your best choice.	If one choice doesn't work, the student should try another one.

Suggested Situations
  School: You are left out of a group game at recess.
  Home: Your brother or sister is leaving you out of an activity with his or her friends.
  Peer Group: A group of friends are going to a movie or a birthday party, but you weren't invited.

Comments
It may be important to discuss the types of feelings that might result from being left out (feeling angry, hurt, or frustrated). When discussing this skill, the teacher might emphasize that it is important to deal with being left out through these skill steps, rather than to continue to feel angry or hurt.

Reprinted with permission from Research Press. Ellen McGinnis and Arnold P. Goldstein. *Skillstreaming the Elementary School Child.* Champaign, IL: Research Press, 1984.

In one resource class, the auditory teacher asked the regular education teacher to choose three hearing students who needed additional support in social skills. These three students met with the auditory teacher and a hearing-impaired student once a week during the resource period. Skills from *Skillstreaming the Elementary School Child: A Guide for Teaching Prosocial Skills* (McGinnis et al. 1984) were taught and practiced during these sessions. The obvious benefits were that all four students learned new ways of interacting with others. An additional benefit was the friendship that developed between the hearing-impaired student and the other three students (Hunt 1989). The structured teaching of prosocial skills both at home and at school facilitates the mainstreaming of our hearing-impaired students.

SUMMARY

We have looked at four critical areas that have an impact on the psychosocial development of hearing-impaired youngsters. Some programs

Table VI.   Skill 35: Dealing with Being Left Out (adolescent level)

Steps	Trainer Notes
1. Decide if you are being left out.	Are you being ignored or rejected?
2. Think about why the other people might be leaving you out of something.	
3. Decide how you could deal with the problem.	You might wait, leave, tell the other people how their behavior affects you, or ask to be included.
4. Choose the best way and do it.	

Suggested Content for Modeling Displays
   School or Neighborhood: Main actor tells teacher of disappointment after not being picked for committee.
   Home: Main actor asks sibling to include him in planned activity with other friends.
   Peer Group: Main actor is left out of plans for party (Goldstein et al. 1980).

Reprinted with permission from Research Press. Arnold P. Goldstein, Robert P. Sprafkin, N. Jane Gershaw, and Paul Klein. *Skillstreaming the Adolescent.* Champaign, IL: Research Press, 1980.

focus on these issues intensively while others do not. When we evaluate and judge mainstreaming programs, we might ask if we have done all that we can in: (1) providing clear access to communication and providing appropriate and adequate resources to help with communication; (2) providing ongoing parental support throughout the educational careers of our students; (3) providing realistic opportunities for participation in extracurricular activities; and (4) teaching our students acceptable social behaviors that will facilitate their success in the everyday world.

We hope to find more and more students reporting satisfaction—both academically and socially—with their educational experiences. As with every other aspect of education, there is no one perfect way to educate all children, but all children deserve to be educated to their individual potential in all areas.

APPENDIX A   RESULTS OF SURVEY AMONG
TEACHERS* IN HEARING-IMPAIRED AND REGULAR CLASSROOM

Question: What Skills Do Hearing-Impaired Students Need to Succeed in the Mainstream?

Characteristics of the Individual

Is responsible.
Is independent.
Is self-motivated.
Is cooperative.
Exhibits self control.
Is self-reliant.

Demonstrates initiative.
Is willing to take risks.
Has self-confidence.
Has a positive attitude.
Asks for help when needed.

Communication Skills

Is able to use an interpreter well.
Is able to use communication skills fully.

Is able to monitor and use amplification systems well.
Has good attending skills.

Socialization Skills

Is comfortable with peers.
Interacts successfully with peers both in and out of school.

Is involved in extracurricular activities with hearing friends.
Has supportive parents.

Academic Skills for Success in the Mainstream

Is on grade level in *reading*, language, and math.
Has appropriate classroom behavior—sits still, raises hand to be recognized, and follows directions.
Has good organization skills.
Has good study skills.
Has good fine motor skills.
Has realistic view of strengths and weaknesses.

Understands vocabulary used.
Has good writing skills.
Is able to take notes or use note-taker skillfully.
Stays on task to completion.
Completes homework.
Is able to do appropriate problem solving.
Is comfortable in large group instruction.

---

*Teachers in Montgomery County, Maryland Public Schools

Question: How Can Parents Help Hearing-Impaired Students Succeed in the Mainstream?

Parental Relationship with Child

Learn the communication system the child is using in school.

Include the student in *all* family discussions.

Be realistic about the child's strengths and weaknesses.

Model good listening skills.

Encourage appropriate risk taking behaviors.

Teach manners.

Have consistent consequences for inappropriate behaviors.

Have a positive attitude about the child's hearing impairment and use of amplification.

Accept the child unconditionally.

Make the child feel successful.

Ensure adequate rest.

Encouraging Socialization

Invite both hearing and hearing-impaired friends to your home.

Provide before- and after-school transportation for clubs and sports.

Encourage participation in church, synagogue, and youth-related groups with hearing and hearing-impaired peers.

Rehearse new or doubtful situations at home *before* the encounter.

Supporting Academic Growth

Read with and to your child

Sit with your child and read to yourself while he or she is reading.

Take turns reading—you read a page, he or she reads the next.

Build vocabulary—keep a notepad in your car and on the refrigerator, jot down unfamiliar words, use them frequently throughout the day.

Discuss world events from the newspaper and from television.

Provide a captioner for your television set so that programs and news are available.

Give directions for home tasks and expect completion of them.

Encourage use of an interpreter other than parents for extracurricular activities.

Teach the vocabulary of extracurricular activities.

Provide transportation so that child can stay after school for extra help from teachers.

Don't do homework for the child.

Encouraging School-related Behaviors

Encourage student to ask for help when needed.

Encourage getting school supplies ready the night before.

Provide a multitude of experiences.

Encourage the child to bring in related items to share with class about school topics.

Take the child to museums, plays, sporting, and cultural events.

Provide adequate language for these experiences.

Reinforce objectives taught in school through outside activities.

Help the child become an independent learner.

Encourage use of resources, such as the library.

Have a TDD (telephone device for the deaf) so the child can make his or her own contacts.

Review the day's work.

Provide a study place and time free from distractions.

REFERENCES

Anita, S. D. 1982. Social interaction of partially mainstreamed hearing-impaired children. *American Annals of the Deaf* 127(1):18–25.

Blatt, B. 1985. Friendly letters on the correspondance of Helen Keller, Anne Sullivan, and Alexander Graham Bell. *Exceptional Children* 51(5):405–409.

Burdette, T. 1989. Montgomery County Public School. Personal Communication.

Doctors, S. 1989. Supervisor, Auditory Programs, Montgomery County Public Schools. Personal Communication.

Fagen, S. 1989. Montgomery County Public Schools. Personal Communication.

Farrugia, D. 1980. A study of social-emotional adjustment patterns of hearing-impaired students in different educational settings. *American Annals of the Deaf* 125(5):535–41.

Fernandez, J. M. 1989. Montgomery County Public Schools. Personal Communication.

Foster, S. 1987. *Life in the Mainstream: Reflections of Deaf College Freshman on their Experiences in the Mainstreamed High School.* Office for Postsecondary Career Studies and Institutional Research. Washington, DC.: Department of Education.

Garrettson, M. 1977. The residential school. *The Deaf American* 29:19–22.

Gershowitz, S. 1989. Montgomery County Public Schools. Personal Communication.

Goldstein, A., and Sprafkin, R., with Gershaw, N. J., and Klein, P. 1980. *Skillstreaming the Adolescent.* Champaign, IL: Research Press Company.

Green, R. R. 1976. Psycho-Social Aspects of Mainstreaming for the Child and Family. In *Mainstream Education for Hearing-Impaired Children and Youth.* ed. Gary Nix. New York: Grune and Stratton.

Gregory, D. 1989. Montgomery County Public Schools. Personal Communication.

Gresham, F. M. 1982. Misguided mainstreaming: The case for social skills training with handicapped children. *Exceptional Children* 48(5):422–32.

Hunt, F. 1989. Montgomery County Public Schools. Personal Communication.

Johnson, L. M. T. 1989. Montgomery County Public Schools. Personal Communication.

Ladd, G. W., Munson, H. L., Miller, J. K. 1984. Social integration of deaf adolescents in secondary-level mainstreamed programs. *Exceptional Children* 50(5):420–28.

Lee, C. 1989. Montgomery County Public Schools. Personal Communication.

Markides, A. 1989. Integration: The speech intelligibility, friendship and associations of hearing-impaired children in secondary schools. *The Journal of the British Association of Teachers of the Deaf* 13(3):63–73.

McGinnis, E., and Goldstein, A. P., with Sprafkin, R., and Gershaw, N. J. 1984. *Skillstreaming the Elementary School Child: A Guide for Teaching Prosocial Skills.* Champaign, IL: Research Press Company.

Meadow, K. P. 1980. *Deafness and Child Development.* Berkley, CA: University of California Press.

Meadow-Orlans, K. P. 1986. Autonomy for deaf adolescents: Facilitative environments. In *Innovations in the Habilitation and Rehabilitation of Deaf Adolescents.* eds., G. Anderson and D. Watson. University of Arkansas. Rehabilitation Research and Training Center on Deafness Hearing Impairment.

Mertens, D. M. 1989. Social experiences of hearing-impaired high school youth. *American Annals of the Deaf* 134:15–19.

Moore, C. 1989. Montgomery County Public Schools. Personal Communication.

Rich, D. 1988. *MegaSkills- How Families can Help Children Succeed in School and Beyond.* Boston: Houghton Mifflin Co.

Ross, M. 1978. Mainstreaming: Some social considerations. *The Volta Review* 80(1):21–30.

Salend, S. J. 1984. Factors contributing to the development of successful mainstreaming programs. *Exceptional Children* February: 409–416.

Schwartz, S. 1987. *Choices in Deafness: A Parent's Guide.* Kensington, MD: Woodbine House.

ADDITIONAL RESOURCES

The following list was obtained from "Materials for Educating Non-handicapped Students about their Handicapped Peers" in *Teaching Exceptional Children* 1980, and "Enjoying Each Other's Company" in *Perspectives* 1987.

For Teachers

Education Unlimited. Educational Resources. 1834 Meetinghouse Rd., Boothwyn, PA 19061.

Covers all disabilities. This is a journal for "mainstream" teachers and administrators in regular and special education who work with exceptional children.

Handicapped People in Society: A Curriculum Guide. R. E. Ross and I. R.

Freelander. University of Vermont. Special Education Department, Burlington, VT.

Covers all disabilities. This 178-page curriculum guide contains lesson plans, activities, resources, and evaluations to influence attitudes toward the handicapped (K–12).

Mainstreaming. R. Piazza. Special Learning Corporation. 42 Boston Post Rd., Guilford, CT 06437.

Covers all disabilities. This is a book of readings on the problems and methods of mainstreaming. Also included are case studies, methodologies, and suggestions for teachers.

Mainstreaming Handicapped Students. A. P. Turnbull and H. B. Schutz. Allyn and Bacon, Inc. Dept. 894, 470 Atlantic Ave., Boston, MA 02210.

Covers all disabilities. This 350-page book features chapters on the IEP, instructional strategies, and modifications in all curricular areas.

Mainstreaming Series. T. Fairchild, ed. Teaching Resources. 50 Pond Park Rd., Hingham, MA 02043.

Has individual books on different disabilities. One on the hearing impaired. They are cartoon style books suitable for secondary and adult levels.

Mainstreaming: What Every Child Needs to Know About Disabilities. S. Bookbinder. The Exceptional Parent Press. Room 708, Statler Office Bld., Boston, MA 02116.

Covers blind, deaf, mentally retarded, and physically disabled persons. This 94-page book contains units and lessons about handicaps (two sessions for each handicap). Also included are simulation activities and use of aids and appliances for each disability (Grades 1–4).

Notes from a Different Drummer. B. Baskin and K. Harris. R. R. Bowker Publishers. 1180 Avenue of the Americas, New York, NY 10036.

Covers all disabilities. This is a 375-page comprehensive guide book to the study of the handicapped child in children's literature.

People Just Like You: About Handicaps and Handicapped People (An Activity Guide). M. Jones and M. Stevens. Committee on Youth Development, President's Committee on Employment of the Handicapped, Superintendent of Documents, US Government Printing Office, Washington, DC 20402.

Covers all disabilities. This 36-page book consists of six lessons or sessions on accepting the handicapped. Topics include prejudice, the nature of handicaps, and eliminating social and environmental barriers (K–12).

Strategies for Training Regular Educators to Teach Children with Handicaps

(STRETCH) (Mainstreaming Order #7213). Hubbard. P.O. Box 104, Northbrook, IL 60062.
Covers all disabilities. This thirty-minute color videocassette for teachers examines areas of disagreement about mainstreaming and covers major service models.

For Nonhandicapped Children

Accepting Individual Differences. Developmental Learning Materials. 7440 Natchez Ave., Niles, IL 60648.
Covers mentally retarded, learning-disabled, visually impaired, hearing-impaired, and motor-impaired students. This kit contains four large flip books, an audiocassette, and four booklets. It is suitable for grades K–6.

Be My Friend. Canadien Council on Children and Youth. 323 Chapel, Ottawa, Ontario KIN 722, Canada.
Covers physically handicapped, hearing-impaired, speech-impaired, visually impaired, and mentally retarded students. Stories, games, and illustrations are included in this coloring book for grades 2–3.

Everybody Counts! A Workshop Manual to Increase Awareness of Handicapped People. M. J. Ward; R. N. Arkell; H. G. Dahl; J. H. Wise. The Council For Exceptional Children. 1920 Association Drive, Reston, VA 22091.
Covers all disabilities. This workshop is designed as an initial experiential learning strategy to assist groups toward a fuller understanding of the needs and desires of disabled individuals. It includes a discussion guide for 25 simulation activities that allow participants to feel what it is like to be disabled. Included are an 80-page manual and an audiocassette.

Feeling Free. Human Policy Press. P.O. Box 127, Syracuse, NY 13210.
Covers visually impaired, hearing-impaired, physical- and health-impaired, mentally retarded, and learning-disabled students. Suitable for grades 3–10 this kit contains children's books, educational guides, and six posters.

Getting Through: A Guide to Better Understanding of the Hearing Impaired. Zenith Radio Co. 6501 W. Grand Ave., Chicago, IL 60635.
Suitable for all grade levels, this record contains simulated hearing loss activities, and hints on how to make communication easier.

Kids Come in Special Flavors. The Kids Come in Special Flavors Co. P.O. Box 562, Dayton, OH 45405.
Covers learning disabled, hearing-impaired, mentally retarded,

and visually impaired students, as well as those with cerebral palsy and spina bifida. This kit, which is suitable for grades K–12, contains a book of simulation activities, a cassette, and materials for simulation activities.

My New Friend Series. Eye Gate Media. Jamaica, NY 11435.
Covers hearing-impaired, visually impaired, physically handicapped, and mentally retarded persons. This kit contains four filmstrips and cassettes.

Special Friends. Listen and Learn Co. 13366 Pescadero Rd., La Honda, CA 94929.
Covers physically handicapped, learning-disabled, emotionally disturbed, visually impaired, hearing-impaired, and mentally retarded students. This kit, which is suitable for grades K–3, contains eight lessons of approximately 15 minutes each, accompanied by filmstrips, cassette tape, and a teaching guide.

What is a Handicap? BFA Educational Media. 2211 Michigan Ave., Santa Monica, CA 90404.
Covers orthopedically handicapped, communication-disordered, hearing-impaired, emotionally disturbed, and multiply handicapped students. This kit, which is suitable for grades 4–6, contains six duplicating masters, four cassette tapes, and four filmstrips.

Children's Books about Handicaps

Primary

Jamie's Tiger. J. Wahl. Harcourt Brace Jovanovich. 757 3rd Ave. New York, NY 10017.
As a result of German measles, Jamie loses his hearing but learns to cope at home, in school, and with friends.

Elementary

A Dance to Still Music. B. Corcoran. Atheneum. 122 E. 42nd St., New York, NY 10017.
Margaret finds adjustments to her severe hearing loss very painful, but learns that running away is not the answer.

Junior High

Father's Arcane Daughter. E. L. Konigsburg. Atheneum. 122 E. 42nd St., New York, NY 10017.
Few demands have been made of Heide because of her handicaps. When a long lost sister returns home, the girl is forced to choose between a safe protected existence and one that offers her a

chance to use her talents but necessitates abandonment of her dependent patterns.

The Swing. E. Hanlon. Bradburg. 2 Overhill Rd., Scarsdale, NY 10583. Beth's deafness makes her the object of cruel teasing. Her unsuccessful efforts to protect some wild animals lead her to an important friendship.

Chapter • 10

Mainstreaming Into the Nineties— Are We On Track?

Dorothy Boothroyd-Turner

The educational process of mainstreaming handicapped children in the Province of Ontario, Canada received its formal framework in 1980 with the passage of Bill 82, an Act to amend the Education Act of 1974. The influence and impact of the previously enacted American legislation, Public Law 94-142, on this educational milestone is undeniable. The mainstreaming of hearing-impaired children on both sides of the border, however, had been in progress well before these laws were passed.

This chapter will outline the history of the mainstream support program in Metropolitan Toronto, and describe the delivery-of-service model. Four case studies will be presented, and analysis of these will provide discussion of some of the issues that should be considered when making decisions regarding appropriate mainstreaming. The focus throughout is on the question, "Are we doing the right thing for hearing-impaired children in the mainstream?"

HISTORY

In Metropolitan Toronto, a large multicultural, urban area, Metro-Wide programs for the hearing-impaired (Dewar, Draffin, and Booth-

The author gratefully acknowledges the support of the administration at the Toronto Board of Education and the Metropolitan Toronto School Board, and the contribution to the preparation of this chapter by colleagues on the hearing itinerant staff, especially Jessie Daubney, Ross Fletcher, Denise Meade, and Patricia Warner.

royd 1989) provide a broad spectrum of services to a diverse population ranging from infants in the home to students graduating from secondary school (see figure 1). Placement in the various programs depends on an individual child's needs at any given time. At one end of the spectrum is the mainstream support, or itinerant program as it is known. This service was initiated in 1969 with one teacher and seven students whose hearing losses were moderate or better. Most students with severe and profound losses were still routinely placed in a special school; a very small number was integrated with parental and private tutorial support.

By 1975, students with severe and profound losses were routinely integrated into regular classrooms, and there were eight itinerant teachers tutoring 50 students and monitoring an additional 128. In 1990, 20 specialist teachers of the hearing impaired provide tutorial instruction to approximately 100 students and monitor an additional 280. Of those students receiving regular support, 40% have a severe or profound loss bilaterally.

There are many reasons for the rapid growth of the itinerant program and the changing population it serves. These include early diagnosis, improved hearing aids, and a focus on the use of residual hearing. The introduction of FM wireless hearing aid equipment to the program in 1975 made it possible for more students to be integrated appropriately. Increased parental and professional knowledge and influence are also significant factors. Many parents opt for regular school

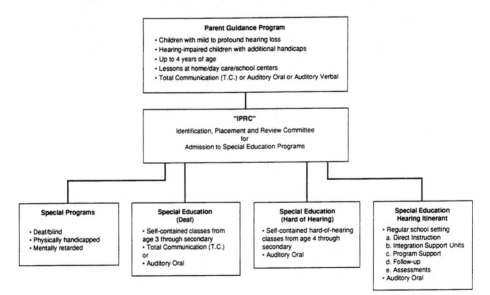

Figure 1. Metro Toronto programs for hearing-impaired children.

placement for their children despite the barriers that must be overcome, since mainstreaming, properly executed, can provide optimal opportunity for the acquisition of normal social and communication skills. Similarly, professionals with accumulated experience now can state confidently that mainstreaming is a viable option for many hearing-impaired children.

PROGRAM DESCRIPTION

The itinerant program serves hearing-impaired students who are integrated in elementary and secondary public schools throughout Metropolitan Toronto. Hearing loss may range from mild to profound.

Itinerant support is provided at three levels of service: *Direct Instruction*, for students who receive tutorial assistance one to four times weekly; *Program Support*, for students who do not require ongoing tutorial support, but who make use of an FM amplification unit; and *Follow-up*, primarily for students with mild or unilateral losses who may or may not be aided, and who are monitored two or three times annually.

Included under Direct Instruction are Integration Support Units (ISUs) (Boothroyd and Draffin 1986). This model of delivery was conceived in 1984 to meet the needs of profoundly deaf students who could not deal with full-time integration, even with maximum support, yet whose parents favored the mainstream option. These students spend each morning with a specialist teacher of the hearing-impaired in a small group setting of three or four. In the afternoon, they are transported to their local school in the home community where they are fully integrated.

Initial educational assessment of new students referred by hospitals, public health clinics, parents, or other agencies is also a large part of the itinerant teacher's work. Results of these assessments assist the Metro-Wide Communications Identification, Placement, and Review Committee in determining the most appropriate placement of a hearing-impaired child within the array of services available in Metropolitan Toronto (see figure 1). This process is frequently complicated by the fact that English may not be the first language of the home, necessitating the use of interpreters to explain programs and procedures to parents, and multicultural assessments to determine whether a child's communication needs are primarily a result of his or her hearing loss, or of the English as a Second Language (ESL) factor.

The objectives (Dewar, Draffin, and Boothroyd 1989) of the itinerant program are:

To help hearing-impaired students achieve their full potential in a regular school setting;

To assess auditory, speech, language, and reading levels using observational techniques, as well as a variety of assessment instruments normed on both hearing-impaired and hearing populations;

To establish developmental needs and realistic goals;

To use appropriate teaching strategies to achieve these;

To provide assistance in specific subject areas in an effort to keep students at the level of their class, particularly at the intermediate and secondary levels;

To provide and help students and teachers effectively use FM amplification equipment if it has been prescribed by an audiologist;

To monitor the use of this equipment through consultation with an on-site educational audiologist, and to arrange for necessary repairs by trained school board employed technicians; and

To counsel students, parents, and teachers and to provide liaison among them and other professionals at hospitals, social service agencies, and educational institutions.

The auditory-verbal or auditory-oral approach is the mode of communication for the itinerant program, and optimal use of residual hearing is stressed at all times.

Many hearing-impaired students are integrated at the junior kindergarten level (age four), and spend their entire school career in regular classes. Others may spend two or three years in self-contained classes for the deaf or hard of hearing before they are integrated. Some are integrated as late as the intermediate or secondary years. An example of each of these possibilities is illustrated in the case studies that follow. The progress of all students in the itinerant program is reviewed annually to ensure that they are best placed to suit their individual needs and abilities.

CASE STUDIES

The following anonymous case studies have been specifically chosen to illustrate the wide variety of students served by the itinerant program. Intentionally absent are examples of students who have progressed through their academic career in the mainstream with no major difficulty. This omission does not arise from lack of pride in their considerable achievements, but from a desire to concentrate in this chapter on those students who might not initially appear to fit the mold of highly appropriate or obvious mainstream candidates.

Andrew

Andrew is an example of misdiagnosis, late diagnosis, and appropriate mainstreaming that was postponed until grade 10. Born in 1966, he presents with a severe to profound bilateral sensorineural hearing loss of unknown etiology (see figure 2). When Andrew's speech and language were noted to be severely delayed as a young child, doctors in the rural area where the family lived suggested such explanations as emotional problems, autism, or mental retardation. At age five, his substantial loss was finally diagnosed in a large urban hospital, and he was fitted with hearing aids binaurally.

Following this late diagnosis, Andrew and his family received one year of help through a monthly visit by a teacher from an outreach program. The family moved to Toronto when Andrew was six, and he attended oral classes at the School for the Deaf for three years. He then transferred to a class for the hard of hearing for grades 4 through 8, and was enrolled in a secondary program for grade 9.

Despite the recommendation from a formal review committee that Andrew remain in this last setting, he transferred to the mainstream in grade 10 at his parents' insistence. He received a substantial amount of itinerant support to preview and review class material, and to prepare assignments. Three years later he earned his secondary school graduation diploma with respectable marks in the seventies. It should be noted that the highest reading level he ever achieved on a standardized test was the equivalent of grade 5.9.

Socially, Andrew now enjoys the company primarily of hearing

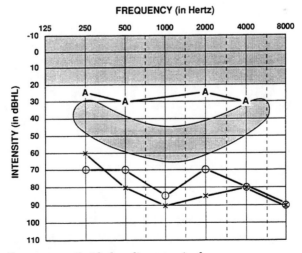

Figure 2.   Pure-tone and aided audiogram: Andrew.

friends. He is successfully and happily employed as an apprentice electrician.

Annie

Annie is a profoundly hearing-impaired child born to a non-English speaking family who had immigrated to Canada from Spain not long before her birth. Her parents did not complete secondary school. Spanish is still the first language spoken in the home.

Born in 1974, Annie was diagnosed as having a profound sensorineural hearing loss at the age of 14 months (see figure 3). Etiology is possibly hereditary as there is some history of deafness on the mother's side of the family. Annie was binaurally aided with body aids immediately following diagnosis. She and her mother participated in a home-based parent-infant program for almost two years. Annie's mother's English was very limited, and she started learning a second language at the same time her daughter was learning her first.

At the age of three years, Annie entered an oral preschool class at the School for the Deaf. After two years of thriving in this setting, her teachers recommended that she be fully integrated in a senior kindergarten, and use an FM system in her local school. Annie has received maximum itinerant support weekly from that time until the present. She is now in grade 10. For the first two years in the mainstream, Annie's mother attended every tutorial session so that she could provide appropriate and meaningful carryover at home. The family also partici-

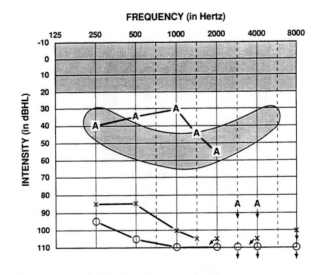

Figure 3. Pure-tone and aided audiogram: Annie.

pated in weekly auditory-verbal therapy sessions in a clinical setting. Annie's speech and auditory skills are excellent.

Annie has followed a regular academic curriculum, with the exception of French, all through school. Standardized testing shows that her growth in reading comprehension has been consistent and close to grade level. She recently scored at the 96th percentile for hearing-impaired students on the Stanford Achievement Test (SAT-HI). She has always been a voracious reader, and excels at subjects related to the humanities.

The transition from elementary to secondary school presented some difficulties, as with many hearing students, mostly because of the variety of subjects, number of teachers, and increased expectations and workload. While class work is fine, test and exam results have been low, partly as a result of anxiety and inexperience in dealing with the format and language of formal testing procedures. Annie will be allowed extended time on future examinations in an attempt to alleviate this problem. She will continue to require ongoing, careful monitoring by her secondary school and itinerant teachers, her parents, and herself.

Annie has had several close hearing friends over the years. As a teenager she began expressing a desire to socialize with hearing-impaired peers as well, and she has learned some sign language. With both hearing and deaf friends, she has recognized herself as a person comfortable in both worlds.

Mary

Mary is a hearing-impaired child who followed an indirect route to appropriate mainstreaming. Born in 1976, she presents with a profound hearing loss of unknown etiology, possibly secondary to illness at the age of 1 year (see figure 4). She was diagnosed at the age of 20 months, and was binaurally aided with two ear-level hearing aids. Mary and her parents attended an auditory-verbal therapy program in a clinical setting until the end of grade 5 when her school workload became too heavy. Speech is generally intelligible to an unfamiliar listener, and auditory skills are above average for age and degree of loss according to a recent Test of Auditory Comprehension (TAC).

Mary entered junior kindergarten at her local school at age four, with an FM system and four hours of itinerant support weekly. By the end of grade 2, it became evident through subjective and objective assessment that she required more direct intervention from a specialist teacher of the hearing impaired. Her parents, however, were very reluctant to remove her from the mainstream.

After months of negotiation and persuasion, it was agreed that

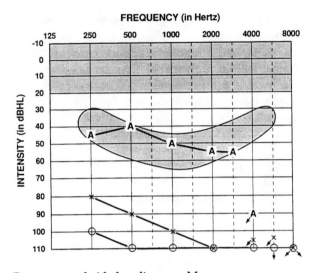

Figure 4. Pure-tone and aided audiogram: Mary.

Mary would enter an Integration Support Unit (Boothroyd and Draffin 1986). This model of delivery was new that year, and offered something unique to students who were experiencing difficulty with full-time integration. Mary spent the next four years attending her unit program each morning with two other hearing-impaired students and a specialist teacher of the hearing impaired. The focus of their work was on auditory, speech, language, and reading development. In the afternoon, she returned to her local school where she continued in the regular program.

Mary repeated grade 2 her first year in the Unit. By the end of grade 5, she had progressed to the point where it was felt that she could again be fully mainstreamed with maximum itinerant support. In addition, Mary visits the school's Learning Center daily for extra help in math, organizational skills, and classroom work. She follows the regular curriculum, with the exception of French. While the other students are in French class, she is with the itinerant teacher working primarily in the areas of speech, audition, language, and reading.

Before Mary entered the Integration Support Unit at age eight, the Grammatical Analysis of Elicited Language (GAEL-S) indicated a language level of a preschooler. Growth since that time has been consistent. She is now within 18 months of grade level in reading comprehension, and recently scored at the 90th percentile compared to other hearing-impaired 13 year olds on the Stanford Achievement Test (SAT-HI). She can deal comfortably and functionally with her grade 7 program.

Mary has many hearing friends. She is involved in extra-curricular activities, especially sports, at school. Other than her former class-mates in the Integration Support Unit, she does not have any hearing-impaired friends. This is circumstantial, not intentional.

Mary's achievements can be attributed to a number of factors. Her parents have always provided her with a wide range of experiences outside of school, and have encouraged her to be a very interested, interesting, and well-rounded person. She has always been an enthu-siastic reader, a fact that has helped her overall vocabulary and lan-guage development. The principal of her school has been a very sup-portive figure from the time it became apparent that the Integration Support Unit would be advantageous, until recently when he did ev-erything possible to facilitate the transition back to full integration.

Bill

Bill is an example of inappropriate mainstreaming. Born in 1973, he is the youngest of three children of a university educated, professional, upper-middle class family. English is not the first language of his par-ents, but has always been consistently and proficiently used at home.

Diagnosis of severe to profound hearing loss, etiology unknown, occurred at two years (see figure 5). Bill was binaurally aided, and audi-tory-verbal therapy was initiated in a clinical setting.

Bill entered junior kindergarten in his local school at age four with maximum itinerant support and an FM system. By the end of senior kindergarten, placement in a self-contained oral class for the hearing impaired was recommended by the itinerant staff, but categorically re-jected by the parents and school principal. This continued to be the pattern throughout the elementary years. Bill was noted to be an ex-ceptionally pleasant and cooperative student, but a very reluctant com-municator. His speech was fairly intelligible to known and/or trained listeners, but not to others. Psychological testing indicated above aver-age ability nonverbally, yet Bill fell well behind his hearing peers at school, and the gap widened annually. In grade 5, the Grammatical Analysis of Elicited Language (GAEL-S) placed him well below the normal range for hearing children four and one half to five years of age.

When Bill reached grade 6, a new principal arrived at the school and was horrified by the state of affairs surrounding Bill's language and achievement levels and routine annual promotion. He attempted to bring the issue to a head through a series of meetings and by refus-ing to promote Bill to grade 7. Bill's mother remained adamant about rejecting full or even half-time self-contained placement in a class for the hearing impaired, and insisted that Bill would attend the local se-nior public school on full rotating schedule with his hearing peers. Fi-nally a compromise was negotiated whereby Bill repeated grade 6 at a

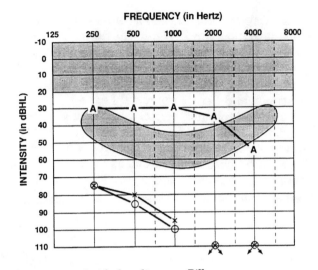

Figure 5.   Pure-tone and aided audiogram: Bill.

different school that included classes from kindergarten through grade 8, and had no rotating schedule.

In grade 7 Bill spent half his time in a special education class and received four hours of itinerant support weekly. He lacked self-confidence, and was understandably a child who was neither happy nor thriving in his academic or social environment. One must ask, "Was this appropriate mainstreaming? Was the sacrifice to a so-called ideal worthwhile?"

By the end of grade 7, through a process of ongoing data collection and frequent meetings, Bill's family finally agreed, albeit reluctantly, to place him in an Integration Support Unit, which had been offered for the past three years. At the age of 14 Bill had never met or interacted with another hearing-impaired person before, as his parents considered that this would exert a negative influence on him.

Very early on, both his parents and his local school reported that Bill was much more relaxed and happy in his new placement. He loved being with his hearing-impaired peers, and immediately began to thrive in all respects in an environment that met his cognitive, communication, and social/emotional needs.

Not surprisingly, Bill was not able to reenter the mainstream full-time for high school. Despite much initial resistance by the family, Bill was placed in a self-contained oral secondary program for the hearing impaired. Bill is now a happy, self-confident, and self-actualizing adolescent. Even his parents are happy—indeed relieved.

Bill will most likely attend community college following high school graduation, and pursue a career in the area of art. His path has been uphill all the way. His parents initially felt that placement outside the mainstream signified failure for Bill and for them. It took many years to convince them that success or failure was never the issue, but that appropriate placement in a setting where their child would thrive, was.

DISCUSSION

The term *appropriate* has become central to the concept of mainstreaming handicapped children in the United States and the Province of Ontario, Canada. The degree of confusion surrounding the intent and impact of the word (Tucker 1984) appears to be similar on both sides of the border. Is a handicapped child, or more specifically in this context, a hearing-handicapped child, entitled to receive only an appropriate education, or is he or she entitled to receive the most appropriate education available? And what if the most appropriate is not available? Is the most appropriate the best? Does it in fact sometimes mean least inappropriate?

It is not the intent here to engage in a legalistic debate about the meaning of the term *appropriate*, although more specificity regarding its use would be beneficial (Board comments 1989). In this chapter *appropriate* is employed in its broadest sense to mean suitable, fit, proper (Gove 1976), and most enabling for the child.

For the record it should be noted that I strongly support the theory and practice of mainstreaming hearing-impaired children. However, what is essentially obvious, although not always popular, must also be stated: mainstreaming is not for everyone. It is one of several educational options (Gjerdingen 1987; Dewar, Draffin, and Boothroyd 1989). It is critical that parents and professionals not "sacrifice" any child to what is often considered to be the ideal, namely educating all hearing-impaired children exclusively with their hearing peers. The whole child must be the focus of attention. The mere presence of a hearing-impaired child in a regular classroom does not mean that effective mainstreaming has been accomplished (Ross 1978; Osguthorpe, Whitehead, and Bishop 1978; Gjerdingen 1987). His or her ability to thrive emotionally, socially, and academically must be considered when making decisions regarding appropriate placement.

Central to the issue of such decisions is the concept that each hearing-impaired child must be placed and educated according to his or her individual needs at any given time. This refers to communication modality as well as specific placement in a self-contained or mainstream setting. Since nothing in education is carved in stone, what may be appropriate for a child one year, may no longer be so the next (Ross, Brackett, and Maxon 1982).

The primary factor in placement decisions must be informed parental preference (Gjerdingen 1987; Board comments 1989), for in the final analysis it is families who must live with their choices, not educators. *Informed* parental preference is stressed, however, for despite what some parents may want to hear, it remains the responsibility of educators to inform them of students' levels, needs, and options on an ongoing basis. The preparation of the annual Individualized Education Program (IEP) or Special Education Plan (SEP) in Ontario, and subsequent annual review procedures, allow this dialogue between parents and educators to occur in a meaningful context. The issue of good subjective and objective performance tracking of students is of the utmost importance to educators, for they are accountable to the population they serve.

At the time of diagnosis, school entry, and even later, parents and educators alike would be happy to engage in a little crystal ball gazing into the future. The uniqueness of each child's hearing and intellectual potential, learning style, family situation, and social/emotional needs makes generalized predictive statements very difficult.

Various criteria or characteristics that would appear to be good indicators of appropriate mainstreaming have been put forward by such authorities as Northcott (1973, 1979), Reich, Hambleton, and Houldin (1977), Bishop (1979), Pflaster (1980, 1981), and Ross, Brackett, and Maxon (1982) among others. These include, but are by no means limited to, such factors as:

Early identification and intervention;
Appropriate and consistent amplification with active emphasis on the use of residual hearing;
Intelligible speech, as well as good ability to understand speech and to communicate using spoken and written language;
Supportive, at least high school educated, English speaking parents;
At least average intelligence;
Reading at grade level;
A good acoustic environment and the appropriate use of FM wireless amplification equipment;
Sufficient and appropriate support services offered by specialists in hearing impairment;
Strong student motivation and determination.

While these criteria are acknowledged as important, the preceding case studies illustrate the fact that such factors need not all be present for appropriate mainstreaming to occur. Our experience suggests that the following points also be considered when trying to make informed placement decisions.

1. Strong and suitable academic support is a prerequisite for mainstreamed students (Osguthorpe, Whitehead, and Bishop 1978; Ross, Brackett, and Maxon 1982). Yet there is a downside to withdrawing the child from the classroom; he or she then misses the classwork. The amount of withdrawal support time must be carefully monitored to ensure that it does not occur more frequently than is absolutely necessary. Otherwise the original intent and benefits of mainstreaming are seriously compromised.

In response to this dilemma, it is necessary to be flexible and creative in establishing tutorial times, for example, before and after school, or during lunch hour and spare periods. The itinerant teacher might also spend part of the assigned time in the student's classroom, observing what is required, providing coping strategies, and perhaps even team-teaching. Needless to say, this depends on the extent to which the classroom teacher and other resource personnel are prepared to cooperate.

2. Students undoubtedly enjoy more success when the school administrator exhibits and instills in his or her staff a philosophy of cooperation and positive, yet realistic, advocacy for the student (Hinkle and White 1979; Pflaster 1980). This was obvious in the case of Mary, who might not have fared as well on her return to full mainstreaming without the encouragement of the principal. It was also evident in the case of Bill, whose first principal did not want to upset the parents and the status quo, yet whose subsequent principals insisted on doing just that for the sake of the child.

3. Parents must be committed partners in educating their child at any given time (Bruce 1973; Pflaster 1980, 1981; Dewar, Draffin, and Boothroyd 1989). They do not necessarily have to be English speaking, well-educated or upwardly mobile for their child to be in the mainstream. They must, however, be prepared to consult with educators before making their decisions, and be as realistic as possible in their choices and expectations.

4. Older students must be given the opportunity to have some input into how they are educated. They should be part of the decision-making process, for they are the ones who must live with the results. This includes choice of communication modality. The desire of a student in the mainstream, who has previously had only hearing friends, to meet other hearing-impaired people and possibly learn some sign language should be regarded as a positive recognition and acceptance of his or her full identity.

5. Students who are appropriately placed in the mainstream may not always be reading within a year of grade level. Yet they are

enthusiastic, independent readers whose *functional* reading level allows them to manage the material they need.

6. It is essential to consider the overall potential of each student when making recommendations and decisions about the future. Not all hearing-impaired graduates from a mainstream program are appropriate college or university candidates. Community or junior college, or a skills program, may be a far better choice. To this end, good counseling must be a key component of any secondary student's program prior to graduation.

7. Tutorial support is usually deemed most necessary for those students who are experiencing some difficulty with education in the mainstream. It should be considered every hearing-impaired student's absolute right. Many students in Metropolitan Toronto, even several who have profound losses, could certainly manage without itinerant help. They may well be intellectually gifted, and they have a fine work ethic. Yet they probably are achieving their full academic potential only because their programs are enriched through ongoing tutorial support.

8. The advantages of FM wireless amplification equipment for profoundly hearing-impaired students in the mainstream are well-documented (Ross, Brackett, and Maxon 1982). Some older students, however, feel uncomfortable wearing these systems, and may in fact refuse to do so. Yet many of these same students can manage without them, despite the fact that an optimal acoustic environment is not present. The pros and cons of each student's situation must be weighed with respect to this issue.

9. I suggest that if a child in the mainstream is doing as well as a comparable peer in a self-contained class, the mainstream is probably the appropriate setting. Assuming that quality support and little frustration exists, he or she will likely thrive in an environment where pragmatics, social skills, and academics are learned alongside his or her hearing peers.

10. Pflaster (1980, 1981) emphasizes the importance of personality factors in identifying students who are appropriate mainstream candidates. If any one of the criteria and considerations discussed in this chapter deserves more attention than the others, it may be this: the child who really wants to make it in the mainstream, through sheer determination, probably will.

SUMMARY

There are, needless to say, many other issues that can be addressed when discussing the concept and reality of educational mainstreaming for hearing-impaired children. This chapter emphasizes that main-streaming is just one of several options available to hearing-impaired students and their families. It is an ongoing process (Bishop 1979) that can commence at various times during a child's academic career. The individual needs and learning style of each child always must be taken into account when considering educational placement. No value judgment should enter into the decision; the value of the placement lies in its appropriateness.

Mainstreaming is never an issue of success or failure; it is an issue of appropriate placement and support. If parents and educators remain flexible, objective, and sensitive to the overall needs of hearing-impaired children, we can feel confident that as we mainstream into the nineties, we are indeed on track.

REFERENCES

Bishop, M. E. (ed.). 1979. *Mainstreaming: Practical Ideas for Educating Hearing-Impaired Students.* Washington, DC: The Alexander Graham Bell Association for the Deaf.

Board comments on COED recommendations 1989. *Newsounds* 14(1):1–3.

Boothroyd, D. R., and Draffin, G. S. 1986. Integration support units—an alternative model of delivery for the hearing impaired. Paper read at the Alexander Graham Bell Association of the Deaf Convention, June 1986, Chicago.

Bruce, W. 1973. The parent's role from an educator's point of view. In *The Hearing Impaired Child in a Regular Classroom: Preschool, Elementary, and Secondary Years*, ed. W. H. Northcott. Washington, DC: The Alexander Graham Bell Association for the Deaf.

Dewar, D., Draffin, G. S., and Boothroyd, D. R. 1989. *Review of Deaf Education.* Toronto: The Metropolitan Toronto School Board.

Gjerdingen, D. 1987. Putting mainstream education into perspective. *Newsounds* 12(8):3.

Gove, P. E. (ed.). 1976. *Webster's Third New International Dictionary.* Springfield: G. and C. Merriam Co. Publishers.

Hinkle, W., and White, K. R. 1979. Assessment and Educational Placement. In *Mainstreaming: Practical Ideas for Educating Hearing-Impaired Students*, ed. M.E. Bishop. Washington, DC: The Alexander Graham Bell Association for the Deaf.

Northcott, W. H. (ed.). 1973. *The Hearing Impaired Child in a Regular Classroom: Preschool, Elementary, and Secondary Years.* Washington, DC: The Alexander Graham Bell Association for the Deaf.

Northcott, W. H. 1979. Implications of mainstreaming for the education of hearing-impaired children in the 1980's. Colloquium address at National Technical Institute for the Deaf, 1979, Rochester.

Osguthorpe, R. T., Whitehead, B. D., and Bishop, M. E. 1978. Training and managing paraprofessionals as tutors and notetakers for mainstreamed deaf students. *American Annals of the Deaf* 123(5):563–71.

Pflaster, G. 1980. A factor analysis of variables related to academic performance of hearing-impaired children in regular classes. *The Volta Review* 82(2):71–84.

Pflaster, G. 1981. A second analysis of factors related to the academic performance of hearing-impaired children in the mainstream. *The Volta Review* 83(2):71–80.

Reich, C., Hambleton, D., and Houldin, B. C. 1977. The integration of hearing impaired children in regular classrooms. *American Annals of the Deaf* 122(6):534–42.

Ross, M. 1978. Mainstreaming: Some social considerations. *The Volta Review* 80(1):21–30.

Ross, M., Brackett, D., and Maxon, A. 1982. *Hard of Hearing Children in Regular Schools.* Englewood Cliffs, NJ: Prentice-Hall, Inc.

Tucker, B. P. 1984. Legal aspects of education in the mainstream: The current picture. *The Volta Review* 86(5):53–70.

Chapter • 11

Recognizing Heterogeneity: Increasing Educational Opportunities Through Mainstreaming

Donald McGee

Mainstreaming can offer opportunities for learning, integration, and social growth that are not usually afforded hearing-impaired students in schools devoted exclusively to their education. Placement in the least restrictive environment can offer an instructional setting in which students are likely to experience success in school. The disagreement among some professionals about the value of educational mainstreaming of the hearing impaired derives from the erroneous concept that mainstreaming and least restrictive environment are synonomous. The mainstream is part of a larger continuum of placement options that may be appropriate for hearing-impaired students. Within the mainstream is a continuum of options that may or may not offer a least restrictive environment. It should be emphasized that least restrictive environment does not mean the easiest program for a student with hearing impairment, but rather one that

Thanks to Carol Ann McBride, Principal, Total Communication, and to Connie Rahill, Principal, Auditory/Oral and Cued Speech, for reviewing this manuscript.

challenges the student while providing the supports that permit and foster learning. Furthermore, even though programs and schools for the hearing impaired meet the criteria for appropriateness under the regulations governing Public Law 94-142, they may nonetheless be deficient in the quality and scope of services they offer. Meeting these regulations does not mean that students will be prepared adequately for the adult world of competition, dependence on technology, and need for flexibility and adaptation to changing roles and situations.

This chapter describes the program for hearing-impaired students of the Fairfax County (Virginia) Public Schools. The development of our auditory/oral program was described earlier (McGee 1976). Since that time the total communication option has been expanded, a cued speech component has been added, and a variety of support services have been added or enhanced.

Our observations, based on the experiences of our students in Fairfax County over the relatively short period of twenty years, include the following:

The average reading achievement of our graduates is dramatically above the national average of hearing-impaired students reported by the Commission on Education of the Deaf (*Toward Equality* 1988).

Access to the mainstream classroom offers the typical hearing-impaired student the opportunity to develop and refine competency in English, to be exposed to the same curricular information as hearing students, and to form relationships with hearing, as well as hearing-impaired, peers.

Extensive specialized support to students is required, beyond the minimum specified by P.L. 94-142.

The resources needed to provide the necessary support are trained teachers of the hearing impaired, audiologists, interpreters, social workers, administrators who are trained in deafness, state-of-the-art amplification equipment, and involved parents who can work cooperatively toward shared goals.

Intensive, direct intervention with hearing-impaired infants and their parents, in contrast to consultative models with infrequent contact, provides the greatest opportunity for later school success.

Options and alternatives in programming need to be available to complement student capabilities and learning styles.

Parents must be active participants in making informed program choices for their children based on knowledge and observation of the diverse population of students with hearing impairment.

POPULATION CHARACTERISTICS

The following demographic information will help the reader develop a perspective for interpreting the structure and details of the program for hearing-impaired students.

Our school division is one system that serves an area of 400 square miles, with a population of 765,000 people.

The school enrollment is 128,000, making it the tenth largest school system in the United States.

The general education program is offered in 185 schools.

There are significant ethnic and minority populations; some 75 different languages are spoken by the residents.

The criteria for eligibility for the program for hearing-impaired students include (1) a documented hearing loss that has an impact on the student's ability to profit from an unmodified general education program, (2) delay of language development due to hearing loss, and/or (3) a history of repeated middle ear infections that may have retarded the development of language during a student's formative years. The structure of the program is as follows:

Some 380 students are enrolled, from infancy through age 22. An additional 35 students attend schools outside the county.

The program offers intensive, center-based services in three communication modalities, and operates in seven centrally located schools.

The program offers less-intensive, neighborhood-school based services in approximately 70 schools; these services are provided by itinerant teachers of the hearing impaired.

The representation of ethnic and minority hearing-impaired students is significantly greater in the program than in the general school population.

Students with secondary handicaps are served within the program if hearing impairment is the primary disability. Otherwise, multiply handicapped hearing-impaired students are served in special centers with support from specialists.

Figure 1 indicates the distribution of students within the various program offerings. More than half are in their neighborhood schools receiving services from an itinerant teacher of the hearing impaired from two to five times per week. Of these 210 students, about 10% were in a center-based program when they were younger, and since have returned to their neighborhood schools.

ITINERANT SERVICES IN NEIGHBORHOOD SCHOOLS (210)

AUDTORY/ORAL (90)

TOTAL COMMUNICATION (60)

CUED
SPEECH
(20)

PERCENTAGES OF PROGRAM MEMBERSHIP

CUED SPEECH	TOTAL COMMUNICATION	AUDITORY/ORAL	ITINERANT SERVICE
5%	16%	24%	55%

TOTAL SCHOOL POPULATION 128,000
COUNTY POPULATION 765,000
LANGUAGES SPOKEN 75

Figure 1.   Array of 380 hearing-impaired students receiving services.

Approximately 25% of students served are in the auditory/oral, center-based program. Unlike the cued speech and total communication programs, which serve only severe-to-profound and profoundly hearing-impaired students, the auditory/oral program enrolls severely hearing-impaired students (60%) as well as those who are severe-to-profound and profound (40%). A high percentage of the severely hearing-impaired students come into the auditory/oral program at an early age for one to three years of intensive language and speech development to allow them to profit later from the mainstream education in their neighborhood schools. The remaining 20% of students are enrolled in total communication and cued speech programs. At least 90% of these students are profoundly deaf by audiogram, and the rest are severe-to-profound.

Figure 2 indicates the distribution over grade levels of the center-based students. It is of interest to note that the auditory/oral program has been used for twenty years, the total communication for fifteen, and the cued speech for ten.

COMMUNICATION MODALITY

Many, if not most, public school programs for the hearing impaired have elected to offer a single method of communication to their students. Our program goals have been to increase the options available to hearing-impaired students, rather than to limit them from the outset. We agree with Quigley and Kretschmer (1983):

PARENT/INFANT (PIP) AND PRESCHOOL (24)	ELEMENTARY (56)		INT. (5)	HIGH (5)

AUDITORY/ORAL (90)

PIP AND PRESCHOOL (8)	ELEMENTARY (25)	INT. (8)	HIGH (18)

TOTAL COMMUNICATION (60)

PIP AND PRESCHOOL (4)	ELEMENTARY (12)	INT. (2)	HIGH (2)

CUED SPEECH (20)

Figure 2.   Distribution of center-based students by grade level.

> There is no clear evidence for the superiority of any form of communica-
> tion or language input over all others for all (or even most) deaf children.
>   We simply do not yet know how to realize fully the educational po-
> tential of deaf children, although a thousand different voices might dis-
> agree and protest in favor of their particular approaches (pp. 27 and 107).

Likewise, in our work with parents of hearing-impaired students, we emphasize that hearing impairment is not a singular category that determines their child's future. Children have diverse and divergent characteristics that must be explored, rather than limited. As Clarke and Leslie (1980) have put it, " . . . no one has yet clearly demonstrated that it is always possible to select reliably the method that will work best for a particular hearing impaired child . . . " (p. 216). In choosing an appropriate communication modality, we work toward arriving at an informed consensus among parents, diagnosticians, and service providers. The guidelines we use for discussion are as follows:

1. Does the audiometric work-up tell us enough about useful hearing or do we need additional diagnostic information from our own audiologists?
2. Have reliable aided thresholds been determined and has appropriate amplification been identified and accepted by the student?
3. Are there compelling reasons (e.g., late identification) why the infant or preschooler should not try an auditory/oral program initially to explore auditory/verbal responsiveness?
4. Have the parents had the opportunity to observe children using various communication modalities?
5. If the staff believes the parent is in error in choice of modality, has there been an earnest effort to counsel the parent and present objective information?

Our experience has been that parents typically come to the school system with a firm belief about the best modality for their child. As they learn more about hearing impairment and the options available to their child, they are able to modify their views in consideration of the needs of the child. One of the strengths of our program is our ability and willingness to change a student from one component to another if adequate progress in language acquisition is not made. We stress this flexibility to the parents of newly enrolled students so that they will not feel locked into a modality, and so that they will be aware that a change in modality may be necessary for their child in the future.

LEAST RESTRICTIVE ENVIRONMENT

There never seem to be enough points along the continuum of placement and service options to satisfy the wide diversity of individual needs. The unique needs of individuals who happen to be hearing impaired often defy our efforts to fit them into descriptive categories (originally used to influence legislatures and raise the consciousness of society, not to describe the educational needs of hearing-impaired children).

One of the advantages of a large program is the availability of a number of classrooms; there is a greater chance to find an appropriate climate for a particular child. Within each communication modality are parent/infant teaching programs, preschool, elementary, intermediate, and high school classes. The auditory/oral, total communication, and cued speech programs are physically separated from each other in different buildings. As soon as we bring children into class groupings— between the ages of two and three—we provide them with hearing peers. By kindergarten age, all students participate with hearing peers in some activity each day, whether or not they can participate in the academic mainstream program. Teachers of the hearing impaired participate as team members with general education teachers at their grade level. The goals and objectives of the regular curriculum are followed in classrooms for both the hearing and the hearing impaired. Since the two programs are truly integrated, the scheduling of students and teachers in the school as a whole is intricate, time-consuming, and interdependent. In some components, all teachers in the building see both hearing and hearing-impaired students every day. At each grade level there is a continuum between the classroom for the hearing impaired and the mainstream classroom.

At intermediate and high school levels, school-based resource teachers offer support to students for one to two periods per day. Their liaison with mainstream teachers is essential to student success.

In spite of our firm belief in the advantages of learning in the mainstream, there are a variety of immediate needs of some hearing-impaired children, needs which work against the value of a local, mainstream placement.

Some children may need to live away from home due to abuse or neglect, or they may have other extraordinary needs that might be addressed by living in a residential environment.

Some children may need wholly self-contained instruction with significantly modified curricular goals and materials, and need the reinforcement of hearing-impaired peers.

Some children have parents who believe that hearing-impaired children should be educated only with other hearing-impaired children.

AUDIOLOGICAL SUPPORT

The necessity of active, daily audiological support in our center-based programs is a given. Perhaps the least understood tool in education of the hearing impaired is the hearing aid or amplification unit. While the behind-the-ear hearing aid looks much as it did in the mid 1970s, its internal characteristics are dramatically different and able to deliver the power and frequency response useful to profoundly hearing-impaired students.

In addition to personal hearing aids, the mainstream student typically utilizes a personal FM unit in the general education classroom. The challenge that faces the school system is to keep amplification equipment operating within the manufacturers' specifications, and to eliminate the downtime endemic to electronic equipment.

We have found it necessary and extraordinarily beneficial to students to have a full-time educational audiologist at each center-based program. These four audiologists have no assigned responsibility for clinical testing; they spend one hundred percent of their time in support of the component to which they are assigned. They operate amplification maintenance programs providing continuous support to teachers and instructional aides on the care of amplification units and the recognition of problems to be referred for trouble-shooting. Each morning before classes begin, the school-based audiologist receives a report from each teacher of the hearing impaired indicating any problems detected in the morning hearing aid check, with either personal hearing aids or personal FM systems supplied by the school. The audiologist makes the rounds of classes in which problems were found and also receives students sent by their teachers to get help with a repair or to have back-up amplification provided. No student is without appropriate amplification for much longer than an hour.

The remainder of the audiologist's time is spent working with individual students in auditory assessment and training. One of the greatest benefits of the school-based audiologist is the time that can be made available to the individual student who is having an audiologically related problem or whose amplification is "not quite right." Typically this is an infant or a preschooler who has not adjusted to an initial hearing aid fitting, does not like binaural amplification, or is having middle ear problems. Amplification problems tend to disappear as a major concern when an audiologist is available to do what is needed, whether it is daily impedance testing, extensive work with the student to identify subtle hearing-related problems or with the parents to discuss management problems, or changing the hearing aid fittings. We have known for a long time that children reject amplification when it is not pleasant or rewarding to them. The school-based audiologist provides the talent and the time to help students achieve an optimum, positive amplification status. At the present time, 98.5% of our students are able to benefit to some degree from the use of amplification.

In addition to four school-based audiologists, we have a special education diagnostic center with an audiology suite staffed by two full-time clinical audiologists. As a part of their service, they provide the annual rechecks of the hearing-impaired students in the program, as well as extraordinary referrals and hearing aid evaluations. Insertion gain measurements are taken on each student. The audiology suite is open to the four educational audiologists if they wish to assist in testing a particular student from their building or if they wish to do their own testing for some reason. Over the past few years, there has been a tendency for our audiologists to rotate among the clinical and educational settings, so that they are familiar with the scope and quality of our offerings. This has permitted the educational program to rely heavily on the clinical audiologists' recommendations for new students being identified for the first time. These audiologists also begin the educational counseling process with parents at once, and maintain contact with the parents through the eligibility process until placement occurs.

Our experience is that when parents are first told of their child's hearing impairment, they need immediate, professional guidance and referral—someone to talk through the trauma with them. Waiting two or three weeks for an appointment at some school or institution to find out about deafness can leave the parents too traumatized to respond effectively to their child's needs. The clinical audiologists help fill this void.

The center-based educational audiologists also select a group of hearing-impaired students within their building whom they see on a regular basis, often twice per week. These are typically students who demonstrate auditory problems or who respond most poorly to auditory stimuli. The audiologists have developed a sequential array of auditory tasks (*Auditory Skills Curriculum* 1984) that are cross-referenced with the general education *Program of Studies* so that auditory goals and objectives can be integrated into the daily curriculum.

As we have followed students of various backgrounds through our program from infancy to graduation, observing their successes and failures, noting their individual differences and wide diversity, we have concluded:

That damaged or incomplete auditory systems must be habilitated in infancy and early childhood to be of maximal use to the child. The habilitation requires intensive work and use of resources, not token efforts.

That structured, intensive, appropriate efforts to stimulate a damaged or incomplete auditory system *usually* produce an internalized and habitual channel of reliable input that the child can use in language learning and communication.

That optimum amplification must be provided to achieve the development of useful hearing and to maintain it throughout life.

That it is possible to find ways for parents to afford the extraordinary expenses associated with amplification.

That it is necessary to provide intensive educational and therapeutic programs in which hearing-impaired children can be taught to use their auditory skills on a continuous basis.

That the present costs of amplification equipment and programming are justified by the huge payoff to the child in the future.

INTERPRETERS

The inestimable importance of classroom interpreters in total communication and cued speech programs is obvious if students are to have access to the mainstream curriculum afforded hearing students.

Approximately 65 of our students use educational interpreters in the mainstream. Some 22 full-time and part-time interpreters serve these students. Our interpreters are contracted employees who meet professional interpreting standards. They report to lead interpreters who schedule and supervise their work as well as provide feedback and evaluation.

The status of educational interpreters with professional and certifying organizations remains somewhat problematic due to their classification as educational interpreters. Codes of ethics and traditional modes of service appropriate for adults are seldom appropriate in public school settings. Public school systems in general have been at a significant disadvantage in finding models and guidelines to inform their Boards of Education and leadership administration about the specialized nature of *educational* interpreting (Castle, McGee, and Rosenstein 1985).

As public school consumers, we owe a debt of gratitude to leaders such as Dr. Diane Castle, Dr. Joseph Rosenstein, Dr. Winifred Northcott, and others for their considerable efforts in focusing national attention on the role and needs of the educational interpreter, and helping to overcome institutional inertia.

PARENT INVOLVEMENT

The close relationship of the teacher of the hearing impaired, the audiologist, and the parent during the parent/infant phase of the child's education leads naturally to parental involvement in later years. A wide variety of programs, seminars, meetings, lectures, demonstrations, mothers'-day-out, sibling programs, and other activities are provided throughout the preschool and elementary years. Those who appreciate the necessity of working closely with parents know that sometimes the needs of the parents are greater than the needs of the student. Two half-time social workers help the staff in working with parents and intervening in crisis situations.

Aside from the relationship between school and individual parent, the involvement of parents in organized, cooperative associations devoted to support and improvement of the program is essential. While there will always be a few parents who can deal with schools only in an adversarial way, the great majority of parents are willing to work for positive change in cooperation with the schools. The cohesiveness of that majority can often contribute significantly to the quality of the program their children receive. We have found that the more accurate information and sophistication that parents have about deafness, the greater their influence can be in affecting changes in program quality and resources.

We also find that parents are dismayed, confused, and disheartened by much of the information available to them. Parents of children newly identified as hearing impaired are perhaps at the greatest disadvantage in trying to make choices that will affect their child's entire life.

If we put ourselves in the place of a parent who knows nothing about hearing impairment, but who actively is seeking to learn by reading recent material, it is hard to imagine the possible effect of such statements as these:

We also use the term *Deaf* to refer to all persons with hearing impairment, including those who are hard-of-hearing, those deafened in later life, those who are profoundly deaf, etc. (*Commission on Education of the Deaf* 1988).

Material presented in spoken English is inaccessible to any deaf child, including even those with less than profound hearing losses (Johnson, Liddell, and Erting 1989, p. 3).

The naive parent might conclude that the child with a 90 dB loss that has been aided to a 25 dB level has no chance of learning language naturally through the ear and eye. Parents of other children with less hearing loss might conclude that the level of disability is far beyond what it actually is.

We find that efforts to help hearing-impaired individuals to break out of the stereotypes of the past are being neutralized by public information that may have some validity for a very small percentage of hearing-impaired children and youth, but that does not address the status of the great majority of the public school hearing-impaired population.

The achievements of our students reject the notion that hearing-impaired individuals all should be treated the same educationally.

OUTCOMES

As we diversified and enhanced our program by adding components, crossing categorical boundaries where appropriate, letting students try what they thought they could achieve, and providing as many resources as we could garner, we gave up the notion of having all students' progress assessed on the same test. We cannot compare components or sub-groups as to similarity of achievement. Special education programs in general do not lend themselves to yielding very meaningful data. According to Reynolds, Wang, and Walberg (1986):

. . . It has not been possible to date to construct a research base for categorical programs because the categories have been ill-defined and unreliable. In addition, the boundaries have shifted so markedly in response to legal, academic, and political forces as to make professional diagnostic constructs less and less meaningful. Accountability to children has become unclear because the categories do not define clear targets, and total programs have tended to be judged increasingly in procedural rather than substantive terms (p. 18).

What is success? Several years ago, we identified a hearing-impaired high school student in our neighborhood school component who was barely passing his academic classes. We saw him as "struggling" with school. We strongly suggested that he transfer to our center-based component where he could receive intensive services from school-based teachers of the hearing impaired, use an interpreter if he

liked, and have the services of an audiologist who might be able to find
out why the student did not wear his hearing aid very often. His itinerant teacher of the hearing impaired told us that he would not transfer.
He was captain of the football team, he was one of the most popular
students in the school, his parents considered him to be exceptionally
well adjusted, and the school had no intention of referring him since it
saw no problem. In our zeal to provide students the rich resources that
are available, we have to remember that we must not live their lives
for them.

Generally we think of academic achievement in terms of scores on
standardized tests. But those scores do not tell us the whole story of a
student's success or lack of it. The student who may have come from a
foreign country at age nine with profound deafness, having no language, and an inability to remember material, might be considered a
success when he or she graduates from school with a fourth grade
reading level. This success may pale when compared to an advantaged
deaf student who graduates with a reading level well beyond the upper
limit of the reading test, but it is nonetheless "success."

Table I summarizes the reading achievement (at 12th grade) of all
our graduates over the past three years (N = 35). Scores were obtained
using the Woodcock-Johnson Psycho-Educational Battery, the Woodcock-Johnson Reading Mastery, or the Stanford Achievement Test-HI
(Advanced).

Table II summarizes the post-secondary choices of all our graduates over the past three years (N = 35). Some of the choices reflect the
local Vocational Rehabilitation Service preference to pay for tuition
only at institutions for the deaf. Only one student per year did not go
on to higher education.

A second aspect of success is the personal adjustment of the hear-

Table I. Summary of Reading Scores at 12th Grade for 35 Graduates in 1989, 1988, and 1987

Reading Levels	1989 (N = 14)	1988 (N = 9)	1987 (N = 12)	% Total
Grade 12 and above	4	3	4	31
Grade 11		1	1	6
Grade 10				
Grade 9			2	6 ·
Grade 8	7	1		23
Grade 7	1	2	2	14
Grade 6	1	2	2	14
Grade 5				
Grade 4	1		1	6

Table II. Summary of Post-Secondary Institutions Chosen by 35 Graduates in 1989, 1988, and 1987

Institutions	1989 (N = 14)	1988 (N = 9)	1987 (N = 12)	% Total
California State University			1	3
Community Colleges (VA, MD, NJ)	4	2	1	20
Gallaudet University	4	3	1	23
George Mason University (VA)			1	3
Lenoir-Rhyne (NC)		1	1	6
National Technical Institute	2		5	20
Old Dominion University (VA)	2			6
Rochester Inst. of Technology		1		3
Sheppard College (WV)		1		3
University of Virginia	1		1	5
Employed	1	1	1	8

ing-impaired student. In a highly academic school system located in a geographical area without the vocational opportunities that industrialized areas provide, do hearing-impaired students develop the confidence and strength to compete with highly academic hearing students? A doctoral study (Bozik 1985) examined the students in our total communication and auditory/oral secondary centers. They were assessed for level of ego development, patterns of social interaction, and identity status. Some of Bozik's conclusions were as follows:

Levels of ego development among this sample of hearing-impaired adolescents are higher than would be expected of a normal adolescent population.

The pattern of identity status and peer relationships does not differ significantly from that of the general population.

Their social and emotional development is much more favorable than found in previous research with the hearing impaired.

They do not appear to have experienced significant isolation or rejection in their mainstreamed environment.

No significant relationship was found between level of ego development and degree of hearing loss (p. 83).

Bozik suggested that perhaps programs studied in previous research were "not adequate implementations of the concept of mainstreaming" (p. 84).

CONCLUSIONS

The prevalence of single-faceted models of education for hearing-impaired children and youth reflects long-established traditions, long-held beliefs, and, in many cases, limited allocations of funds and resources.

No program can appropriately accommodate all students. The concept of a continuum of services implies the cooperation of agencies and jurisdictions in new and creative ways. The more options that can be developed in offering habilitation and education to hearing-impaired students, the better their individual needs will be served and their talents and abilities developed.

In Fairfax County, we believe that access to mainstream education offers opportunities to hearing-impaired children and youth that are unique. We agree that the influence of school culture is intertwined with what is learned. If English is to be mastered, the mastery is most likely to come from its daily, habitual use in settings where others use it too, whether they are signing in English, utilizing cued speech, or using listening and speech reading exclusively.

> . . . Knowledge is situated, being in part a product of the activity, context, and culture in which it is developed and used (Brown, Collins, and Duguid 1989, p. 23).

However, it is not enough to offer merely a mainstream environment for most hearing-impaired children. They require extensive and intensive supports that permit them to develop language appropriately as they grow. They require specialized teachers who can differentiate between limitations imposed by deafness and limitations imposed by being a child. They require the specialists necessary to insure that they can make daily use of the hearing they have available to them. They require educational interpreters who can work in non-traditional roles; speech and language clinicians who are skilled in teaching methods developed for the hearing impaired; and administrators who are sensitive to the needs of the hearing impaired.

Our experience in Fairfax has led us to believe that the mainstream setting is an appropriate setting for most hearing-impaired children *if all the necessary supports are provided.*

REFERENCES

Auditory Skills Curriculum. 1984. Fairfax, VA: Fairfax County Public Schools.

Bozik, J. 1985. A study of ego development and psychosocial adjustment in mainstreamed hearing-impaired adolescents. Ph.D. diss., University of Pittsburgh.

Brown, J., Collins, A., and Duguid, P. 1989. Situated cognition and the culture of learning. *Educational Researcher* Jan–Feb:32–35.

Castle, D., McGee, D., and Rosenstein, J. 1985. Oral interpreting in the United States: Educational issues. Paper read at International Congress on Education of the Deaf, August, 1985, Manchester, UK.

Clarke, B., and Leslie, P. 1980. Environmental alternatives for the hearing handicapped. In *Implementing Learning in the Least Restrictive Environment: Handicapped Children in the Mainstream*, eds. J. Schifani, R. Anderson, and S. Odle. Baltimore: University Park Press.

Commission on Education on the Deaf. 1988. *Toward Equality.* Washington, DC: U.S. Government Printing Office.

Johnson, R., Liddell, S., and Erting, C. 1989. Unlocking the curriculum: Principles for achieving access in deaf education. Washington, DC: Gallaudet Research Institute.

McGee, D. 1976. Mainstreaming problems and procedures: Ages 6–12. In *Mainstream Education of Hearing Impaired Children and Youth*, ed. G. Nix. New York: Grune & Stratton, Inc.

Quigley, S., and Kretschmer, R. 1983. *The Education of Deaf Children*, Baltimore: University Park Press.

Reynolds, M., Wang, M., and Walberg, H. 1986. Reflections in research and practice in special education: A case of disjointedness. Occasional paper in press.

Chapter • 12

Supportive Mainstreaming From A Residential School

David Manning

The Education for All Handicapped Children Act (P.L. 94-142) of 1974 ushered in the current version of educational integration in this country. Although it was certainly not a new idea, this was the first time the public school system in the United States took responsibility for all of its disabled children. The concept of "mainstreaming" that drew so much popular attention was familiar to the staff of The Clarke School for the Deaf in Northampton, Massachusetts. Our school was founded in 1867 by a group of parents and friends whose express purpose was to prepare hearing-impaired students to enter the mainstream. The Oral Method (speaking the English language and lipreading) was chosen as the means to accomplish this. From that time until the present, Clarke School has educated and mainstreamed thousands of students. A survey of our graduates in 1981 showed that 92% of those responding had graduated from regular high schools. (Clarke School's program ends at the ninth grade level.) Fifty-nine percent had gone on to post-secondary programs, many of them earning bachelors', masters', and even doctorate degrees.

This chapter will describe the origin and philosophy of The Mainstream Center at Clarke School, lay out the steps our transitional program follows, discuss the follow-up supervision, and conclude with a brief outline of the work yet to be done.

ORIGIN AND PHILOSOPHY

Clarke School for the Deaf is a private residential and day school. It accepts hearing-impaired students between the ages of 4 and 17 from anywhere in the world. The school's mission is to instill in hearing-impaired children a belief in their own capabilities and self-worth, to provide a strong educational background, and to prepare the students to participate as independently as possible in a society that speaks and uses the English language for communication. Present enrollment is 116 students, with 35% of the students coming from outside Massachusetts. Most of the current and previous students are profoundly hearing-impaired. The academic program purposely ends at the ninth grade so that the students can have the opportunity to complete their education in regular schools with hearing students.

The Mainstream Center officially began in 1977 in response to requests from many alumni. In describing some of the difficulties encountered in going to regular schools, they indicated a lack of readiness on the part of the receiving school. It would have been helpful, they commented, to have had the assistance of a teacher of the deaf in planning their programs, in orienting teachers to deafness, and in helping schools resolve whatever difficulties developed. They felt prepared to do their part as students, but did not feel prepared to advise and counsel teaching professionals about the best ways to accommodate them in their classrooms.

It was clear from the graduates' stories that people in regular schools simply did not have the information they needed about deafness. With the recent passage of Public Law 94-142, it was also clear that there would be an increased number of these students in mainstream classrooms. A consulting service was needed to help schools manage their mainstreaming efforts. Thus, the Center began in September 1977, available to any former Clarke School student who was enrolled in a regular school. Since then, most of the students we have assisted have been in high school, but the number of younger students leaving our school and entering regular schools in the lower grades has continued to grow, as has the number of students we serve who have been only in the mainstream.

Once a hearing-impaired student has acquired the fundamentals of language, speech, lipreading, use of hearing, reading, and writing, our staff believes that it is realistic and desirable to consider mainstreaming. At the same time, we realize that the decision to mainstream a particular student becomes a highly individual undertaking. We do not use a simple checklist or a formula. We strive to arrange an educational program that is as normal as possible, while providing whatever assistance is needed to enable the student to achieve success in the mainstream.

We also believe in the parents' ability to oversee their child's education, provided they have access to information about the experiences of other students, a way to get answers to their questions and concerns, and up-to-date information about their child's performance, ability, and interests. Our program requires the active participation of the parents in making all decisions.

Experience has also convinced us that the staff of a regular school has the ability to deal effectively with hearing-impaired students if it has adequate knowledge about the handicap, if it has a clearly defined and smoothly functioning support system, and if it devotes enough time and attention to the task. At the same time, we realize that integrating a deaf student into the life of a school requires much hard work from people who already are heavily burdened with the needs of other students with widely varying disabilities.

From the beginning, the program developed by The Mainstream Center has assisted students, parents, and new teachers in a way that requires them to make all of the important decisions. We do not take mainstreaming out of the hands of the parents or the schools. We do not teach or tutor the students. Instead, we consult with everyone involved in the mainstreaming process to help them understand the disability and what its effects are on an individual's educational and social experiences. We provide them with information concerning the experiences of other students who have gone before, and we encourage them to make their own decisions.

THE TRANSITIONAL PROGRAM

The Student

Experience has shown us that "an ounce of prevention is worth a pound of cure," and so our program is heavily focused on preparation for mainstreaming. We begin working with the students when they enter their final year at Clarke School. Our immediate goal is to become completely familiar with each student's background, personality, academic profile, and family life, so that we can provide him or her with appropriate guidance and advice. This familiarity is achieved by consulting school records, holding frequent discussions with the family, observing classroom behavior, and discussing the student with teachers.

At the same time, the students begin meeting with our guidance counselor, who is a graduate of Clarke School and of a regular mainstream high school. He knows what it is like to attend a school with hearing students, and he can anticipate many of our students' questions and concerns. He is also a good role model for them as he goes about his professional career. The meetings he has with the students are intended to help them understand all aspects of the transition to the new school. During the fall, some of the questions he discusses with them are:

1. What is mainstreaming?
2. What kind of regular school programs are there?
3. What are your individual educational needs?
4. What are support services?
5. What services do hearing-impaired people usually need?
6. What kind of educational program is "right" for you?
7. What should you look for when you visit a prospective school?
8. What are your responsibilities in mainstreaming?
9. How can you become involved socially?

The students' questions and feelings about the changes they are experiencing are the sole focus of these meetings. Knowing that the guidance counselor has gone through the experience makes it easier for them to talk about their questions and fears.

Concurrently, the consultants in The Mainstream Center also hold discussions with the students. Where the guidance counselor's meetings are more informational and general, the conferences in The Mainstream Center deal with identifying personal goals, locating and investigating potential schools, making the final selection, and then making preparations for the next year. Our staff works in concert with the guidance counselor's program, basing our activities on topics the students are currently discussing, and feeding information back to the guidance counselor from students who are already out in the field. We find this to be a time of remarkable growth in the students, since they must look at themselves candidly to plan for their future. Each student must decide with his or her parents which school he or she will attend.

The Parents

We begin discussions with parents during the summer prior to the students' final year at Clarke School by sending each family a packet of information about special education laws, terminology, and the experiences of previous graduates. Also included are an outline to help them begin their planning effort, information about locating both public and private schools, and general information about alternatives after high school.

Since the parents have the primary responsibility for choosing the next school, they must begin by making sure they are fully informed about the student's academic and social status. In conjunction with the supervising teacher of our upper school, a mainstream consultant reviews the student's recent performance with the parents to see what implications there are for the selection of the future school. Considerable time is spent doing this, so that everyone understands what type of program the student will need and what support services will be required. During this discussion, we talk about the different types of schools available in both the public and private sectors. We are also interested in finding the best of whatever alternatives exist so that the student has the greatest opportunity to succeed. All of this points to the need for parents and student to investigate carefully the total program offered at a school. This includes learning about the dress code, sports activities, and extra-curricular activities, in addition to the academic offerings. About 80% of our alumni choose a public school, but private schools offer very attractive alternatives for many others. In all cases, we are looking for programs in which the student will be challenged to achieve.

Often during these separate discussions with the student and with the parents, we learn that they have different ideas concerning the next school. When this happens, we all meet together to resolve the differences. The search and selection cannot move forward without common agreement among family members.

The Teachers and Houseparents

The mainstream consultants meet with the teachers and houseparents of each student who will be mainstreamed. We have developed particular questions to highlight the underlying strengths and weaknesses of each student. We discuss skills that are important for successful mainstreaming and determine whether the student has developed these skills sufficiently to function in the new school. When important skills are found to be weak, we may reconsider the type of school under consideration or the amount of support service a student will receive. In a few cases, we have discovered that the teachers and houseparents have entirely different views of a particular student. The discussions resulting from this discovery usually lead all of us to a better understanding of the student.

At the same time we are gathering this information, the psychologist, audiologist, speech coordinator, and language evaluator are busy completing their final evaluations of the students. The results of these tests are forwarded to The Mainstream Center to aid in the transition planning. Later, these results will be forwarded to the new school.

When we have gathered all of the pertinent information about a student and have analyzed it, we then recommend a particular type of school and program for the next year. This recommendation is based not only on the information at hand but on our experiences with hundreds of other students we have placed and then followed into the mainstream. With this recommendation, the parents and the student contact prospective schools and arrange for a visit and an admission interview. At this point, we expect the parents to be familiar enough with their child's academic strengths and weaknesses to be able to discuss them in general terms. We will assist them in preparing to visit a school by presenting them with questions typically asked by school officials and by aiding them in formulating their own set of questions about the school's program and requirements. After the scheduled visit, we discuss their impressions, help get them into perspective, and compare their conclusions with the needs of their son or daughter. In some cases, we will also make a visit to the same school to examine it from a more technical point of view.

Autumn is a busy time for our students and their families. In addition to the regular academic and social activity here on our campus, the students and parents are deeply involved in the preparation and planning for the transition to the new school. If, during the discussion and planning, it becomes apparent to any of us that mainstreaming is not a realistic alternative for a particular student, this information is brought into the open and discussed. The atmosphere in these discussions is free of negative judgments, and the focus is always on the future of the student and what he or she needs in order to be successful in the next school. The vast majority of our graduates have elected to enter regular schools with hearing students. Fourteen percent, however, have decided to enter programs for the deaf because they felt those programs would better meet their needs. By requiring all options to be investigated and discussed, our program has insured that each decision was reasonable and deliberate. In every case, the students and their parents made the final selection and, as far as we know, were satisfied they made the appropriate decision at the time.

In midwinter, we bring the parents together and ask them to start looking ahead to the following September when their son or daughter will enter the new school. We ask them to consider what program, information, and services they want to be in place for their child on the very first day. Parents typically say they want everyone in the school to know who the student is and to know a little about deafness; to have the tutor (if one is needed) on hand and ready to begin work; and to have any special equipment, such as an FM hearing aid, available and ready for use. After outlining this wish list, we ask the parents to think about the proper time to request it. It quickly becomes apparent that a meeting—we call it the Orientation Conference—should be held at Clarke School for representatives from the new schools, to educate them about the needs of their new student. This meeting is usually scheduled for mid-April and the parents usually have a leading role in it.

From our point of view, the Orientation Conference at Clarke School serves as a precursor to individual placement meetings that will be held at each school during the late spring. The program for the Orientation Conference is packed with activities that provide a basic orientation to hearing loss and to special education: the experiences of previous alumni are shared. We also offer activities for the students, including a panel of mainstreamed alumni. The parents hear from a panel of parents whose children already are in the mainstream, giving them a first-hand perspective on the regular school experience. At the close of the day, we distribute to the school representatives two copies of a bound book containing the important records of the student they will be receiving the following fall. Included in the book is a copy of the student's health record; most recent audiological, psychological, speech, academic achievement, and language test results; and a detailed description of each course the student is taking, including materials used, typical assignments given, the student's strengths and weaknesses in the course, recommendations for the next year, and samples of uncorrected written work. We ask the school representatives to have the head of each academic department in their high school read the book prior to the student's placement meeting.

The Placement Meeting

This meeting is held at the student's new high school for the purpose of reviewing all of the records, setting up the student's program of courses, choosing academic levels, determining support services to be provided within the school, and arranging for support services from outside the school. It is attended by the special education director, the principal, guidance counselor, heads of academic departments, the school nurse, the student and parents, and representatives from The Mainstream Center. By prior agreement, the special education director of the student's new school allows the first half of the meeting to be conducted by our mainstream consultant. An outline for a typical meeting is shown below.

Placement Meeting for John Smith
May 5, 1989

I. Introductions

    A. Names and responsibilities of school staff are made known to the student and parents

    B. Student- and parent-centered meeting
(Since we are discussing this student's future, it is important for him or her to understand the meeting as it goes along. We, therefore, ask that all remarks be directed to the student and that the student respond to them or ask for further clarification. Although this increases the length of the meeting, it insures that the student and the parents understand all of the decisions being made.)

    C. Brief conversation between student and mainstream consultant so group may see and hear communication process
(During this discussion, we deliberately create situations where either the student or the mainstream consultant does not understand something the other has said. Our purpose in doing this is to show people how to handle a communication block.)

II. Student's Special Abilities and Interests
(A new student will have an easier time integrating socially if he or she is introduced as someone with a special ability or interest instead of as someone "who can't hear." We make certain the key people in the new school know about a student's special talents.)

III. Communication Factors

    A. Comments about the student's speech, lipreading, and hearing abilities
(We mention this during the meeting to demonstrate to people that these are matters that can be discussed openly.)

    B. Comments about how hearing loss affects language development
(Although this is acknowledged, there is a wealth of information in the student's placement book that goes into this topic in greater detail.)

IV. Background Information from Upper School at Clarke

    A. Student's oral, written, and reading language abilities
(Questions are directed to the student during this discussion to

demonstrate that the student understands the impact his or her hearing loss has had on his or her language performance.)

B. Summary of student's academic performance while at Clarke
(Questions are directed to the student to demonstrate that he or she understands the quality of his or her academic performance.)

C. Social/emotional experiences while at Clarke
(During this discussion, we try to highlight the student's desire to develop friends at his or her new school.)

D. Recommended grade and program placement
(We make an official recommendation for grade placement based on the student's performance at Clarke School and the program offered in the receiving school. This is intended to discourage misguided attempts to place the student in a grade simply on the basis of chronological age. Our students routinely enter from one to three years below other students the same age.)

V. Discussion of Support System

A. Specific support services recommended by The Mainstream Center
(Our recommendations are based on reports from the classroom teachers at Clarke School, on the services we know the new school can provide, and on the experience we have had with other students in the mainstream.)

B. Availability of outside support from The Mainstream Center
(Monitoring and troubleshooting services are suggested.)

(The Special Education Director chairs the meeting from this point on.)

VI. Course Selection for Next Year

A. Major courses and possible electives

B. Choose level for each course
(Where possible, we ask the heads of departments to bring a copy of the textbooks with them so that we can make a brief check of the language used in them. We have sometimes found that college textbooks are used in a high school course.)

C. General suggestions for choosing teachers

VII. Discussion of Social Mainstreaming Issues

A. Possible involvement of hearing students who have visited Clarke School
(See a discussion of this below.)

B. Discussion of ways to promote social integration

VIII.   Future Steps

    A.   Plans for orienting teachers
       (The Mainstream Center is available to provide this service. If the school does not contract with us, we still ask them to set a date for providing a staff orientation. Experience has shown that without this commitment, the meeting is often not held.)

    B.   Student/tutor/teacher interaction before September
       (Where possible, we encourage informal interactions so that everyone can become more comfortable.)

    C.   Any other pending questions

We go over the entire agenda for this meeting with the student a few days before it actually happens. Often the student will have things to say, or questions to ask, and this preview of the meeting helps us decide when to bring up these points. On the day of the meeting, we meet the parents for a private run through of the agenda in a relaxed setting. This gives them a chance to ask questions and to bring up matters they think ought to be discussed. It is a fact that many parents are intimidated at school meetings. This preview enables them to go into the official meeting with a clearer understanding of the information that will be presented.

Student Exchange Program

We have observed that it is easier to make new friends if it can be done on safe territory. For this reason, we invite one or two students from the new school to come to our campus for a two-day exchange visit. The guidance counselor usually selects the visitors from the same grade level as our student. Background information about Clarke School and the Exchange Program is then sent in order to alleviate any concerns the visitors might have. The students arrive at Clarke School on the appointed day and deliberately are placed in classes with the deaf students, with very little introduction. From that moment on, they attend all of the classes and functions with the student who will be entering their school. Taking part in a variety of activities during the remainder of the day allows these guests to develop some insight into the way Clarke School operates.

Before the students leave the following day, we meet with them to discuss their observations of their visit. What we hear is usually the same: "This visit has been great! When I first arrived yesterday, I didn't know what it would be like and I was nervous. I didn't know if I would be able to understand the kids' speech or if they would want to be friends with me. But once I got started, I found I could understand pretty fast." "Some of the kids are easier to understand than others, but I can understand most of them. I like the small classes and I wish we had them at our school. The kids here seem to be such good friends with each other. And they really seem to care about their school and the dorm."

This meeting gives us a chance to clear up some of the obvious misunderstandings they may have about deafness and to point out to them that the nervousness and fear they felt as they entered our school will be felt by the deaf student who enters their school in the fall. All of them assure us that they will do everything they can to help the student find a place for himself or herself in the life of the new school. Despite these assurances, we find that the social side of mainstreaming is the single most difficult element to resolve during the time a student is mainstreamed. There are many reasons for this, and some students learn to handle it quite well. We must report, however, that a large number of students find mainstreaming to be a lonely time.

The transition year concludes with graduation from Clarke School. Just prior to the graduation ceremony, we hold a final group meeting with all of the parents to assure them that the feelings they have as their children leave Clarke School really are quite normal and to remind them that The Mainstream Center will be working with them throughout the high school years. We also talk to them about the range of feelings and moods their son or daughter will experience during the course of the summer. These range from elation after the Clarke School graduation to nervousness and anxiety during the days before the new school begins. Experience has shown us that parents go through many of these same feelings. We encourage them to contact the special education director toward the end of the summer to be sure that everything that is supposed to be ready is actually in place. We also invite them to call us if they just want to talk. They are facing a significant change, and it is normal for anyone in that situation to have feelings of anxiety. We offer them support as they move from a familiar and trusted world to a new and uncertain one. This entire transitional program is provided to each student as part of the regular Clarke School program.

FOLLOW-UP SUPERVISION

Once graduation is over, we complete the year by sending a copy of the student's transcript to the new school along with a contract for the support services we have agreed to provide. The monitoring and follow-up services offered by The Mainstream Center are:

1. Comprehensive educational evaluation of students
2. On-site consultation with schools
3. Orientation of professional staff in client schools
4. Classroom observation and teacher consultation
5. Fall conference on mainstreaming (held at Clarke)
6. Periodic telephone checks with school, student, and family
7. Special meetings (yearly IEP meetings, coordinating meetings)
8. Tutorial service (academic and communication therapy)
9. Audiological services (basic management, audiological outreach program, and equipment leasing)
10. Post-high school planning with student and family
11. Requests for information

Any or all of these services are provided through contracts with the receiving school or, in the case of private schools, with the parents. The services in each contract come from deliberations by a student's Individualized Education Program (IEP) Team so that each contract is developed according to the needs of the student and the school. Although our services are primarily consulting services, we do provide a limited amount of tutoring for students who live near Clarke School.

Services that warrant special mention:

"The Mainstream News" is a monthly newsletter on mainstreaming that was an outgrowth of a survey we did several years ago. In that survey, teachers opted for a newsletter instead of a year-long series of meetings about deafness. This publication is mailed to schools throughout the United States and several foreign countries. It provides teachers with interesting and practical tips for mainstreaming a student. It also serves as a monthly reminder that there is a deaf student in the class. (See Appendix A)

The Fall Conference on Mainstreaming was started in 1979 and is held each year at Clarke School. Open to anyone who is working with a mainstreamed hearing-impaired student, teachers, speech pathologists, guidance counselors, audiologists, tutors, interpreters, and special education directors from around the Northeast attend each year.

The Audiological Outreach Program was begun in 1988 because we found a great deal of equipment in the regular schools that was not operating properly. Further investigation showed that the teachers in regular school classrooms do not have the experience or training to be able to troubleshoot the equipment properly. The Audiological Outreach Program provides for three appointments each year. On two occasions, an audiologist goes to a client's school to do an electroacoustic check of the student's equipment and to answer teachers' questions. A third appointment is scheduled at the Clarke School testing center for a complete audiological evaluation and a third electroacoustic check of the equipment.

Equipment leasing was suggested to us by several special education directors who were reluctant to invest in expensive FM hearing aid equipment when the student would be in their school for only two or three years. The leasing program enables us to place an FM system in a school and have it under our supervision for as long as a school wants it. Once the student graduates, the school can return it and not be left with unused equipment sitting on a shelf gathering dust.

Special aspects of our program include:

1. Our philosophy about mainstreaming for qualified hearing-impaired students. We understand that mainstreaming requires the effort and commitment of a variety of people; that once they have acquired the needed information and guidance, people involved in mainstreaming have the ability to make their own decisions; that the chief contribution The Mainstream Center can make to mainstreaming is to share Clarke School's years of knowledge about educating hearing-impaired students. This philosophy is very important to us because it enables us to evaluate our performance and assists us in planning for the future.

2. The steady flow of information we provide to the people with whom we are working in the mainstream. In turn, we encourage a steady flow of information about the experiences of students and professionals back to us from the mainstream. This enables us to share valuable information with our own school to be used in preparing future students for the mainstream.

3. The student's Placement Book containing formal evaluations, suggestions for mainstreaming, course summaries, and samples of the student's written work in each subject area. This has been well received by every school. (See Appendix B)

YET TO BE DONE

We are not yet satisfied with the degree to which our students have been able to integrate socially in their new schools. Social integration depends to a great extent upon the personality of the particular student; but we believe that more can be done to facilitate this aspect of integration, and this is a goal we have set for ourselves for the future.

We are not satisfied with the quality of our communication with individual classroom teachers. Until recently, all information has had to go through the guidance counselor in each school. Experience has shown that these people are very busy and information is not always passed on. Striving for more direct communication, we began our monthly newsletter.

We believe there needs to be more counseling offered to the hearing-impaired students in their new schools. These students face a significant daily challenge as they attempt to complete their education in regular classrooms, and they often need the opportunity to talk about their frustrations. They also need regular encouragement to keep trying. Hearing people, busy with their own lives, often forget just how difficult the challenge is. There needs to be a better system that allows the student to receive regular attention in this regard.

CONCLUSIONS

The Mainstream Center's program is based on the idea that for most people, hearing and hearing-impaired alike, personal fulfillment comes through participation in the world at large. To achieve this, individuals must be able to communicate with their peers, contribute to society at a meaningful level, and share in the camaraderie of group effort. Since society is designed for people with normal hearing, people with hearing losses find many impediments to achieving their potential. In keeping with Clarke's overall mission, The Mainstream Center serves as a facilitator between individuals with hearing losses and the rest of society, providing information and guidance to help them live, learn, and work together. To this end, we provide services for hearing-impaired persons of all ages, parents, educators, and co-workers. Taking into account the various options available to our clients, we advocate placements that are appropriate to the individual abilities and needs of the students. Our experiences have demonstrated that the mainstreaming of even profoundly hearing-impaired students can be successful, provided that it is prepared adequately, implemented sensitively, and supervised carefully.

APPENDIX A

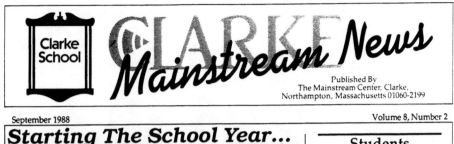

Published By
The Mainstream Center, Clarke,
Northampton, Massachusetts 01060-2199

September 1988 · Volume 8, Number 2

Starting The School Year...

ARE YOU READY?

**Coordinators · Students · Parents · Tutors
Teachers · Speech Pathologists**

COORDINATOR

☐ Does each member of the student's Support Team know who the other members are?

☐ Have you told them you are the Coordinator of the student's program?

☐ Have you told them they should notify you if they have questions, problems, or concerns?

☐ Have you set up a time with the student for a weekly conference with you to see how he feels his program is working?

☐ Have you arranged for an orientation to hearing impairment for the Support Team?

☐ Have you made the student's cumulative file available for the teachers to read?

☐ If the student is returning this year, have you arranged for the new teachers to talk with those who worked with him last year?

☐ Have you checked to be sure that the tutor has an adequate place to work with the student, including all of the equipment and materials he or she needs?

☐ Have you checked to be sure that the tutor is aware that he or she is expected to have a regular meeting with each teacher every week or so throughout the school year?

☐ Have you ordered the "Note-Writer" Notetaking System, or made arrangements for the student to get a copy of the class notes?

☐ If the student is using FM hearing aid equipment, is it on hand and ready to use? Has someone shown the teachers how to use it?

☐ Have you made arrangements for the student to be able to follow during assemblies or other group meetings?

Students

Elementary Level

At the elementary level, the Support Team should agree on what it expects the student to learn about his or her handicap during the year. If the child has any usable hearing, he or she should be expected to indicate when his hearing aid is not working. An older child can be expected to learn how to put on and take off his hearing aid equipment. Learning to change the hearing aid battery is useful, as is learning to clean the earmolds. Telling you when he or she is not able to understand what is being discussed in class is yet another good habit to develop. Each year, one or more of these should be added to the list of skills that the child has mastered.

Secondary Level

A secondary student should learn what arrangements need to be made at the beginning of each *to page 2*

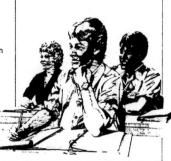

APPENDIX B

Each student's Placement Book contains approximately 100 pages of information, including:

Student profile, written by the Mainstream Consultant
Student profile, written by the parents
Medical and health history
Audiological evaluation
Speech profile and recommendations
Psychological assessment
Achievement test results
Explanation of the oral and written language development of the
    student
Results of language assessment
Student autobiography (corrected and uncorrected)
Description of the upper school program
Report cards (first and second terms)
Course summary for each subject (includes teacher recommendations
    for the receiving school)
Samples of the student's written work (several for each course)
Recommendation for grade placement
Description of follow-up services available from The Mainstream
    Center
Photographs and descriptions of Clarke School
Additional pages about such things as communication, lipreading,
    and written test questions

Chapter • 13

Mainstreaming and NTID

William Castle

BACKGROUND INFORMATION

The National Technical Institute for the Deaf Act was one of the first pieces of United States Congressional legislation passed by Congress in 1965 (Public Law 89-36, 1965) designed to bring disabled persons into the mainstream of society.

The Bureau for Education of the Handicapped was not created until two years later. The Amendments to the Vocational Rehabilitation Act, which created what has come to be called Section 504, were not passed until the early 70s (Public Law 93-112, 1973; Public Law 93-516, 1974). The Education for All Handicapped Children Act was passed in 1975 (Public Law 94-142, 1975); and the new Americans with Disabilities Act, the most thoroughgoing civil rights legislation regarding disabled persons, was passed in 1990. Thus the National Technical Institute for the Deaf (NTID) serves as a vanguard in our society's efforts to provide equal educational and employment opportunities to its disabled population.

The concept of a national technical institute for the deaf was first introduced to the literature in 1930 (Peterson 1930). It came into consideration again in the 1960s when the report of a special advisory committee on education of the deaf (Babbidge 1964) was submitted to the Secretary of the Department of Health, Education, and Welfare (DHEW).

In 1964 the national deaf community, parents of deaf children, educators of deaf students, vocational counselors of deaf clients, and organizations serving deaf people lobbied Congress about the impor-

229

tance of an NTID. At this time, most deaf persons were either underemployed or unemployed because they did not have a spectrum of post-secondary educational opportunities equal to that which prepared their hearing peers for employment in the mainstream, i.e., in business and industry.

Congress, therefore, passed the National Technical Institute for the Deaf Act. The Act specified that the National Technical Institute for the Deaf must be established as an integral part of an already existing institution of higher learning that offered, at a minimum, the baccalaureate degree. The law did not specify that the deaf students who entered NTID must be integrated (i.e., mainstreamed) with respect to all aspects of their education. In fact, NTID could have been established on the campus of Gallaudet University where there is limited opportunity for integration or educational mainstreaming for undergraduate students. However, Gallaudet University did not have any interest in becoming the host institution for NTID.

Because the law also specified that the Secretary of DHEW was responsible for finding an appropriate host institution, the Secretary sought an institution that was designed primarily to serve hearing students, thus setting the stage for a significant level of mainstreaming. The Secretary put in place, as required by law, a special National Advisory Board that wrote the guidelines for the establishment of NTID and eventually chose the host institution. These guidelines did not suggest that the deaf students who entered NTID must be integrated, i.e., mainstreamed, in all aspects of their education. Instead, the guidelines specified that the students admitted to NTID must have general educational achievements of eighth grade or better. This meant, of course, that many deaf students at NTID would not have the ability to pursue the academic programs at the host institution that were designed for hearing students and, therefore, that they would be in classes with other deaf students only.

In 1966 the Rochester Institute of Technology (RIT) was chosen to be the host institution for NTID. At that time there were 2,600 institutions of higher learning in the United States that offered, at a minimum, the baccalaureate degree. In all, only 12 of these institutions submitted proposals for consideration by the special National Advisory Board. From among these institutions, RIT, the University of Illinois (Chicago Circle), the University of Pittsburgh, and the University of Tennessee were selected as finalists and were visited. After the site visits, RIT was unanimously recommended by the Board to the Secretary of DHEW as their choice for the following reasons:

1. RIT had a long history of providing a vast array of technical programs to hearing students and showed strong potential for preparing deaf students for working in the mainstream;

2. RIT had a long history of providing cooperative work experiences in business and industry (i.e., in the mainstream) for its students, having done so since 1912; and
3. RIT was the only institution among the four that planned to have all the deaf students take all of their courses on its own campus; and thus would provide the students with the best opportunities for being educationally and socially mainstreamed.

A GENERAL DESCRIPTION OF NTID AT RIT

RIT was contracted officially by DHEW in December of 1966 to establish NTID on its campus; and in September of 1968, the doors of RIT opened to the first 70 deaf students to be sponsored by NTID. At that time, NTID had no academic programs of its own; therefore, all 70 deaf students matriculated as full-time students into one of the other colleges of RIT for their first RIT academic experiences. Thus, they were fully mainstreamed for their classes. At the same time, the deaf and hearing students shared the same dormitories, ate in the same dining facilities, and used the same recreational facilities. From this description, it would appear that all the deaf students were fully integrated in all aspects of campus life and that ideal educational and social mainstreaming was occurring. However, by the time the 1968–69 academic year was completed, a different circumstance was clearly evident. During the first quarter of that academic year it became clear that 50% of the deaf students were not capable of successfully pursuing any of the courses in the major programs that they had chosen and that many others needed some remedial work in English, mathematics, or the basic sciences. Therefore, in the second quarter NTID established an extensive remedial program called the Vestibule Program, and a majority of the deaf students were placed in classes for deaf students only. It was also observed that in both the dormitories and the dining halls the deaf students tended to stay together as a group for their socialization.

For more than six years, there were no buildings on the RIT campus that were devoted to the several special purposes of NTID. By the 1974–75 academic year, five new buildings were in place on the RIT campus to symbolize the presence of NTID, and in 1983 a sixth one was added. These include three dormitory structures, a dining commons, and two academic buildings. The academic buildings house the certificate, diploma, and associate degree programs that are designed to provide technical training for those deaf students who are not able to pursue or are not interested in pursuing the baccalaureate and master's degree programs offered in the other colleges of RIT.

The academic buildings also are designed to accommodate special courses for the personal and social growth of the deaf students; special courses for improving the reading, writing, speaking, speechreading, listening, and manual communication skills of the deaf students; programs for training new professionals to work with the deaf population; programs of applied research; programs for public affairs; programs related to recruitment, admissions, and job placement; and administrative support services. To some students and administrators, these academic facilities have become a symbol of segregation because their chief purpose is to serve the special needs of deaf students and the particular needs of the faculty and staff of NTID. The counterbalancing symbols of integration (i.e., mainstreaming) are not readily recognized by the casual observer. For instance, every year hundreds of RIT's hearing students use these academic facilities for their work study or cooperative work experiences and participate in the NTID performing arts programs in music, dance, and theatre. In addition, as is true of all the other dormitories and dining facilities at RIT, those constructed because of the presence of NTID are used by both hearing and deaf students. Furthermore, currently over 20% (about 250) of the deaf students are pursuing baccalaureate and master's degree programs in the other colleges of RIT while another 50% (about 625) take some of their courses in those other colleges; and to support these deaf students who are competing academically with hearing students on a daily basis, a large number of NTID faculty and staff (about 150) have their offices in the other colleges of RIT.

NTID students who are majoring or taking some of their courses along with hearing students in the other colleges of RIT are called cross-registered students. They are not required to take a College Board examination, e.g., the Scholastic Aptitude Test. They pursue their major programs or take specific courses in the other colleges on the recommendation of NTID faculty who feel they can succeed so long as they are provided with all the appropriate support services, including interpreting (simultaneous, manual, or oral), notetaking, tutoring, and special academic advising. Data now show that the recommendations of the NTID faculty regarding deaf students who major in another college at RIT are quite valid—74% of the deaf students who pursue baccalaureate or master's degree programs in those other colleges successfully complete them (*NTID Annual Report* 1989). This is in contrast to a 50% completion rate for the hearing students in those same colleges.

The bottom-line measures of RIT's success in preparing its deaf students to function in the mainstream are the data about job placement of the graduates. Of the 80% of deaf graduates who enter the labor force, 96% are employed; 94% are in jobs commensurate with their training; 70% are in business and industry, 5% are in education, and 25% are in government; 80% are in white collar jobs in contrast to 52% of the entire labor force and 26% of all deaf people who are in the labor force. As a rule, then, they are employed in the mainstream, working side by side with hearing people and earning comparable wages (*NTID Annual Report* 1989).

NTID can be thought of as the epitome of educational mainstreaming for a large population of students with a specific disability because there is no other institution like it in the entire world. In a usual year there are 1,200 deaf students on the RIT campus with over 11,000 hearing students.

THE COMPLEXITIES OF EFFECTIVE
EDUCATIONAL MAINSTREAMING AT RIT

There are a number of factors regarding the mainstreaming of deaf students at RIT that deserve special attention: assessment of abilities and interests, program selection, principles for providing interpreting services, principles for providing notetaking and tutoring services, how to orient the faculty of the other colleges of RIT, how the faculty can have an impact on a student's personal and social growth, how to deal with improving communication skills, and how to accomplish some degree of reverse assimilation.

Assessment

The admissions criteria for NTID are quite flexible. Students who are eligible for admission to NTID must show evidence of the following:

1. The student should have attended a school or class for the deaf and/or have needed special help because of being deaf.
2. The student must have a hearing loss that seriously limits the chances for success in a regular college or program for the hearing. There is general agreement that an average hearing loss of 60 decibels (ASA) or 70 decibels (ISO), or more, across the 500 and 2,000 Hz range, is a major educational handicap.
3. The student's educational background must show that there is a probability for success in a program of study at NTID. Admitted students will have an overall 8th grade achievement level or above.
4. Information from a student's references should suggest that the applicant has the personal and social maturity to enter the type of program offered by NTID.
5. The NTID program is designed for students who have finished a high school educational program. A student may be considered for admission before completing a high school program if school au-

thorities, who know the student well, feel he or she would profit more from the NTID program than by remaining in high school. Age and personal social maturity would need to be given special consideration under such a condition.

In addition, applicants currently or previously enrolled in other post-secondary educational programs will be considered for admission if one or more of the following conditions are met:

6. There is clear evidence that support services provided by NTID are required for success and that these services are or were not available in the educational institution(s) where enrolled.
7. Support services are or were available to the student but the applicant has changed career goals, and the program desired is or was not available.
8. The student has or will be completing the post-secondary program and it is felt that advanced training in his or her major would be of value.

Placement in specific technical programs at RIT, including the certificate, diploma, and associate degree programs of NTID or placement in remedial programs or core programs designed to prepare deaf students for entry into specific majors at RIT, require that the deaf students undergo a very thorough assessment. This assessment for all new students occurs during what has come to be called a special Summer Vestibule Program (SVP), which takes place for a five week period immediately prior to each fall quarter. During these five weeks the students are tested to determine their overall communication skills, their academic skills, and their personal/social skills, the three categories of skills considered by most experts on integration to be the most important (Bitter, Johnston, and Sorenson 1973).

In terms of communication skills, the students' hearing losses are measured with standardized and consistent procedures designed and implemented by the American Speech-Languge-Hearing Association (ASHA)-certified audiologists employed by NTID. These audiological assessments provide a consistent approach to validating the audiological records that are submitted by the students at the time of application for admission to NTID. They offer the audiologists the bases for advising the student about optimal use of any residual hearing that may be present. As Ross and others have pointed out, the degree of hearing loss and the ability to make use of residual hearing is one good predictor of the academic performance of most deaf students (Luterman 1974; Ross 1976). In addition the students are given a battery of tests to measure their speechreading capabilities with or without sound, their abilities to receive manual communication with or without speech, their abilities to read, their speech intelligibility, their abilities to communicate manually with or without speech, and their writing abilities. Except for the reading test that is used, these tests were all designed at NTID and are described in the August, 1976 edition of the *American Annals of the Deaf* (Johnson 1976).

The students are evaluated for their performance IQ with results obtained from the Wechsler Intelligence Scale for Children (Wechsler 1949). Although there are measurement instruments for helping to define personal/social skills, most evidence suggests that they are not valid for the deaf students at RIT (Hinkle and White 1979). Through NTID, each deaf student is assigned to a personal/career development counselor who makes judgments about and counsels the student about the personal/social skills that are important for dealing with the RIT environment.

Educational Placement

By the time the fall quarter begins, judgments have been made, based on the assessment program, regarding which programs each new student may pursue. Some are admitted directly into the baccalaureate and master degree programs of the other colleges at RIT. Some are placed in one of several pre-baccalaureate preparatory programs. Some are admitted directly into the certificate, diploma, and associate degree programs of NTID; others are placed in core curricula that are designed to prepare the students for entry into given majors, and still others are put into programs for remedial mathematics, science, and English.

There are two types of associate degree programs within NTID: the Associate of Applied Science and the Associate of Occupational Studies. The former requires that five courses be taken in the College of Liberal Arts. The latter does not have such a requirement; instead, the students are required to take a battery of general education courses designed specifically for deaf students, some of which are described later. The courses in the College of Liberal Arts demand that the students have reading and writing skills of a higher level than those required for the NTID general education courses. Because the verbal skills of many NTID students do not match the requirements of the College of Liberal Arts, the Associate of Occupational Studies and the diploma and certificate options are designed to develop the technical, personal/social, and communication skills needed for employment in business and industry and for dealing with society in general.

Mainstream Placement

As mentioned earlier, over 20% of the deaf students are placed in baccalaureate and master degree programs of the other colleges of RIT.

Nearly 50% of all other deaf students take some of their courses in those colleges, especially in the College of Liberal Arts. Students are placed in these courses and major programs based on the judgment of NTID professionals who believe the students can pursue these courses and major programs if they are provided with a well-organized program of educational support services, including interpreting, notetaking, tutoring, and special academic advising.

Interpreting. In 1968, when the doors of NTID were first opened, educational interpreting was not prevalent. As a general rule, classroom teachers with hearing-impaired students in their classes communicated with those students without an intermediary. However, at RIT and at other post-secondary institutions in which deaf students are educationally mainstreamed, this general rule does not apply. Classroom teachers at NTID who provide the courses designed specifically for deaf students are expected to learn how to communicate for themselves. In the other colleges of RIT, however, sign language and oral interpreters are provided in accordance with the communication needs of the deaf students in a particular class.

Today educational interpreting is prevalent. Since NTID established the first program for training persons to be educational interpreters in the summer of 1969, educational interpreting has become a profession in its own right. There are now over 150 post-secondary programs for the deaf in the United States, all of which use educational interpreters (Rawlings, Karchmer, and DeCaro 1988); and because of increased mainstreaming of deaf children at the elementary and secondary levels of education, the demand for educational interpreters in our public schools has increased dramatically. There are now more than 76 programs for training educational interpreters in the U.S. and Canada (Stuckless, Avery, and Hurwitz 1989).

The number of full-time educational interpreters currently at NTID is 65; this number is insufficient to cover all of the needs. Therefore, NTID must hire free-lance educational interpreters on an hourly basis and must remain flexible about scheduling deaf students into study sections for which interpreters can be provided. Regretfully, some interpreting needs still go unmet.

Effective management of an educational interpreting program as large as that of NTID includes: a good management team; effective and efficient scheduling; a good understanding on the part of the interpreters, the classroom teachers, and the deaf students of their respective roles in the interpreting process; and opportunities for the interpreters to obtain whatever professional development is pertinent to their certification by the national Registry of Interpreters. Details regarding these principles are provided by Hurwitz and Witter (1979) and by the report of the National Task Force on Educational Interpreting.

During the 1988–89 academic year, approximately 50,000 hours of interpreting were provided in classrooms and another 9,000 were provided for students outside of classes.

Notetaking/Tutoring. Although it is common practice for college students to take notes for themselves, it is not an easy thing for a deaf student to do in the usual classroom situation because the deaf student must focus attention on the lecturer, on an interpreter, or on other media. Often deaf students require tutoring as a backup to what occurs in the classroom. Initially, NTID depended upon its mainstreamed deaf students to seek volunteer notetakers and tutors from among their fellow students; it was soon learned that this was not the best way to use these two support systems. Now the institute seeks hearing students and pays them to undergo a training program. This program emphasizes techniques for tailoring notetaking and tutoring to the specific characteristics and communication skills of individual deaf students. Osguthorpe and Whitehead (1979) have pointed out that these notetaker/tutors

> "become familiar with the unique personal and educational effects of deafness on students they support. By the close of our training period tutor/notetakers have:
>
> 1. Established a working relationship with their support manager
> 2. Practiced tutoring and taking notes
> 3. Had follow-up diagnostic evaluations
> 4. An understanding of the individual students they will be supporting
> 5. Learned which classes they will cover
> 6. Set up regular meetings with their manager for purposes of skill" (p. 152).

Osguthorpe and Whitehead (1979) go on to say,

> . . . at NTID the paraprofessionals must be prepared to deal with a variety of content areas, for they may be assigned to a different course each quarter. Efforts are made to place tutor/notetakers in courses they have already taken or to place them in courses closely related to their area of expertise. Because college courses include a broad range of content areas and the skill level of the paraprofessional is relatively high, structured teaching materials for each course are not provided for tutor/notetakers to use when working with deaf students. Emphasis is placed on training tutors to encourage and facilitate students' self-learning efforts, rather than going through a fixed series of lessons with the student (p. 152).

As has been pointed out by Osguthorpe and Hurwitz (1979),

> In the NTID tutor/notetaker program, each major area of study has a different support manager. This person, in each case, is a full-time professional with other responsibilities, including teaching. During the 30-hour

training program . . . managers become closely acquainted with the tutor/notetakers who will be serving under their direction. Managers participate in the training program as trainers, tailoring some sessions to the unique needs of students in their area. For example, since different content areas pose different notetaking problems, each manager exposes tutor/notetakers during the training program to the types of classes in which they will serve.

Following the training program, managers meet regularly with each of their tutor/notetakers. During these meetings, managers discuss the quality of notes being taken and suggest improvements. The manager also discusses the tutoring contacts the tutor/notetaker has had, and the progress each student is making in the course. These student contacts should be reported to the manager on Tutor Logs filled out by the tutor/notetaker following each tutoring session. As the manager gains confidence that the tutor/notetaker's skills are well developed, meetings are initiated less frequently. Managers are encourged, however, to observe tutoring sessions and to continually monitor the quality of notes being provided to students. Record keeping is built into the support system to allow managers to keep track of each tutor/notetaker and all of the students receiving service (pp. 172–174).

During the 1988–89 academic year a total of 37,000 hours of notetaking and 12,000 hours of tutoring were provided by trained notetaker/tutors to the mainstreamed deaf students. Such numbers of hours are not considered atypical.

Academic Advising.   In each of the other colleges of RIT, other than the College of Continuing Education, there is a team of NTID professionals who manage the educational support services for the deaf students who take courses in that college. These professionals sometimes take notes or tutor. One among them manages the interpreter services for that college, another manages the notetaking and tutoring done by students in that college. Some teach specific courses in that college. Most provide a certain amount of academic counseling to students who are taking their major programs in that college. It is this academic counseling that helps the student determine how best to sequence his or her academic courses; which sections of a given course to take for best assurance of interpreting, notetaking, and tutoring services; which professors to avoid because they are not particularly happy to have deaf students in their classes; how to seek out special help from the classroom instructor; and how to become more independent.

RIT Faculty Orientation.   Another responsibility of the NTID professionals who are housed in the other colleges of RIT is to help orient the faculties of the colleges to the special needs of hearing-impaired students. Thorough treatises have been written that can be shared with these faculty members, e.g., *Suggestions for the Regular Classroom Teacher* by Culhane and Mothersell (1979). NTID has published its own brochures on "do's and don'ts" regarding communicating with the hearing-impaired students, the use of interpreters, and how to deal with the several myths about deafness. These are shared readily with the faculty of the other colleges, but just as important is the day-to-day presence of the NTID professionals as resources to those who have deaf students in their classes.

TEACHING PERSONAL, SOCIAL, AND COMMUNICATION SKILLS

The foregoing has made it clear that RIT provides the deaf students who are sponsored by NTID with substantial opportunities to be educationally mainstreamed. It is also important to emphasize that NTID is ready to prepare its deaf students to enter the mainstream of society once they graduate from RIT. To do that, the graduates need to be well-adjusted, successful, and productive citizens. Such a citizen is one who has a good self-image; is able to interrelate with other people on a positive basis; is well-prepared to enter the world of work; understands about career ladders; uses his or her energies to be an active citizen, both on and off the job; and is one who earns money and pays taxes rather than being dependent upon welfare.

Knowing that most persons lose their jobs because of poor personal and social skills, NTID has instituted expansive opportunities for students to grow personally and socially, including opportunities to improve communication skills.

To this end NTID has a number of courses for credit in general education, in the social sciences, in the fine arts and humanities, in theater, and in speech, language, and listening. In addition the deaf students have opportunities to participate in extracurricular activities along with hearing students in such areas as physical education, sports programs, the performing arts, and special seminars. Courses available include:

1. *Learning Strategies*—designed to help students evaluate their strengths and weaknesses and to improve their learning efficiency and effectiveness through appropriate training. Students have the opportunity to improve their learning skills in areas such as reading, test taking, questioning, and general study habits.
2. *Personal Development*—helps students learn about themselves. They learn to understand their actions, their needs, their desires, and their relationships with other people. Topics include personal goals, planning time, choosing friends, and choosing a career.
3. *Leadership Development*—assists students in developing managerial and leadership skills. Topics include one- and two-way communication, group leadership and fellowship, styles of leader-

ship, delegating responsibility, planning skills, helping behaviors, establishing goals, and problem-solving techniques.

4. *Drug and Alcohol Usage*—designed to give a general overview of various drugs that are commonly used among college-age populations. Upon completion of the course, students are able to identify and describe the effects on the body from using each drug that is covered, including dependence and tolerance. The students study social impact, peer pressure, the economy of drugs, and personal values related to drugs.

5. *Introduction to Outdoor Living*—teaches students about decision making, group interaction, and environmental awareness.

Courses that relate to career and job development are also taught. These include:

1. *Interpersonal Relationships on the Job*—teaches about employer/ employee relationships, co-worker relationships, and how work relationships affect job satisfaction.

2. *The World of Work*—teaches students about the many skills important to success at any job.

3. *Job Search Process*—designed for students to learn about resumé writing, job application letters, interviewing, and ways to find a job.

4. *Life After College*—provides information about budgeting, housing, birth control, and keeping a job.

5. *Psychology and Your Life*—emphasizes the psychological aspects of emotional, self-concept, and interpersonal relationship development. Students are helped to identify important life issues for themselves and others and to develop a better understanding of their own behavior as well as the behavior of children, teenagers, parents, and older adults.

6. *Community Service courses*—give students opportunities for volunteerism, for investigating and reporting on community and social problems, and for learning how their personal goals and values can affect a community.

7. *Law and society course*—assists students in understanding the basic rules and applications of practical law as it applies to personal rights and responsibilities. Some topics included are how laws affect a society, civil rights, legal rights, marriage, family relations, and criminal law.

There are also courses that teach about individuality. These are:

1. *The Human Experience: An Individual Life*—introduces the students to the major challenges faced by human beings throughout the life-cycle. It explores the factors that affect healthy and unhealthy

adjustments to the circumstances of an individual's life, including biological inheritance, thoughts, feelings, and environment. Students examine contemporary issues related to the challenges of adolescence, adulthood, and old age in order to understand how unconscious adjustment and conscious decision making help in attaining and maintaining psychological health. Alternative solutions to life's challenges are generated, shared, and evaluated by students. Through the experiences of this course students are introduced to the knowledge, communication skills, and critical thinking skills important to making responsible decisions throughout their adult lives.

2. *The Human Experience: The Individual and Society*—focuses on the individual's relationships with others, starting from a study of primary groups and moving through a study of secondary groups (peers, school, work, and citizenship groups) to a study of world awareness and responsibility. The course involves the perception and evaluation of values, morals, ethics, human rights, and responsibilities.

3. *The Individual and Technology*—examines the social, political, economic, and ethical dimensions of the relationship between the individual and technology in modern society. The course reflects on the nature of science and technology, the role of human values in determining the course of scientific inquiry and the social uses of technology, and some major areas of controversy in this field.

As an especially creative technique for bringing deaf and hearing students together, fifteen different courses for credit are offered in theatre, including acting, public theatrical performances, sign mime, dance, a music practicum, costume design, scenery construction, prop collecting, make-up, and stage lighting.

The speech department at NTID offers no less than thirteen courses for credit that emphasize the importance of developing interpersonal relationships through the use of speech. These courses are complemented with other courses that offer speech therapy, vocabulary development, pronunciation, and self-monitoring skills.

The audiology department at NTID offers twenty-two courses for credit for providing the students with renewed opportunities to improve their speechreading abilities and to gain optimal use of residual hearing. These courses include orientation to hearing aids and listening, telephone communication, and the use of the experiential learning approach to help students improve their abilities to understand other people in technical/on-the-job situations.

NTID's English department offers thirty-eight credit courses that are designed to improve the reading and writing capabilities of the deaf students; these include a course that examines the various types of letters, memos, and reports that students will encounter in the work place.

In addition to what is provided through NTID, many additional courses in the social sciences, in language and literature, and in the fine arts and humanities are offered through the College of Liberal Arts.

Social adjustment is achieved by many of the deaf students by virtue of their participation in intramural and varsity sports, in student government, in student television productions, in producing a yearbook, in organizing fraternities and sororities, and inserving as officers of various student clubs.

In addition, if the emotional needs of the deaf students require them, the services of a psychologist and/or a psychiatrist need to be made available.

It seems quite clear that strong efforts must be made to foster healthy socialization for severely and profoundly hearing-impaired students with their hearing-impaired peers, with their hearing peers, and with other hearing and hearing-impaired adults.

CONCLUSION

The experience of 22 years of the NTID at RIT prompts a number of conclusions about deaf persons and mainstreaming. Not all deaf persons want to be a part of the mainstream during every aspect of their education, employment, and community life, and some may want never to be. Also, not all parents of deaf children want to have their children mainstreamed at every point of education; some may believe rightfully that the least restrictive alternative for their child is a residential school for the deaf; some may believe rightfully that the least restrictive alternative is an oral school for the deaf. In the first 10 years of NTID, the majority of students came from residential schools for the deaf; today 67% come from mainstream programs. Yet the basic educational characteristics of the entering students as a group are quite the same now as they were 10 years ago.

Not all deaf persons can be mainstreamed during every aspect of their education, employment, and community life; and some can never be mainstreamed. Thirty percent of today's NTID students go only to classes that are exclusively for deaf students; nearly 50% more have most of their classes with deaf students only; and nearly all the remaining 20% have some classes that are for deaf students only, such as classes devoted to the development of communication skills.

Educational mainstreaming of the deaf, if properly done, is very costly. It requires that deaf children at all levels of their education have teachers who are fully trained to deal with them or who have received extensive in-service training. It requires that deaf children at all levels of their education have specific and thorough attention from language specialists, speech pathologists, audiologists, and guidance counselors; and that they be given tutors, notetakers, interpreters, and special counseling, including psychological counseling when needed.

Educational mainstreaming of the deaf, if not properly done, is also very costly. If many of the patterns of mainstreaming that have been used in the past continue, deaf children will be cheated in the same ways that they always have been, and a great deal of time and money will have to be spent in later years to make up for it. A case in point is that deaf children taught in regular high schools by subject matter specialists who do not know how to teach the deaf are generally no better off than deaf children taught in residential high schools by teachers of the deaf who are not subject matter specialists.

For deaf persons to be mainstreamed in the most ideal sense, i.e., making a living and living a life on par with and among hearing persons, they do not have to be mainstreamed during every aspect of their education, employment, and community life. In this case, "to be mainstreamed" is a goal; it is not necessarily a means to that goal!

REFERENCES

Babbidge, H. 1964. *Report of the Advisory Committee on Education of the Deaf.* Washington, DC: U.S. Government Printing Office.

Bitter, G. B., Johnston, K. A., and Sorenson, R. G. 1973. *Project Need: Facilitating the Integration of Hearing Impaired Children Into Regular Public School Classes* (Technical report). Salt Lake City, UT: University of Utah, Department of Special Education.

Culhane, B. R., and Mothersell, L. L. 1979. Suggestions for the regular classroom teacher. In *Mainstreaming: Practical Ideas for Educating Hearing-Impaired Students* (1st ed.), ed. M. E. Bishop. Washington, DC: The Alexander Graham Bell Association for the Deaf.

Hinkle, W., and White, K. R. 1979. Assessment and educational placement. In *Mainstreaming: Practical Ideas for Educating Hearing-Impaired Students* (1st ed.), ed. M. E. Bishop. Washington, DC: The Alexander Graham Bell Association for the Deaf.

Hurwitz, T. A., and Witter, A. B. 1979. Principles of interpreting in an educational environment. In *Mainstreaming: Practical Ideas for Educating Hearing-Impaired Students* (1st ed.), ed. M. E. Bishop. Washington, DC: The Alexander Graham Bell Association for the Deaf.

Johnson, D. D. August, 1976. Communication characteristics of a young deaf adult population: Techniques for evaluating their communication skills. *American Annals of the Deaf* 121:409–424.

Luterman, D. M. 1974. A comparison of language skills of hearing-impaired children in a visual oral method and auditory method. Unpublished manuscript. Boston: Emerson College.

Osguthorpe, R. T., and Hurwitz, T. A. 1979. Organizing support services. In *Mainstreaming: Practical Ideas for Educating Hearing-Impaired Students* (1st ed.), ed. M. E. Bishop. Washington, DC: The Alexander Graham Bell Association for the Deaf.

Osguthorpe, R. T., and Whitehead, B. D. 1979. Principles of tutoring and note-taking. In *Mainstreaming: Practical Ideas for Educating Hearing-Impaired Students* (1st ed.), ed. M. E. Bishop. Washington, DC: The Alexander Graham Bell Association for the Deaf.

National Technical Institute for the Deaf Annual Report. 1989.

Peterson, P. N. 1930. A dream and a possibility. *The Vocational Teacher* 1.

Public Law 89-36. 1965. *The National Technical Institute for the Deaf Act.* Washington, DC: U.S. Congress.

Public Law 93-112. 1973. *The Rehabilitation Act.* Washington, DC: U.S. Congress.

Public Law 93-516. 1974. *The Rehabilitation Act Amendments.* Washington, DC: U.S. Congress.

Public Law 94-142. 1975. *The Education for All Handicapped Children Act.* Washington, DC: U.S. Congress.

Rawlings, B., Karchmer, M., and DeCaro, J. J. (eds.) 1988. *College and Career Programs for Deaf Students.* Washington, DC: Gallaudet University.

Ross, M. 1976. Assessment of the hearing-impaired prior to mainstreaming. In *Mainstream Education for Hearing Impaired Children and Youth,* ed. G. W. Nix. NY: Grune & Stratton.

Stuckless, E. R., Avery, J. C., and Hurwitz, T. A. 1989. *Educational Interpreting for Deaf Students.* Rochester, NY: National Technical Institute for the Deaf.

Wechsler, D. 1949. *Wechsler Intelligence Scale for Children.* NY: Psychological Corporation.

Chapter • 14

Post-Secondary Mainstreaming in a State College: Akron, Ohio

Carol Flexer and Denise Wray

People who experience hearing loss have the same range of interests and abilities as do persons with normal hearing; thus they should have access to a range of options for post-secondary education. One option that is available to persons with hearing loss is attendance at a regular college or university.

Success in college may be a tenuous proposition for any student who needs to rise to the demands of a new and often stressful learning environment. College can be a time of expanding horizons, determination of self-identity, reaching out to new people, learning self-discipline, developing independent living skills, and accepting responsibility for personal decisions. For many students who experience hearing loss, the meaning, impact, and management of that hearing loss is woven throughout the college experience.

Because individuals do not "outgrow" their hearing loss, many need as much or more support service in college as they needed in elementary or high school. College may not be the time to "go it alone." There are many support services available to all college students, and several special services that can be made available to students with hearing loss. The trick is to know when, where, and how to get access to these services before one feels defeated by the demands of a college environment. Said in a positive way, there is much that can be done, in a proactive fashion, to facilitate success in college.

DESCRIPTION OF COLLEGE STUDENTS WHO EXPERIENCE HEARING LOSS

Before appropriate support services can be prescribed, it is important to highlight some general characteristics of the population of students with hearing loss who attend state universities. What will emerge through the following description is that most students with hearing loss, like other freshmen, enter the university in a very confused state, but one that has been intensified by the difficulties that accompany hearing loss.

Hearing Loss and Amplification

The majority of students with hearing loss who have attended the University of Akron are functionally hard-of-hearing rather than deaf. Consistent with national data that show over 92% of the 20 million persons with hearing impairment in this country to be hard-of-hearing, most of the students had mild to severe hearing losses (Diedrichsen 1987).

A pretest given verbally to 20 college students who had experienced hearing loss all of their lives and who had worn amplification for an average of 17 years, showed the following results (Flexer, Wray, and Black 1986):

1. Fifteen students could not demonstrate an understanding of the type and degree of their own hearing loss, aided or unaided. In fact, several did not know that their hearing loss was symmetrical, but thought that they had a dead ear. Eighteen students could not interpret their own audiogram, and ten did not have any idea where to begin.

2. When asked about hearing aids, only the earmold, battery, and volume control could be identified by all of the students. In addition, only ten students could recognize the telecoil switch, and seven had never used it even though their hearing aids were equipped with one. None of the students knew very much about assistive listening devices, even telephone amplifiers. Only one student was aware of "those auditory trainers," and all felt that they were doing just fine in class without any special equipment.

3. When audiometric and hearing aid assessments were performed, it was found that not one student had appropriate amplification. Only seven of the 20 students had binaural amplification, none had acoustically tuned earmolds, and most had hearing aids that were at least five years old. Further, most students did not have basic hearing aid trouble-shooting skills (Flexer and Wray 1984). When college students brought their hearing aids into the University of Akron's Speech and Hearing Clinic for repair, in three instances the battery was dead, and in another, the earmold was plugged with cerumen.

An interesting observation was that many of the students believed that their academic difficulties were unrelated to their hearing loss. That is, because they had not experienced any alternative amplification models, they felt that they heard fine, their hearing aids were suitable, and they did not need FM units. Their skewed perceptions and lack of knowledge about hearing and technology was not due to low intelligence, but rather due to lack of information and experience. Their information deficit prevented them from independently managing their hearing, and thus the students continued to experience unnecessary barriers. Because most of the students resisted changes in amplification and use of assistive technology, such changes became a focus of the support-information group.

Academic Preparation

Unfortunately, many of the students had been channelled into vocational programs in high school. That is, many primary and secondary schools do not offer an array of options for the appropriate education of students with hearing loss (Ross, Brackett, and Maxon 1982). When in elementary or high school, the college students had been treated as either "deaf" or as normally hearing, and neither placement was suitable (Blair and Berg 1982). As a result, many of the college students had not received appropriate preparatory coursework, services, and counseling, and arrived at the University with immediate deficits.

Approximately 75% of the students with hearing loss at The University of Akron were enrolled in non-credit remedial courses because of their low scores on college entrance examinations (Flexer, Wray, and Black 1986). Specifically, 60% needed to take developmental courses in English, 40% needed to take the developmental math course, and over one-third of the students needed to take remedial courses in both math and English.

Many of the students were surprised by their lack of preparation for a college curriculum. In addition, difficulties with reading and writing as well as the rapid pace of college classes, prevented most students from successfully taking more than 12 hours per semester.

Emotional Issues

Many of the students had been mainstreamed throughout their primary and secondary school years, and had not met another youngster who was hearing impaired. Thus, even though they had friends who had normal hearing, many students felt that additionally they would like to associate with a special group of peers who understood their unique needs and frustrations. Further, most of the students were still hiding their hearing loss, embarrassed to have classmates know about their disability, and reluctant, even terrified, to tell teachers. Many had never really discussed their hearing loss with friends or family members. While a few students accepted their hearing loss as easily as they accepted their blue or brown eyes, most appeared ashamed and victimized.

All of the deficits and problem areas highlighted thus far in this chapter indicate that many college students with hearing loss display an array of educational and emotional needs that must be addressed. The identified difficulties need not prevent students from entering or from succeeding in college. Potentially troublesome areas for each student should be identified and managed in order to provide an opportunity for him or her to grow as an individual and to compete in a university setting.

SUPPORT/INFORMATION GROUP FOR
COLLEGE STUDENTS WITH HEARING LOSS

In view of the multiple social-emotional, audiological, speech-language, and academic needs evidenced by the college student with hearing loss, a support group appeared to offer a medium for addressing the areas of concern (Berg 1972). There was already a community self-help group available—SHHH. However, for the most part, the members of this SHHH group were older, already in the work force or retired, and had acquired their hearing losses later in life. A special group designed to address the unique needs of college students could serve as a unifying force and an efficient way of providing resources and services.

Development of the Support/Information Group

The Department of Communicative Disorders at the University of Akron was in a position, for several reasons, to spearhead the development of a support group. First, there were two faculty members committed since the early 1980s to the preparation of preschool children with hearing loss for mainstreamed placement into regular classrooms. Because one faculty member was an audiologist and the other a speech-language pathologist, a comprehensive "whole hearing" and "whole language" program was already being implemented. Working with two extremes of the school continuum proved to be insightful, with one group's needs shedding light on the other's.

Second, many students with hearing loss were already being seen for audiological evaluations as a result of referrals from the Bureau of Vocational Rehabilitation. One of the audiological recommendations that could be made was referral to the support group.

A third and most important reason that the Department of Communicative Disorders was successful in organizing a support group was that the support group had a strong advocate outside of the Department, i.e., the Director of Handicapped Student Services. To explain, on college application-for-admission forms, students could choose to disclose any disability that they had, including hearing loss. All applications that had disabilities noted were given to the Director (also called Advisor) of Handicapped Student Services. The Advisor personally met with all students who had designated that they had a disability. As a result of numerous discussions between members of the faculty of the Department of Communicative Disorders and the Advisor of Handicapped Student Services, the Advisor strongly suggested that all students with hearing loss meet with her as well as contact the University's Speech and Hearing Center. Thus, students received comprehensive support services in compliance with Federal law.

Organization of the Support/Information Group

Once the need for the group and its concept and purpose had been identified, the task of promoting interest and recruiting members became the next goal. The Director of Handicapped Student Services agreed to inform all incoming students with hearing loss of the existence of the group, and to refer them to the Department of Communicative Disorders for details. Attendance was voluntary. However, if a student was experiencing difficulty in school, the Director could make group attendance a prerequisite to the continued receipt of assistance from the student services office.

Meetings were established at one specific time every semester, in order that the students might work the sessions into their schedules. The meetings lasted two hours and were conducted twice per month. Over twenty-five students have been involved as their schedules would permit, with between four and ten students attending every meeting.

The "kick-off" meeting of the semester was promoted by means of telephone calls to students whose names had been provided by the Office of Handicapped Student Services. The calls were made by intern clinicians from the Department of Communicative Disorders, and subsequent meetings were announced by mailing flyers. Refreshments, always an enticing feature, were served at all meetings.

Once again, it must be emphasized that the entire support/information group project has involved teamwork and cooperation between two separate departments on campus. Either department working alone would not have had sufficient information or resources to provide comprehensive services.

Goals of the Support/Information Group

Following an assessment of the needs of each new group participant, potential goals for each semester were generated, always with input from the students themselves. Problem areas were addressed by having guest speakers, group discussions, role playing, simulations, and social activities.

Information and support that would enable students to remain in college received the highest priority and included: appropriate hearing aids and assistive listening devices; information about hearing and hearing loss; academic accommodations managed through Handicapped Student Services; speech-language therapy including writing skills and vocabulary development; and emotional support (Flexer, Wray, and Leavitt 1990).

One activity that was instrumental in promoting the use of personal FM units was a study comparing personal hearing aids to assistive listening devices, involving all of the students in the group (Flexer et al. 1987). Prior to the study, none of the students used the personal FM units that were purchased through the Office of Handicapped Student Services and managed through the Department of Communicative Disorders. The study demonstrated that the students experienced better and easier word identification skills with personal FM units than they did with their own hearing aids, even in a quiet classroom with front row seating. The safe practice environment provided by the study convinced the students to try the FM units in class. Furthermore, word quickly spread among the students with hearing loss that a personal FM was technology worth trying.

A skeptical graduate student, who had been severely to profoundly hearing impaired since age three, tried an FM unit as a result of peer pressure prompted by the study. Following a day of using the FM unit, he reported his observations to the support/information group; he stated that the teachers' speech was so clear that for the first time he could take notes and listen at the same time; he could even hear a teacher over the hum of the slide projector; for the first time that he could remember, he did not have to take a nap due to the exhaustion induced by the intense concentration required in class. He has become one of the strongest supporters and will not let new group members leave a meeting without promising to take an FM unit to class.

Raising student awareness of the accommodations to which they are entitled has been a continual struggle and consequently a major goal of the group. As incoming freshmen, students were often intimidated by the university environment and reluctant to ask questions. While many have been recipients of services from the Bureau of Vocational Rehabilitation, most students did not realize that the University could provide additional assistance. The support/information group emphasized available services offered by Handicapped Student Services by inviting the Director to speak to the group. The discussions that followed the presentation allowed students to share experiences that they had with various accommodations such as notetakers, FM systems, tutoring, extended test-taking time, and preferential class scheduling. Students often experimented with new services and equipment as a result of the group interaction, testimony, and support.

Timely use of tutors was another result of group meetings with the Director of Handicapped Student Services. Often, a student would request a tutor toward the end of the semester when little could be accomplished to raise a failing grade. With increased awareness, students asked for academic help early in the semester when there was more opportunity for improvement.

Interestingly, many of the college students have become motivated to improve their speech skills. Even though most had not had speech-language therapy since elementary school, new friends and demanding environments prompted many to request individual sessions to refine speech skills. The students reported being more aware of their responsibility to be clearly understood. Initially, they had preferred that new acquaintances believe them to be from another state or country, rather than to think that something was "wrong" with them.

The need to improve language skills has not been as clearly understood by the college students as the need to improve speech skills. The impact of language on academic performance has been discussed at group meetings. Those students who experience difficulty comprehending vocabulary, reading texts, or composing themes in English class, were encouraged to enroll in individual language therapy. Once persuaded to try therapy, many students have made significant gains in writing skills (Wray, Hazlett, and Flexer 1988).

An activity of the support/information group that has received the most enthusiasm is an altruistic endeavor called the Community Outreach Program (Flexer and Wray 1989). Two different populations were the focus of the Outreach Program. One of the target populations was junior and senior high school students with hearing loss who are primarily in mainstreamed situations. The college students were intrigued by the notion of meeting and participating in a panel to answer questions posed by the younger students with hearing loss. The college students expressed the opinion that a support group during the turbulent years of junior high and high school would have been a welcome source of strength for them.

Parents and family members of the toddlers and preschoolers with hearing loss who attended the University Clinic were the second targets of the Outreach Program. The parents of these very young children had questions about hearing loss and parenting, and also questions about their children's perspectives that they could not ask their preschoolers; but these questions could be and were asked of the college students. Questions were asked about over-protection by parents, ridicule from peers, and refusal by the child to wear amplification. The college students, many of whom could not initially admit that they had a hearing loss, would stand in front of a group of strangers at an Outreach meeting and talk about their private feelings, experiences, and values. They would give encouragement and offer hope. Members of the community would leave the Outreach meetings refreshed. Parents of the preschoolers were heard to say, "I hope my child grows up to be like those college students." And the college students, many of whom were so timid they would not give their names at the first group meeting, have served as mentors and as sources of information and strength.

Additional goals for the support/information group were lower priority yet still of significant interest to the students. These included development of telephone skills, conversational strategies relating to pragmatics, idiomatic expressions, figurative language, career opportunities, job interviewing techniques specific to persons with disabilities, legal rights, and listening to guest speakers—themselves successful community members—who had been hearing impaired since birth. Each semester, group members decide the particular goals that they would like to target. The intern clinicians and supervisors play a facilitory role only. Appendix A is a checklist of possible goals for a support/information group (Flexer, Wray, and Leavitt 1990).

SUPPORT SERVICES FOR COLLEGE STUDENTS WITH HEARING LOSS

As previously mentioned, the creation of a support group for college students with hearing loss was an effort that coordinated services from two separate departments on campus. The contributions made by the Department of Communicative Disorders have been discussed in the previous section. However, services for students were not confined to that department. Other forms of accommodation were more appropriately delivered by Handicapped Student Services.

The first need of the student with hearing loss who is contemplating entering higher education involves selection of a suitable institution. There are many considerations that face the student with hearing loss, and Handicapped Student Services (or an office with a different name but a similar function; perhaps just the Office of Student Services) should be contacted at each institution that the student is considering. The student should determine if the prospective university has any organized accommodations available. Will the student be going into a supportive environment with a network of services in place, or will the student need to arrange for everything alone? Not all colleges and universities offer easy access to appropriate accommodations.

One of the first forms of assistance that Handicapped Student Services can provide has to do with scheduling and course selection, i.e., advising. Thoughtful advising is invaluable to a freshman who does not yet understand the university system. The advisor can provide accurate information regarding requirements for a student's major, course prerequisites, curriculum, recommended credit hours, and load per term.

Additional accommodations for the student with hearing loss may include, but not be confined to: tutoring, note takers, priority registration, oral or manual interpreting, telephone amplifiers, TTY/TTD, loan of FM systems, personal counseling, career planning, health services, and on-campus job placement while one is in school. In many, but not all universities, these services are available free of charge to the student with hearing loss. The extent to which these accommodations might be required will vary from student to student and from term to term. Appendix B provides a summary checklist of those accommodations that have proved to be the most beneficial for students enrolled at The University of Akron (Flexer, Wray, and Leavitt 1990).

Students attending our University are encouraged to view accommodations as survival strategies. Such strategies are not forms of "cheating" or means of attaining a college degree the "easy" way. All are services to which the student with a disability is entitled as mandated by federal law. To capitalize upon the availability of services is to enhance the student's pursuit of an education that will allow access to a quality life as a contributing citizen.

CONCLUSION

Clearly, the student with hearing loss cannot afford to function as an "island" in a university environment, and cling to the hope that things will work themselves out as they may have in high school. As the pro-file data suggest, most students with hearing loss enter the university with significant deficits. The purpose of this chapter has been to dis-cuss accommodations that can be useful in overcoming those deficits and in facilitating success in college.

A support/information group can be a means of organizing the service delivery system. In an accepting atmosphere, students can learn to identify their own areas of need, and seek—even demand—the necessary accommodations. College can be a time of growth and accomplishment. A thoughtful provision of services can allow students with hearing loss the opportunity to compete successfully in state universities.

APPENDIX A

Checklist of Possible Goals for a Support/Information Group
_____ Arrange for audiological and hearing aid assessments
_____ Have hearing aid trouble-shooting sessions
_____ Have discussions about hearing, hearing loss, and the impact of hearing loss in a college environment
_____ Arrange demonstrations and hands-on experience with as-sistive communication technology
_____ Arrange for individual speech and/or language therapy ses-sions as appropriate
_____ Discuss idiomatic expressions that are currently in use at the university
_____ Share fears, concerns, and experiences with hearing loss
_____ Provide information about funding for college and for ampli-fication devices
_____ Have guest speaker discuss legal rights
_____ Have guest speaker from Handicapped Student Services
_____ Have guest speaker from the Bureau of Vocational Rehabili-tation
_____ Have guest speaker from the Placement Office discuss career options, interviewing, etc.
_____ Have a psychologist speak about assertiveness
_____ Invite guest speakers with hearing loss who are successful members of the community and college graduates
_____ Have discussions and practice sessions dealing with telephone amplifiers, and strategies for communicating on the phone
_____ Discuss demanding social/listening situations and role play problem solving techniques
_____ Establish a Community Outreach Program

_____ Arrange social activities
_____ Anything else the group wants to do

APPENDIX B

Useful Services for College Students with Hearing Loss Provided through the Office of Handicapped Student Services

_____ Information regarding financial assistance for education and amplification devices
_____ Academic advising
_____ Academic tutoring
_____ Arranging for the student to take developmental or remedial courses which will allow the student to be competitive in regular college courses
_____ Personal counseling
_____ Notetakers
_____ Oral or manual interpreters
_____ Loaner personal FM systems
_____ Part-time on-campus employment while a student
_____ Closed-captioning of instructional materials
_____ Fire alarms equipped with strobe lights in the dorm room

Services Available through the Department of Communicative Disorders

_____ Audiological and hearing aid assessments and management
_____ Speech/language therapy
_____ Support/information group
_____ Community Outreach program
_____ Amplified telephones on campus or access to a TTY

REFERENCES

Berg, F. S. 1972. A model for a facilitative program for hearing impaired college students. *The Volta Review* 74:370–75.
Blair, J., and Berg, F. 1982. Problems and needs of hard-of-hearing students. *Asha* 24:541–46.
Diedrichsen, R. 1987. Towards the acquisition of basic rights and services for persons who are hard-of-hearing. *SHHH* 8(2):3–4.
Flexer, C., and Wray, D. 1984. Congenitally hearing-impaired college students: The forgotten group. *Hearing Instruments* 35:20–49.
Flexer, C., and Wray, D. 1989. Role models: Hearing-impaired college students reach out to the community. *The Volta Review* 91:157–62.
Flexer, C., Wray, D. F., and Black, T. S. 1986. Support group for moderately

hearing-impaired college students: An expanding awareness. *The Volta Review* 88:223–29.

Flexer, C., Wray, D., and Leavitt, R. (eds). 1990. *How the Student with Hearing Loss Can Succeed in College: A Handbook for Students, Families, and Professionals.* Washington, DC: Alexander Graham Bell Association for the Deaf.

Flexer, C., Wray, D. F., Black, T. S., and Millin, J. P. 1987. Amplification devices: Evaluating classroom effectiveness for moderately hearing-impaired college students. *The Volta Review* 89:347–57.

Ross, M., Brackett, D., and Maxon, A. 1982. *Hard of Hearing Children in Regular Schools.* Englewood Cliffs, NJ: Prentice-Hall.

Wray, D., Hazlett, J., and Flexer, C. 1988. Strategies for teaching writing skills to hearing-impaired adolescents. *Language, Speech, and Hearing Services in Schools* 19:182–90.

Chapter • 15

Implementing an In-Service Training Program

Antonia Brancia Maxon

The number of hearing-impaired children in regular education classrooms and/or on the caseloads of public school special educators has grown considerably since 1976. The advent of Public Law 94-142 resulted in both regular and special educators being required to meet the individual, often unique, needs of children with all types and degrees of handicapping conditions. For many direct service personnel, this mandate was overwhelming and resulted in difficulties, particularly when they were expected to take on new responsibilities without having received appropriate training. Although a free education was provided for all children, many were receiving "special services" that were provided by professionals who were not prepared to meet their unique needs.

Acknowledging that problems were inevitable for hearing-impaired children in the regular classroom, the "UConn Mainstream Project" was developed in 1976. Originally conceived and designed by Mark Ross, the in-service training project was housed at The University of Connecticut and supported by funds from the Bureau of Education for the Handicapped, Federal Department of Education. With the influx of hearing-impaired children into the mainstream, it was assumed that direct service personnel would have difficulties in managing these children because of the diverse nature of hearing impairment and its concomitant problems.

That hearing-impaired children are a heterogeneous group can be seen from the data in table I. These data were collected during the six

Table I. Descriptive Data on Hearing-Impaired Children (N = 165) in Public School Settings (Brackett and Maxon 1986)

Performance	Mean	Range
Hearing Levels (dB HTL) Better ear pure tone average	70.1	5–110
Receptive Speech Discrimination (%) Unaided better ear at MCL	78.0	0–100
Aided Receptive Speech Discrimination (%) Amplification, normal conversation		
Auditory only	58.4	0–100
Visual only	44.0	0–98
Combined (auditory + visual)	86.2	8–100
Receptive Single Word Vocabulary (PPVT) Deviation from chronological age (years)	−3.3	−10.8–+4.8

years that the UConn Mainstream Project was in existence and the sample reflects the fact that children who were in regular education (i.e., mainstream) classes in the Connecticut public schools (1976–1982) had a wide range of potential, abilities, and skills. As a sample, these children are considered to be representative of the hearing-impaired children found in mainstream classes since the inception of P.L. 94-142 (Brackett and Maxon 1986).

Although not the major focus of this chapter, these data are important because they serve to make the point that children vary considerably with respect to hearing and communication skills. Therefore, their ability to function in the classroom will vary also. As can be seen in table I, the mean degree of hearing loss was in the severe category; however, it is important to note that the degree of loss ranged from normal hearing in one ear (unilateral hearing loss) to bilateral profound hearing loss. How well could these children use residual hearing? Both the receptive speech discrimination scores and the aided receptive discrimination scores indicate that some could make no use of hearing for perception of speech (0%) while others could rely on it readily (100%). The combined aided receptive scores are quite revealing when considering what classroom personnel face in terms of a wide range of skills. In general, when using their amplification (either personal hearing aids or wireless FM systems) and receiving both auditory and visual cues, mainstreamed hearing-impaired children could readily perceive the various speech sounds (Mean = 86.2%). This mean score is misleading, however, since the range of scores demonstrates that some children in regular education classes, under optimal listening conditions, could correctly perceive only two of twenty-five words (8%) presented. The final piece of data, which underscores the variation in abilities with which these hearing-impaired children presented, can be observed from the scores of receptive vocabulary. The scores displayed were calculated as deviations from chronological age, and demonstrate that, on the average, hearing-impaired students had a receptive, single-word vocabulary which was more than three years below that of their normally hearing peers. At the upper end of the range there were a few who scored at or above age-level, but at the other end there was at least one child with a delay of almost eleven years.

These data help explain why regular education classroom teachers were overwhelmed with the type, degree, and diversity of problems presented by the children who were suddenly in their classes as a result of the federal law. That diversity made it impossible for a teacher to generalize from one hearing-impaired student to the next. Therefore, even those school personnel who had some experience with hearing-impaired children could not rely on it to provide them with the necessary answers. In some cases, their experience did not give them an advantage over those professionals who had none. The heterogeneity issue was compounded by something that cannot be seen from these data: correlational analyses showed that vocabulary deficit and use of residual hearing were not directly related to the degree of hearing loss (Maxon and Brackett 1987). That is, the children with the poorer auditory skills and lower vocabulary levels did not necessarily have the greater degrees of hearing loss. Therefore, even the direct service personnel who were knowledgeable about audiograms and clinical data could not predict from the child's hearing loss the type of problems a particular child might exhibit.

In summary, the heterogeneity of the population of hearing-impaired children in regular classes, the lack of training of both regular education and special education personnel, and the inability to predict the type of problems an individual child might have, made appropriate educational management quite difficult. Therefore, the preparation and implementation of an appropriate Individualized Education Program (IEP) was an overwhelming task. Just as the children varied in skills and needs, the professionals working with them also had a wide range of knowledge, abilities, and needs. For example, the classroom teacher would have to know how hearing loss affects skills in a regular education classroom, and the speech-language pathologist would have to know what impact the hearing loss had upon the ability to communicate in various types of situations.

THE UCONN MAINSTREAM PROJECT

Recognizing this variance in the needs of hearing-impaired children and professionals, the UConn Mainstream Project was developed.

That program of in-service training was provided via the protocol displayed in figure 1. The training was carried out by the project directors (A.B. Maxon, Ph.D., audiologist, and D. Brackett, Ph.D., speech-language pathologist). The project participants were enrolled for one year during which time they received the training outlined in the diagram. The children with whom the participants were working at the time were eligible to receive audiological and amplification evaluations from the project directors. All training and services associated with the project were provided without cost to the school system, the individual service provider, or the child's family.

The goal of the project was to provide in-service training that would meet the specific needs of speech-language pathologists, teachers of the hearing impaired, and audiologists who were involved in direct management of hearing-impaired children. These professionals had different areas of expertise and different orientations to the problems related to managing the children. They all brought particular strengths to the educational setting, but no one group of professionals could be expected to handle all of the components of management for the hearing-impaired children in the mainstream, that is, management of academic, communication, and social interactions (Maxon and Brackett 1983).

The large number (over 74) of professionals who participated in the project recognized a need to increase their competencies in order to provide appropriate services. The perceived gap in training of school personnel was not limited to the geographical area in which the

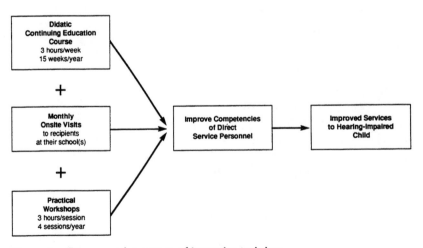

Figure 1. Diagram of program of inservice training.

UConn Mainstream Project was conducted. Requests for workshops and seminars were quite high nationally as well. Often, as a result of those presentations, requests were received for copies of training materials. In all, the experience of working on the UConn Mainstream Project made it clear that there was a gap in available, and perhaps more importantly, usable information about hearing loss with all its manifestations and about the impact of the loss on the child's classroom behavior and performance.

Throughout the duration of the project, the directors were asked numerous questions about appropriate educational management of hearing-impaired children in regular schools. At the end of each project year, the directors elicited questions and evaluations from the project participants. The questions (over 200) could be grouped into nine definite major categories or factors. Table II displays the factors and gives some examples of the questions that were asked. These factors/ categories were considered to show the areas in which participants had the greatest needs. It was assumed that the project participants were a representative sample of direct service school personnel who were working with hearing-impaired children. The final result was the development of informational and supportive audio-visual materials to be used in in-service training.

TRADITIONAL IN-SERVICE TRAINING

Although the primary purpose of polling the UConn Mainstream Project participants was to develop the in-service materials, the polling revealed related information. Aside from indicating their own specific needs, the direct service personnel expressed a distinct dissatisfaction with their traditional in-service training. Of all their concerns, three major problems with traditional in-service training emerged. They were: (1) programs are not "training": information is provided in an informal manner, often "on the run"; (2) the information provided is too general: it is not specifically geared to address the needs of personnel working with an individual child; and (3) the information provided is too theoretical and difficult to use because the person providing it does not really understand it.

Such comments by participants demonstrated that the information was provided, often in hallways or through telephone conversations, in a manner that was too informal. The result was that the interpretation of test scores or explanation of reports from outside sources was given little attention, affording minimal support for classroom teachers and other educational personnel. When efforts were made to imple-

Table II. Questions and Factors Related to the Needs of Hearing-Impaired Children and Direct Service Personnel

Sample Questions/Problems	Resulting Factor
1. If her hearing loss is permanent, why must she have a yearly evaluation?	Audiological Evaluation
The report from the audiologist says that his middle ear function is normal, I thought he was hearing-impaired.	Audiological Evaluation
2. I don't understand why he can hear some speech sounds and not others.	Speech Acoustics
Why does her speech sound so slushy?	Speech Acoustics
3. She seems to be able to communicate pretty well with the other kids, why does she have trouble in class?	Speech/Language Problems
Does he really need to be taken out of class every day to go to speech?	Speech/Language Problems
4. Even with those two hearing aids on, he doesn't seem to follow what I say.	Hearing Aids
I think there's a problem with his earmolds; they have holes in them.	Hearing Aids
5. Does this FM microphone have to be worn all of the time?	FMs
I should make sure that the environmental microphones are always turned off, right?	FMs
6. I think she is just ignoring me when she doesn't respond.	Classroom Acoustics
Why should I have to rearrange my classroom set up? It has been this way for years.	Classroom Acoustics
7. What do you mean she has to have the academic testing done individually?	Educational/Psychological Evaluation
Why not use deaf norms, she's deaf isn't she?	Educational/Psychological Evaluation
8. I can't understand a word he says. What should I do in class?	Classroom Behavior
She always raises her hand to questions, but doesn't know the answers.	Classroom Behavior
9. Why don't you just place him in a hearing-impaired program? Wouldn't he be better off there?	Management
It makes no sense to have so much of her education take place in the resource room if she's supposed to be mainstreamed.	Management

ment formal in-service training, the material was often too general to be applicable to a given child and/or was too theoretical and difficult to understand because of the limited expertise of the person making the presentation. In either case, questions and concerns about a particular child were not addressed, which left the classroom teacher and other personnel still unable to handle the needs of the child with whom they were working.

INDIVIDUALIZED IN-SERVICE PLAN (IIP)

Recognizing these problems and the issue of heterogeneity of the children, the concept of an Individualized In-service Plan (IIP) was developed. This concept was designed to address the fact that one or two in-service programs covering global issues do not meet the needs of school personnel or mainstreamed hearing-impaired children. Just as it is not possible to pull a pre-packaged educational program off the shelf and provide appropriate service to a hearing-impaired child, it is not possible to use a pre-packaged in-service training program and expect it to meet the needs of school personnel.

An in-service plan must be developed in much the same way that an Individualized Education Program (IEP) is developed: that is, the needs and resources of the personnel, the setting, and the child must be assessed before an appropriate plan of management can be implemented. The major considerations for developing an individualized in-service plan are these:

1. The in-service training should be developed in much the same way as an IEP must be developed.
2. There are certain items that need to be addressed for all hearing-impaired children, but there are others that should be very specific to a given child.
3. The in-service materials have to be flexible so they can be adapted by special educators to use with regular educators.
4. In-service training should be based on the specific needs of the group to be addressed. Classroom teachers should be the focal point, but information should be usable with reading teachers, social workers, and others who work with the child.
5. In-service plans should be developed for the families of hearing-impaired children.
6. In-service plans should be developed for peers of hearing-impaired children.

This outline demonstrates that the concept has several basic underlying components: (1) in-service training can and should be conducted by the most knowledgeable professional in the school system; (2) some information is common to all children and professionals, regardless of the individuals being trained; (3) all school personnel who come in contact with the child should receive some level of in-service training; (4) the child's peers should be included in in-service plans; and (5) the child's family should be considered as in-service recipients.

In order for the IIP concept to work, the person who does the planning and, therefore, develops the various types of training must know about the specific child/children with whom the professionals work and about the level of knowledge of those professionals. This individual also must have information and materials that will allow for a comprehensive and adaptable in-service program.

CONDUCTING AN INDIVIDUAL IN-SERVICE PROGRAM

Table II contains nine questions and concerns of direct-service school personnel that are crucial to understanding hearing-impaired children in a mainstream setting. The following is an explanation of the resulting factors seen in table II.

1. Audiological Evaluation: A description of assessment procedures and how to interpret results, especially in regard to educational implications.
2. Speech Acoustics—Perception: An overview of acoustic cues of speech with relational descriptions of how hearing-impaired children can compensate for hearing loss.
3. Speech and Language Problems: A discussion of speech and language problems typically associated with hearing impairments, including educational implications.
4. Amplification—Hearing Aids: A description of how hearing aids work and help, including trouble-shooting.
5. Amplification—FM Systems: A description of how FM systems work and overcome problems of classroom listening, including trouble-shooting.
6. Classroom Acoustics: A description of acoustic problems likely to occur in school buildings and the influence on classroom performance.
7. Evaluation—Educational/Psychological: A description of appropriate assessment procedures for hearing-impaired children, including interpretation.
8. Classroom Behavior: A description of ways of evaluating a child's classroom performance, as well as expected problems.
9. Management: Suggestions for developing appropriate management programs for hearing-impaired children.

Not all of this material is necessary for all in-service programs, but the presenter must be familiar with all of this information so that when specific concerns arise, they can be readily addressed. The presenter should determine the theoretical material necessary for any given presentation and use it to provide information and to answer questions.

In-service training programs can benefit from the use of audio-visual presentations and should include written materials that the participants can take away with them. The audio-visual materials may consist of graphics that have been made into handouts and/or transparencies (e.g., the schematic of an FM system), videotapes to elucidate particular points (e.g., the effects of different types of amplification on speech perception), audiotapes to demonstrate specific points (e.g., the effects of hearing loss on speech production intelligibility), and slides to display equipment and amplification systems. A description of those materials is provided in Appendix A. Handouts, videotapes, etc., are an excellent way to ensure that the personnel attending the in-service program comprehend the rather complex information that is basic to understanding hearing loss and its effect on the school-aged child.

It is possible to maintain the concept of flexibility in developing an IIP and to make use of a set of prepared outlines appropriate for particular children and/or particular personnel. Appendix B contains some suggestions for outlines that may be useful. The outlines are designed to demonstrate different types of in-service workshops that can be selected after determining the needs of a particular group.

The first workshop (I: The Mainstreamed Hearing-Impaired Child) would be applicable as a full-day program that provides general information about hearing impairment and its effects on the school-aged child. Specific information can be included to make such a workshop address particular concerns and/or problems for a given child. A more defined workshop to answer questions that have been asked about the child's need for an FM system, for example, is one on amplification (VIII: Classroom Amplification). The information that is provided can address the questions asked by the group, and discussion can revolve around the child or children with whom they all work.

Using these workshop outlines to examine the concerns of the school personnel will ensure an in-service training program that is specific to a particular child and to the needs of the professionals working with him or her. In that way, the information presented can be readily incorporated into the direct management of the child and, hopefully, reduce the feelings of being overburdened by the demands of teaching a hearing-impaired child.

In addition to in-service training directed toward school personnel, it is important to consider providing information to classmates and families of hearing-impaired children. The development of the IIP for these groups should be very specific to the child and the way in which the child can and will function in the classroom and/or at home.

With respect to classmates, it is important not to make the hearing-impaired child the object of curiosity, but instead to diffuse any derision and feelings of discomfort before they occur. It is not possible to completely protect any child from being on the receiving end of unkind remarks and jokes, but open discussion of hearing loss and amplification is sure to decrease the comments that arise out of ignorance. Most often, classmates have questions about classroom amplification. Frank explanation allows them to find out how it works, why it is necessary, and that the hearing-impaired child needs it in order to function like the rest of them. The presentation can be informal and "hands on," which is particularly helpful in the lower grades. It is often beneficial to carry out such discussion early in the academic year, before negative attitudes have developed. As with any of the other in-service programs, the discussions should be based on the needs of the classmates and the hearing-impaired child. It is also wise to inform the hearing-impaired child that such discussions will take place so any feelings of discomfort can be handled.

Working with the families of hearing-impaired children goes well beyond the provision of factual information. Parents and siblings should have access to a professional who has skills in counseling and knowledge about hearing loss, and who can help the families learn to separate the issues related to hearing impairment from issues or problems that all children face. Difficulty in delineating problems that may be related to the hearing loss may become exacerbated during the hearing-impaired child's adolescence.

Parents will have concerns regarding hearing loss in the classroom that they will want to discuss with school personnel. They typically want a fair and accurate evaluation of their child's performance and potential that includes information about hearing loss and the accommodations that are being made for their child. It is difficult to separate these considerations from the development of the IEP. Parents are often in need of factual information and typically need help when applying it to their child's skills and programming.

Parents should be included in the development of the IIP, in the same way they are involved in the IEP. They should be made aware of the kinds of concerns and questions that school personnel have. They should also be allowed to contribute to the information given to school personnel about their child. Including parents in workshop development and providing them with exposure to the in-service material will be invaluable in ensuring appropriate management for the child.

APPLICATION OF THE IIP CONCEPT

The development of a good in-service program is crucial to successful mainstreaming. It is not an easy task, but one that can be readily managed with the appropriate materials. In order to demonstrate how IIP development can be carried out, three case histories are presented below with pertinent background information and selected questions that were asked by school personnel. Suggestions for appropriate in-service workshop selection are included.

Case 1—JM

Age   JM is a 12-year-old girl.

Hearing   She has a bilateral, severe-to-profound sensorineural hearing loss which is presumed to be congenital. The hearing loss was diagnosed at 3 years of age.

Amplification   JM's personal amplification consists of binaural ear level hearing aids. She was originally provided with amplification at 3 years of age. JM uses a wireless FM system which is coupled to her hearing aids via a teleloop. JM uses school-worn amplification full-time.

Residual Hearing   JM makes good use of her residual hearing. She can effectively combine auditory and visual cues for accurate speech perception.

Speech   Her speech production is generally judged to be intelligible by naive listeners.

Language   JM demonstrates a two to three year delay in language content and form.

Placement   She is presently enrolled in the seventh grade in a junior high school. She takes departmental classes that are taught by different instructors.

Performance   JM's performance is at grade level in all non-language based classes. However, performance in language-based classes is two years below grade level. JM is bright, but her reduced language skills affect her academic performance.

Services   JM has daily academic support from a teacher of the hearing impaired. That educational management consists of preview/review of academic material and vocabulary work related to classroom activities.

Social JM is one of several hearing-impaired children in a small city school. She has both normally hearing and hearing-impaired friends, but she has difficulty with relationships outside of her family. Although the family members are very close and supportive, they are somewhat sheltering.

Personnel Questions and In-service Workshop Suggestions:

Concerns	Area*	Workshop**
She seems to have trouble taking notes and listening at the same time, Why?	2, 3	III, VI, VII
The grammar of her spoken language is worse than in her written language, Why?	3	V, VII
I'm tired of her mother coming in and telling me how to run my class.	8, 9	I, III, VII, IX

*See pages 10–11.
**See Appendix B.

Case 2—BF

Age BF is a 6-year-old boy.

Hearing Loss He has a bilateral, moderate, high frequency sensorineural hearing loss that was diagnosed at 3.5 years of age.

Amplification BF uses binaural ear level hearing aids as personal amplification. He has used these hearing aids since 3.5 years of age. School worn amplification is a traditional, chest-mounted FM system which is worn all day.

Residual Hearing In optimal listening conditions, BF can depend solely on hearing for perception of speech.

Speech BF's speech production intelligibility is excellent. He has an interdental lisp that is unrelated to the hearing loss.

Language All language skills are age appropriate at this time.

Placement BF is presently fully mainstreamed in the first grade.

Performance He is performing at grade level or above in all of his academic subjects. BF is very bright and is very aware of it.

Services BF has speech-language management for articulation and vocabulary on a daily basis.

Social   BF has poor interpersonal skills and is described as a "real loner." He lives in a rural area. He is convinced he is smarter than his peers. His main interest outside of school is reading.

Personnel Questions and In-service Workshop Suggestions

Concerns	Area*	Workshop**
I know this room is noisy, but the other kids do fine. Why does he have trouble?	6, 4, 8	III, V, VII, VIII
Why doesn't he play well with other kids?	8, 9	III, VI, IX
When we work on phonics he has trouble. Why?	2, 6	III, V

*See pages 10–11.
**See Appendix B.

Case 3—ER

Age   ER is a 15-year-old boy.

Hearing Loss   He has a bilateral, severe, sensorineural hearing loss which was diagnosed at two years of age.

Amplification   ER uses binaural ear level hearing aids as personal amplification. He was first amplified at 2.5 years old. School-worn amplification is a traditional wireless FM system, worn waist-mounted. It is used throughout the school day.

Residual Hearing   ER makes excellent use of his residual hearing, needing some visual cues for accurate speech perception.

Speech   His speech is intelligible to naive listeners.

Language   ER has language skills that are one to two years below age level for form and content.

Placement   ER is mainstreamed in the eleventh grade, in an inner city school, for most of the day. He spends two hours in a resource room for the hearing impaired. All regular education classes are departmental.

Performance   ER is functioning one to two years below grade level in all academic subjects.

Services   The resource room in which ER is enrolled is run by a teacher of the hearing impaired. The material used in that class is from a separate published curriculum for the hearing impaired. Therefore, the resource room work is unrelated to that of his regular education classes. No other services are provided.

Social ER interacts quite readily with normally hearing and hearing-impaired peers. He is very good looking and socially "with it." ER hates the FM system because it makes him so obviously different. He has indicated that he would be accepting of a personal FM system that coupled to his personal hearing aids. ER comes from a bilingual home. His parents feel alienated from school personnel because of language and cultural differences.

Personnel Questions and In-service Workshop Suggestions

Concerns	Area*	Workshops**
Should he be getting all this help? He needs to learn to survive on his own.	1, 3, 8, 9	III, IV, V, VII
Doesn't sitting in the front of the room help enough? Why should he use an FM if he doesn't want to?	4, 5, 6	VI, VII, VIII
I use a lot of audio-visual material. Where should he sit so he can hear?	5, 6	VIII, I

*See pages 10–11.
**See Appendix B.

APPENDIX A

Materials that were developed for the UConn Mainstream Project in-service training package (Maxon, Brackett, and Ross 1986).

Contents: Graphics, Videotapes, Audiotapes, Slides

1. Graphics: To be used as overheads and handouts
   Audiological Assessment Procedures
   Sample Audiograms
   Immittance Measurement Results
   Tympanogram Types
   Acoustic Characteristics of Consonants
   Vocabulary Selection for Management
   Communication Assessment Tools and Procedures
   Sample Communication Evaluation Results
   Trouble-shooting Amplification
   Difficult Listening With Hearing Aids

Appropriate Use of FM Systems
Inappropriate Use of FM Systems
Ways to Demonstrate the Need for an FM System
Schematics of FM Systems
Signal-to-Noise Relationships
Classroom Observation
Trouble-shooting the Child's Behavior
How a Hearing Aid Works

2. Videotapes:
   Speech Through Amplification
   Trouble-shooting Amplification
   A Child's Reaction to Amplification
   Speech Discrimination in Different Listening Conditions
   Public School Personnel Ford the Mainstream

3. Audiotapes:
   Speech Through Amplification
   Speech Samples of Hearing-Impaired Children
   Language Samples of Hearing-Impaired Children

4. Slides:
   Audiological Assessment Equipment
   Different Types of Hearing Aids
   Different Types of FM Systems

APPENDIX B

Workshop Outlines that were developed for the UConn Mainstream Project in-service training packet (Maxon, Brackett, and Ross 1986).

   I. *The Mainstreamed Hearing-Impaired Child*
      A. Evaluation: Standardized procedures
      B. Evaluation: Classroom behavior
      C. Management: Audiological
      D. Management: Speech and language
      E. Management: Educational
  II. *Evaluating the Mainstreamed Hearing-Impaired Child*
      A. Hearing: Audiological evaluation
      B. Communication: Speech and language
      C. Educational: Psycho-educational
      D. Educational: Classroom behavior
 III. *Managing Mainstreamed Hearing-Impaired Children*
      A. Audiological
      B. Speech and language
      C. Educational

IV. *Program Planning*
  A. Need for evaluation
  B. Need for management
  C. Support personnel
  D. Classroom modifications
  E. In-service training

V. *Applying Test Results to Program Planning*
  A. Information obtained from the audiologist
  B. Child's primary modality for speech reception
  C. Child's use of residual hearing
  D. Information obtained from the speech-language pathologist
  E. Information concerning psycho-educational factors

VI. *Hearing Loss: An Overview*
  A. What is hearing loss
  B. Type and degree of hearing loss
  C. Amplification
  D. Effects on speech and language
  E. Effects on academics

VII. *Effects of Hearing Loss on Academic Performance*
  A. What is hearing loss
  B. Communication
  C. Hearing

VIII. *Classroom Amplification*
  A. Rationale
  B. Why it is necessary
  C. How the FM works
  D. Classroom use
  E. Trouble-shooting
  F. Ways to demonstrate the need for FM systems

IX. *Classroom Management*
  A. How to accommodate hearing
  B. How to accommodate communication

(Maxon, Brackett, and Ross 1986)

REFERENCES

Brackett, D., and Maxon, A. B. 1986. Service delivery alternatives for the main-streamed hearing-impaired child. *Language, Speech, and Hearing Services in the Schools* 17:115-25.

Maxon, A. B., and Brackett, D. 1983. Inservice training for public school speech-language pathologists in the management of mainstreamed hearing-impaired children. In *Speech of the Hearing-Impaired: Research, Training, and Personnel Preparation*, eds. I. Hochberg, H. Levitt, and M. J. Osberger. Baltimore: University Park Press.

Maxon, A. B., and Brackett, D. 1987. The hearing-impaired child in regular schools. *Seminars in Speech and Language* 8, 4:393-413.

Maxon, A. B., Brackett, D., and Ross, M. 1986. Managing hearing-impaired children in regular schools: Inservice models and materials. Miniseminar presented at the A. G. Bell Association for the Deaf Convention, Chicago, IL.

Chapter • 16

Performance Aspects of Mainstreaming

Ann E. Geers

A review of recent literature regarding the performance of hearing-impaired students in the mainstream indicates that most integrated students have the following characteristics:

1. They have a better unaided ear average of less than 90 dB or are post-lingually hearing impaired (Allen and Osborn 1984; Wolk, Karchmer, and Schildroth 1982).
2. They are integrated with normally hearing students primarily for nonacademic rather than academic subjects (Wolk, Karchmer, and Schildroth 1982; Moores and Kluwin 1986; Libbey and Pronovost 1980).
3. They outperform non-integrated students on standardized achievement tests, even when degree of hearing impairment and age at onset variables are controlled (Allen and Osborn 1984; Jensema 1975).
4. They have better speech and English language skills than non-

Data for this study were obtained from a series of Reading Research Camps that were conceived and implemented by Jean S. Moog, Principal of CID. Without her extraordinary efforts to assemble a large group of orally educated adolescents this research could not have taken place. The contribution of these teenagers and their families is gratefully acknowledged along with that of the examiners from the CID and Gallaudet University staffs. Assistance in data analysis for the mainstreaming portion of this study was provided by Mary Weinstock.

This research was supported by Contract No. NO1-NS-4-2366 from the National Institute of Neurological and Communicative Disorders and Stroke of the National Institutes of Health to Central Institute for the Deaf.

integrated students (Reich, Hambleton, and Houldin 1977; Pflaster 1980).

5. They improve their relative performance in comparison to non-integrated students the longer they remain in the mainstream (Reich, Hambleton, and Houldin 1977).
6. They have well-informed parents who saw to it that their child got a hearing aid at an early age and continually received assistance outside the educational environment (Reich, Hambleton, and Houldin 1977).
7. They exhibit academic delay in comparison to their normally hearing peers (Kodman 1963; Quigley and Thomure 1968; Peckman, Sheridan, and Butler 1972).

These conclusions are based primarily on the performance of hard-of-hearing mainstreamed students. In fact, the recent books and chapters on the subject of mainstreaming focus on those with moderate or severe hearing impairments (Ross, Brackett, and Maxon 1982; Paul and Quigley 1990). However, the conclusions apply even more strongly when data for profoundly hearing-impaired students from total communication programs are examined. This paper examines the applicability of these conclusions to orally educated, profoundly hearing-impaired students.

In the summer of 1986, Central Institute for the Deaf (CID), under contract from the National Institutes of Health (NIH), had the opportunity to evaluate comprehensively a large group of orally educated, profoundly hearing-impaired students. Results of this study are described in a *Volta Review* article by Geers and Moog (1989). This chapter will focus on the functioning of these students in the mainstream, a topic that was not addressed in the *Volta Review* article.

SUBJECT

SELECTION

All subjects were required to meet the following criteria:

1. Sixteen or seventeen years of age (+ or − two months);
2. Better-ear speech frequency pure tone average (500, 1000, and 2000 Hz) greater than 85 dB (re: ANSI 1969);
3. Hearing impairment reported to be congenital or present by age two;
4. Nonverbal intelligence quotient no more than one standard deviation below average (i.e., IQ ⩾ 85);
5. Enrolled in a program that used oral communication exclusively throughout the preschool and elementary school years.

Because the students meeting these criteria were spread throughout the United States and because the test battery required approximately fifteen hours, a decision was made to gather the students in one location to conduct the testing. A Reading Research Camp was created at CID and students were invited to come to the camp for five days during the summer for both testing and recreation. Announcements of the project were placed in publications of the A.G. Bell Association, and directors of oral programs throughout the country were contacted to recommend the program to potential subjects. As a result, 210 students applied, but only 100 met all the criteria listed above. All of these 100 applicants were accepted and attended one of four summer camps conducted at CID. Transportation costs to and from St. Louis and other expenses associated with the camp were paid by the project grant[1] so that participation was not dependent on the family's ability to pay.

Characteristics

The 100 participants in the study represented a broad spectrum of orally educated students. Students came from twenty-six states and three provinces in Canada. There were forty-nine boys and fifty-one girls, ranging in age from 15 years 10 months to 18 years 2 months: four subjects were 15, twenty-nine were 16, sixty-three were 17, and four were 18 years old.

The data reveal that the subjects were alike in a number of ways. Socio-economic status of the families of these subjects generally was above average. Sixty-eight percent of the families had incomes above $35,000, putting these subjects in the middle to upper-middle class stratum. Only 4% had incomes below $15,000. Seventy-five percent had at least one parent who worked in either a managerial, sales, or professional position. Sixty percent of the subjects had at least one parent who had completed college, and 75% had at least one parent who had attended college. All children had at least one parent who had graduated from high school. The parents were, on the whole, highly supportive with 90% or more reporting that they had a good understanding of their child's hearing impairment, helped with correction of speech, language, and academic work, read to their child, and discussed television programs with their child on a regular basis while he or she was growing up. Ninety percent had been fitted with hearing aids by age 2 and 54% were fitted by age 1. The average age first aided was 21 months. Seventy-five percent had been enrolled in some form of

[1]This research was supported by contract number NO1-NS-4-2366 from the National Institute of Neurological and Communicative Disorders and Stroke of the National Institutes of Health to Central Institute for the Deaf.

parent-infant program. Sixty-three percent of the subjects had been enrolled in a special education preschool class by age three.

It might appear from these socio-economic and early intervention data that this is a highly select group. However it is likely that these 100 subjects represent a large proportion of the total population of profoundly hearing-impaired 16- and 17-year olds from oral programs. Based on the 1985–86 Annual Survey of Hearing-Impaired Children and Youth from the Center for Assessment and Demographic Studies at Gallaudet University, there are about 19,000 to 22,000 profoundly hearing-impaired children between birth and 21 years of age. If we assume an approximately even distribution throughout the age range, there are about 1,000 of these children in each age group, so that there were about 2,000 profoundly hearing-impaired 16- and 17-year olds at the time of this study. Since approximately 10% of profoundly hearing-impaired children educated orally (Allen and Karchmer, in press), during 1986 there were about 200 oral 16- and 17-year olds. Therefore this study sampled about half of the total population of orally educated, profoundly hearing-impaired 16- and 17-year olds available. Although this sample is a subset of hearing-impaired children in general, it is likely representative of those who remain in an oral setting.

Although the criteria for inclusion in the sample did not specify mainstream placement and most recruiting was done through schools for the deaf, 93% of the subjects were mainstreamed for all or part of the school day. However, all of the subjects had been enrolled in some form of special education at one time or another. Seventy-five percent began in a parent-infant program where they attended sessions on a weekly basis. Four subjects went directly from a parent-infant program into the mainstream, but the vast majority (96%) enrolled in a special education class that they attended daily from 3 or 4 years of age.

The number of years spent by these subjects in a special education class is depicted in a histogram in figure 1. The group had an average of nine years of special education with 25% spending three or fewer years in a special class. Age at mainstreaming is depicted in the histogram in figure 2. Twenty-five percent were mainstreamed by age 6 and 50% by age 11.

In terms of current educational placement, fifteen of the mainstreamed students had an interpreter for one or more of their academic courses. Another fifteen took one or more of their academic classes in a self-contained setting. Seven of the students were still enrolled in full-time special education. Sixty-three students were enrolled full-time in classes with normal-hearing students with no interpreter.

Many of the mainstreamed students reported receiving support services from their school. In figure 3 the number of hours of support service in the form of therapy, academic tutoring, resource room help,

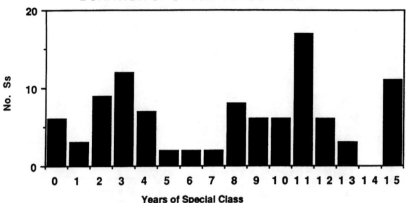

Figure 1. Frequency distribution histogram depicts the number of years enrolled in a special education class for the hearing impaired.

etc. is plotted in hours per week. The mainstreamed group averaged four hours per week of such service, with 25% receiving no support service in their high school.

The mainstream experience of the orally educated students reported here differs in significant ways from that of the students studied in research cited at the beginning of this chapter. While the findings of Allen and Osborn (1984) and Wolk, Karchmer, and Schildroth (1982) suggest that a sample of prelingually profoundly hearing-impaired students would contain relatively few who were educated in the mainstream, 93% of this sample were so classified. Data reported by Moores

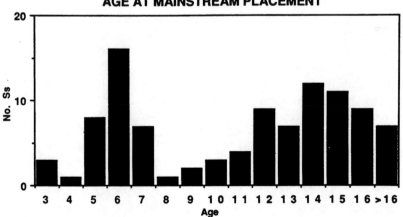

Figure 2. Frequency distribution histogram depicts the age at mainstream placement.

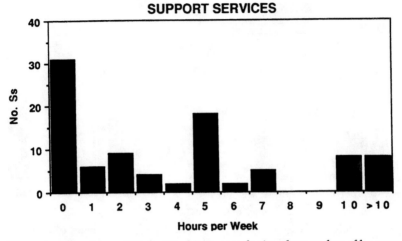

Figure 3. Frequency distribution histogram depicts the number of hours per week of support services provided for the ninety-three mainstreamed students.

and Kluwin (1986) and Libbey and Pronovost (1980) suggest that a sample of profoundly hearing-impaired students would be mainstreamed for nonacademic rather than academic subjects. However, examination of data reported by the 93 mainstreamed subjects in this sample indicates that all of them were mainstreamed for one or more academic subject.

Academic integration data for this sample are compared with data from Moores and Kluwin (1986) and Libbey and Pronovost (1980) in figure 4. Data reported by Moores and Kluwin (1986) were obtained from 185 hearing-impaired students from three large urban high schools. Students were mainstreamed from total communication settings and had sign interpreters for most of their integrated classes. Libbey and Pronovost (1980) obtained data from 221 profoundly hearing-impaired adolescents enrolled in thirty-two different public high schools across the country. Presumably this sample included both oral and total communication students, although results were not analyzed separately. It is apparent from this histogram that a considerably higher proportion of this exclusively oral group from the CID study was enrolled in mainstreamed classes for English, Mathematics, Social Studies, and Science than in either of the other reported samples.

METHOD

For the purpose of examining the impact of mainstreaming on this sample of orally educated subjects, four groups were formed on the

PERCENT MAINSTREAMED BY CLASS

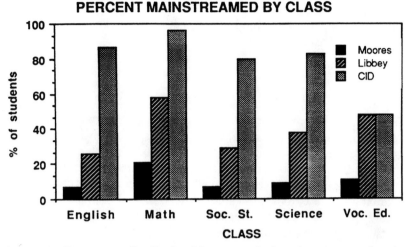

Figure 4. Frequency distribution histogram depicts the percent of main-streamed students integrated with normal hearing students for academic subjects and vocational education courses as reported by Moores and Kluwin (1986), Libbey and Pronovost (1980), and the present study (CID).

basis of age at the time of mainstream placement. Group 1 consisted of the twenty-eight students who spent an average of 2.1 years in special education and were placed in integrated classes at preschool, kindergarten, or first grade (i.e., between the ages of 3 and 6). Group 2 consisted of twenty-seven subjects who spent an average of 6.7 years in special education and were mainstreamed during elementary school (i.e., ages 7–12). Group 3 consisted of twenty-nine students who spent an average of 10.7 years in special education and were mainstreamed in junior high (i.e., ages 13–15). Group 4 consisted of sixteen students who either had just been placed in the mainstream at age 16 or who still were enrolled in all day special education. Group 4 averaged 13.3 years of special education.

To the extent that the students in this sample are representative of those reported by Reich, Hambleton, and Houldin (1977); Pflaster (1980); and Allen and Osborn (1984), better performance should be observed for students who have been mainstreamed longer than for those who entered the mainstream later in their educational experience.

A comprehensive battery of tests was administered to describe the hearing, speech, oral language, cognitive, reading, writing, and sign language abilities of subjects in the sample. This battery was administered by a team of audiologists, speech-language pathologists, psychologists, and teachers of the hearing-impaired, who evaluated each child individually during the camp session. Sign language evaluations were conducted by two researchers from Gallaudet University, one who was skilled in signed English and a deaf adult who communicated in American Sign Language.

RESULTS

Mean scores are presented in table I for each of the four mainstream groups on measures of hearing, intelligence, speech, and communication skill. Analyses of variance were conducted for each of these measures and the F ratio is presented in the last column. When the overall F reached significance at the .05 level or better, differences between individual group means were tested using Fisher's Protected Least Significant Difference Test (Winer 1971). Significantly different pairs are indicated by lower-case italic letters.

Hearing

The better ear averages for the four groups are quite similar, ranging from 97 to 103 dB, but the early mainstream group (3–6 years) has significantly more hearing (98 dB) than the junior high group (103 dB). These differences in auditory skills are more apparent when aided speech perception scores are examined. The aided articulation index (Gittelman and Popelka 1987), a measure of the audible portion of the speech spectrum, is significantly greater for the early mainstream group than for any of the other groups. The index is lower in the junior high group than in any of the other groups. A similar pattern is seen in word recognition scores on the Monosyllable, Trochee, Spondee Test (MTS; Erber and Alencewicz 1976), with students mainstreamed at junior high having the lowest scores. On the Visual Enhancement subtest of the Minimal Auditory Capabilities Battery (Owens et al. 1985), no significant differences were observed in the lipreading alone scores but the aided lipreading scores were significantly better for the early mainstream group (85%) than for the other three groups.

Cognitive Abilities

Both Performance and Verbal subtests of the Wechsler Adult Intelligence Scale (Wechsler 1981) were administered. The Performance IQ is considered a measure of learning potential in deaf students. For a student with a Performance IQ within the normal range, the Verbal IQ is considered a measure of achievement in language in relation to normal hearing individuals. Thus, one might expect to see significantly higher verbal IQ scores in students who had been enrolled in the main-

Table I. Descriptive Measures

	Score	Age Mainstreamed				F
		Group 1 3–6	Group 2 7–11	Group 3 12–15	Group 4 16+	
Hearing						
Better Ear: 500, 100, 2000 Hz	dB, HL	98[a]	99	103[a]	97	3.44*
Aided Articulation Index	Percent	56[a,b,c]	45[a,d]	29[b,d,e]	42[c,e]	8.04***
Monosyllable, Spondee, Trochee	% Recog.	73[a,b]	59[a,c]	44[b,c]	59	5.95***
MAC—Visual Enhancement	% Lipread.	61	57	57	52	1.73NS
	Lip + Aid	84[a,b,c]	74[a]	69[b]	68[c]	4.73**
Intelligence						
Wechsler Adult Intelligence Scale	PIQ	110	109	115	108	1.20NS
	VIQ	92	88	88	85	1.30NS
Speech						
Phonetic Inventory	% Correct	86	85	78	81	2.08NS
Speech Intelligibility Evaluation	% Intell.	91[a]	86[b]	78[a,b]	84	6.01***
Communication Skills						
Language Proficiency Interview	Signed English	0.6	0.7	0.9	1.1	0.67NS
(0 = None; 4 = Excellent)	ASL	0.6[a]	1.0[b]	1.1	1.7[a,b]	3.32*
	Oral	3.7	3.4	3.4	3.2	2.07NS

NS = Not Significant
* = $p \leq .05$
** = $p \leq .01$
*** = $p \leq .001$

a
b } significantly different pairs
c
d } 95% confidence—Fisher PLSD
e

stream longer. However, no significant differences were observed between the mainstream groups in either verbal or performance IQ scores. Furthermore, average verbal IQ scores were within the average range (i.e., >85) for all four groups.

Speech Production Abilities

The CID Phonetic Inventory (Moog 1989) evaluates a subject's ability to imitate fifteen different vowel and twenty-two different consonant sounds in single syllables, repeated syllables, and alternated syllables. No significant differences were observed between groups in this phonetic-level speech skill. The Speech Intelligibility Evaluation (SPINE; Monsen 1981) was used to estimate overall intelligibility. Groups 1 and 2 achieved high speech intelligibility scores of 91% and 86%. Group 3, the junior high group, was rated significantly less intelligible with an average score of 78%. However group 4 students who were not mainstreamed until age 16 or later averaged 84% intelligibility, which was not significantly different from scores obtained by students mainstreamed during preschool and elementary school, a result contrary to results reported by Reich, Hambleton, and Houldin (1977).

Communication Skill

Each subject's language proficiency was rated in three communication modes in a conversational interview with an experienced communicator. The Language Proficiency Interview (LPI) was originally designed by the Foreign Service to assess a candidate's facility with a second language. It has been adapted by researchers at Gallaudet University to assess sign and oral language proficiency. Separate interviews were conducted by a signed English examiner and an ASL examiner, both of whom were from Gallaudet University, and an oral teacher of the deaf. Levels of proficiency were reported on a five point scale, with 0 representing no skill in the language evaluated and 4 representing a high level of proficiency.

Most of the sample knew no sign language at all. Signed English scores remained essentially the same across the four groups. However, there was a significant tendency for ASL competence to increase with years spent in special education. All of the students communicated quite well orally with average ratings of 3 and 4 in all four groups, so no significant differences were observed here either. Oral proficiency ratings at level 3 indicated practical proficiency with oral English. At this level the student can accomplish social formulas with sophistication and precision. His or her vocabulary is broad enough to deal with most topics without groping for words, but complex topics might require circumlocution. The student comprehends at a normal rate, requiring few repetitions. Oral proficiency ratings at level 4 indicate that the subject can converse with sophistication and precision on complex, unfamiliar, and technical topics. The student's vocabulary is broad, colloquial, and idiomatic. Fluency is smooth and always at a rate appropriate to the topic. Mispronunciation is rare and does not interfere with communication. Comprehension is almost never a problem.

Contrary to results reported by Reich, Hambleton, and Houldin (1977), students mainstreamed in junior high and high school exhibited oral proficiency comparable to that attained by those who had been mainstreamed for all or most of their educational experience.

Reading Skills

A reading grade average was obtained for each subject by averaging grade equivalent scores on the following seven subtests:

Stanford Achievement Test	Reading Comprehension
	Spelling
California Achievement Test	Vocabulary
Woodcock Reading Mastery Test	Word Attack
Peabody Individual Achievement Test	Reading Comprehension
Gates-MacGinitie Reading Survey	Reading Speed
	Reading Accuracy

This average reading score ranged from 3rd grade 2nd month to post high school. Average scores of each group are presented in the top row of table II. Group 1, with an average grade equivalent of 9th grade 1st month, scored significantly higher than group 4, with an average grade equivalent of 6th grade 7th month. This is consistent with Reich, Hambleton, and Houldin (1977) who reported better achievement scores in students mainstreamed longer. However, when pairs of means were examined, only group 4 differed significantly from group 1. Average reading scores of groups 2 and 3 did not differ significantly from those of group 1, in spite of the fact that they were mainstreamed at later ages.

Another way of examining these data is to look at the number of subjects in each group who achieve at or near expectation for normal hearing students their age. Since most of these subjects had just completed 9th or 10th grade, an overall reading grade average of 8th grade or higher was considered to be age appropriate. Students with reading grade averages of 7th grade or lower were considered to be below expectation in reading skills.

A chi-square statistic was used to compare the distribution of good and poor readers in the four groups. The distribution is presented in table III. A total chi-square of 8.919 ($df = 3$) was obtained that was sig-

Table II. Reading, Writing, and Spoken Language Measures

	Type	Group 1 3–6	Group 2 7–11	Group 3 12–15	Group 4 16+	F
Average Reading Score	Grade	9.1^a	7.5	8.0	6.7^a	3.03*
Average Syntax Score	% Correct	87	83	83	80	1.6NS
Written Composition (0 = Poor; 6 = Excellent)	Rating	$4.0^{a,b}$	3.2^a	3.5	3.1^b	3.0*
Average Vocabulary Score	Age	$12.9^{a,b}$	11.0^a	11.5	9.7^b	3.4*
Expressive Discourse	DSS	11.8^a	10.5	10.5	9.2^a	3.7**
Receptive Discourse	DAB	$26^{a,b,c}$	22^a	22^b	22^c	2.9*

NS = Not Significant
* = $p \leq .05$
** = $p \leq .01$
*** = $p \leq .001$

a
b
c } significantly different pairs
d   95% confidence—Fisher PLSD
e

Table III. Distribution of Good and Poor Readers by Grade Entering the Mainstream

	Good Readers Grade 8–12	Poor Readers Grade 3–7
Group 1 Preschool	22	6
Group 2 Elementary	13	14
Group 3 Junior High	18	11
Group 4 High School	6	10

$\chi^2 = 8.92$

$p \leq .03$

nificant at the .03 level of confidence. The highest proportion of academically successful students were those mainstreamed at the preschool and junior high levels. Almost 80% of those mainstreamed at age 6 or younger and over 60% of those mainstreamed during junior high demonstrated 8th grade reading skills or better. The good performance of the junior high group is somewhat unexpected in view of their more profound hearing impairment, poorer speech perception scores, and previous research demonstrating poorer performance by children mainstreamed at older ages.

The relatively small proportion of good readers in group 4 (less than 40%) is not surprising since many of them had just entered the mainstream and some had not yet left special education. A more interesting result is that the twenty-seven subjects who had been mainstreamed during their elementary school years were split almost evenly between good and poor readers. A comparison of this result with the higher proportion of successful readers in the junior high group indicates that some of the subjects in group 2 may have been mainstreamed too early, before reading and language skills were firmly established.

Syntactic Ability

Scores on two measures of syntactic ability were averaged to obtain a syntax score. The Test of Syntactic Abilities Screening Form (Quigley et al. 1978) tests the subject's ability to distinguish correct syntactic structures from incorrect versions. The Written Language Syntax Test (Berry 1981) tests the subject's ability to construct a syntactically correct sentence to describe a picture from a set of randomly ordered words.

Average percent-correct scores of each of the four groups are presented in the second row of table II. All of the subjects did well on these tests, scoring 80% or higher. Although group 1 scores are highest at 87% and group 4 scores are lowest at 80%, there is no significant difference between the mean scores of the four groups.

Composition Skill

Each subject wrote an essay that was scored by the Educational Testing Service using a rating system developed for evaluating composition skill in normal hearing students (Mullis 1980). The possible ratings ranged from 0 for an incomprehensible paper to 6 for a superior paper. Ratings encompassed a variety of factors including writing with clarity on the selected topic, imagination and originality, good sentence structure, organization, and mechanical correctness. Although no papers in this sample were rated at level 0 or 1, some were rated at level 2, indicating use of immature sentence structure, poor organization, inappropriate word choices, and frequent mechanical errors. Most of the essays received ratings of 3 and 4. A few essays (those rated 5 and 6) contained considerable imagination and originality. These essays were highly descriptive and used a number of literary devices. Examples of essays rated at various levels are reproduced in figure 5.

Average ratings for each of the four groups are presented in the third row of table II. Paired comparisons using the Fisher PLSD test revealed that the average rating of 4.0 for group 1 was significantly different from the mean ratings of groups 2 and 4, but not significantly different from the average of 3.5 obtained by the junior high group.

Spoken Language

An oral vocabulary score was obtained by averaging age scores obtained on the Peabody Picture Vocabulary Test (Dunn and Dunn 1981) and the Expressive One-Word Picture Vocabulary Test (Gardner 1979). Print was not used with the Peabody so subjects had to rely on their lipreading and listening skills to understand words presented orally. The Expressive One-Word Picture Vocabulary Test presents a progression of pictures that the subject must name. Average vocabulary age scores are presented in table II. The average age score of group 1 is close to the 13-year-old level. This score is significantly higher than the scores of 11.0 years for group 2 and 9.7 years for group 4, but not significantly different than the 11.5 years age score obtained by the junior high group.

In addition to vocabulary, more global measures of receptive and expressive spoken language ability at the discourse level were also obtained. Developmental Sentence Scores (DSS) (Lee and Koenigsknecht

DIRECTIONS

Everybody knows of something that is worth talking about. Maybe you know about a famous building like the Empire State Building in New York City or something like the Golden Gate Bridge in San Francisco. Or you might know a lot about the Mormon Tabernacle in Salt Lake City or the new sports stadium in Atlanta or St. Louis. Or you might be familiar with something from nature, like Niagara Falls, a gigantic wheat field, a grove of orange trees, or a part of a wide, muddy river like the Mississippi.

There is probably something you can describe. Choose something you know about. It may be something from around where you live or something you have seen while traveling, or something you have studied in school. Think about it for a while and then write a description of what it looks like so that it could be recognized by someone who has read your description.

Name what you are describing and try to use your best writing.

Rating 2 = Weak

I went to the waterpark. It have tube floating, water slides, riverpedal boat and pools. It is so great! I could play in pools. My friend played volleyball in a pool. When I went up to the water slides. I could scream and fast. It was so fun! I bet you'll love the greatest waterpark.

Rating 3 = Acceptable

St. Louis South County
That's where I live and there are a lots of new places. It build a lot of stores in Lemay Ferry, but it causes alot of traffic. Also in Lindbergh, there are new stores and restuarests! It is very neat because I can go to some stores around my house instead of travelling way up to north. They were building new two hotels in Lindbergh and also a restuarest named "Bob Evans". It won't open till June 23.

Most friends of mine wanted to work new stores whenever they are done this year. But I got a job already and I don't have to worry about other jobs!

Few years ago, we used to have a drive-in movie by my house. Suddenly it knocked down and now we have Dierburg and other small stores in Lemay Ferry. But Ronnies (movie theater), they build new small stores and a restuarest (Fridays). That place used to be a drive-in movie! There are a lost of changes places!

They are building bigger road so they won't cause lot of traffics in Lindbergh. By Lemay Ferry, it was build bigger road in few years ago. It is much better because there is no traffic.

Rating 4 = Good

Washington D.C.
Washington D.C. is an interesting place to visit during summer vacations. It is located near the Potomac River in the northeast.

Figure 5.   The ETS wholistic rating scale for descriptive essays is illustrated by examples for levels 2 through 6.

There are a lot of interesting museums and homes to see. One of the most interesting homes is "Mount Vernon", where our first president, George Washington, lived. It is located somewhere in Virginia. You could see the Washington Monument, one of the world's third tallest monument, in Washington D.C. There are so many things that you can see in Washington D.C. that I can't put down the places. I'm sure you will have a lot of good time when you visit Washington D.C. sometime in the future.

Rating 5 = Very Good

Florida
Florida would be a nice place to settle in the winter-time. Florida is beautiful—just imagine, a dream house on a beach front with a swimming pool, a garden, and beautiful flowers. There would be green grass around the house with a water sprinkling system. There is alot of pretty, bug boats on the ocean. The water on the ocean looks so fresh. The sky is blue with clouds so white like cotton. There are many sports cars like corvettes, porsches, ferraris, etc. There many small and big homes on and near the beach front. The fish you may catch will look so good to eat for dinner.

Rating 6 = Superior

I enjoy downhill skiing, and one of my favorite places to ski at is Sugar Loaf Mountain Resort in Cedar, Michigan. It is located on the northwest tip of Michigan by Lake Michigan. It is a big mountain by Michigan's standards; as you stand on the top of the mountain, you can see a vast range of environment. On one side, you can see Lake Michigan, which looks like an ocean since it is so big. Several other mountains can be seen in the distance; some of them are other ski resorts. The land around it is diverse, some areas wooded while others are just plain farmland.

As a ski resort, the mountain is mostly open area as a result of trees cleared to make room for skiers, also called "slopes" or "trails". Unlike Colorado, there aren't that many pine or related trees in comparison to other kinds, like oak and maple. The lack of leaves for cover allows one to see through them, providing a more open feel for the area.

No ski resort is complete, obviously, without the slopes. The types of slopes vary in terrain. Some are no steeper than ten degrees but others are more than 45 degrees, to provide a challenge for expert skiers. Sugar Loaf has an easy slope that is a mile long and a slope called "Awful Awful" which is a big challenge because in addition to its steepness, it is like a waffle, containing bumps about three feet high! The resort has about 15 slopes which encircle all around the mountain. The slopes, from a distance, look like white stripes down a black mountain. The contrast can't be missed.

In order for the skiers to go down the mountain, they must get up first, of course. "Chairlifts" serve this function by carrying people seated on benches attached to a cable and spaced about 20 feet

Figure 5 *continued*

apart. Pulleys on the top and bottom hold it tight and moving. They look like Christmas decorations, because of the lines of cable with bright objects on them.

The mountain is so big, you can only see a tiny portion of it while on it, but from a distance you can see half of it. These different view points also have different looks.

Figure 5

1974) were obtained for fifty consecutive utterances transcribed from the oral language proficiency interview described earlier. These scores reflect the complexity of syntax used by the students in conversational exchanges. Average DSS scores are presented in table II. As was the case for vocabulary, students mainstreamed at preschool (group 1) produced significantly more complex sentences than did students mainstreamed at age 16 or older (group 4). However the differences for the intermediate groups were not significant.

The receptive measure of global discourse skills was the Story Comprehension subtest of the Diagnostic Achievement Battery (Newcomer and Curtis 1984). The examiner read aloud to the subject a set of stories of increasing length and complexity. The subject was scored in terms of his or her ability to answer a series of questions about each story immediately after it had been read. Group 1 averaged 26 correct responses out of 32 questions, which is typical performance for normal hearing adolescents and is significantly better than all three of the other mainstream groups.

Background Characteristics and School Adjustment

Extensive background information regarding these families was collected from questionnaires completed by the parents. There was no significant difference between the groups in age first aided or age first receiving special education. There was no significant difference in socioeconomic variables such as parental education, income, and occupation. Parents rated their expectations for and participation in their child's education in various areas. Sample items from this section of the parent questionnaire are presented in figure 6 along with the percentage of ratings in each category.

When ratings were compared across the four mainstream groups, there was no significant difference in parental expectations for or involvement in their child's education. Students in all four groups have well-informed and supportive parents, as was also observed in the Reich, Hambleton, and Houldin (1977) sample of mainstreamed students.

What is the highest level of education you realistically expect your child to complete?

POST GRADUATE DEGREE (lawyer, doctor, etc.) 6%
COLLEGE/UNIVERSITY DEGREE 72%
SOME COLLEGE 12%
HIGH SCHOOL PLUS PROFESSIONAL TRAINING 9%
LEAVE SCHOOL AS SOON AS POSSIBLE................ 0%

How particular would you say you are about the way your child uses English (correct grammar, vocabulary, etc.)?

VERY PARTICULAR.................................... 49%
FAIRLY PARTICULAR 34%
ABOUT AVERAGE 16%
NOT TOO PARTICULAR 0%
NOT AT ALL PARTICULAR 0%

How often do you tell your child how to construct sentences, when to use certain words, and in other ways help with his or her English grammar?

EVERY DAY 36%
JUST ABOUT EVERY DAY 25%
ABOUT THREE OR FOUR TIMES A WEEK 13%
ABOUT ONCE OR TWICE A WEEK...................... 15%
LESS THAN ONCE A WEEK 7%
NOT AT ALL... 3%

How often do you introduce your child to a new word?

EVERY DAY 13%
JUST ABOUT EVERY DAY 28%
A COUPLE OF TIMES A WEEK........................... 33%
ABOUT ONCE EVERY TWO WEEKS...................... 8%
ABOUT ONCE A MONTH 7%
NOT AT ALL OR RARELY 9%

When your child was young, before he or she started school, how frequently did you read to him or her?

JUST ABOUT EVERY DAY 53%
ABOUT THREE OR FOUR TIMES A WEEK 18%
A COUPLE OF TIMES A WEEK........................... 12%
ABOUT ONCE A WEEK 7%
LESS THAN ONCE A WEEK 2%
NOT AT ALL... 7%

Figure 6. Sample items from the parent questionnaire with distribution of observed responses.

Another set of data was collected from questionnaires completed by the students themselves. A few sample items from this questionnaire are also included in figure 7, along with the percent of students responding in each category. These responses indicated no significant difference between groups in their adjustment to the school environment. Most subjects in all groups reported that they often or sometimes understand what happens in class, feel a part of their school, and communicate easily with teachers. There was no significant difference in their report of hearing aid use. Most subjects reported receiving benefit from amplification.

Below are several statements which describe how students feel about their school. Put a check on the line that best fits the statement.

	Often	Sometimes	Seldom	Never
I understand what happens in class.	44%	53%	3%	0%
I feel that I am a part of my school.	57%	33%	9%	1%
My friends help me when I need help with my school work.	44%	32%	19%	4%
I can communicate easily with my teachers.	59%	33%	6%	2%
I feel alone at my school.	4%	22%	27%	46%
I understand the teachers.	43%	52%	5%	0%
I understand class discussion.	30%	52%	15%	3%
Other students are helpful to me.	51%	35%	11%	3%

Try to think back to when you were 12 years old. When you were 12, how much did you wear your hearing aid?

MOST OF THE TIME 87%
SOMETIMES OUTSIDE OF SCHOOL 6%
DURING THE SCHOOL DAY ONLY 7%
ONLY DURING AUDITORY TRAINING 0%
NOT AT ALL 0%

continued

Now think of your present age. How much do you wear your hearing aid?

MOST OF THE TIME 90%
SOMETIMES OUTSIDE OF SCHOOL 4%
DURING THE SCHOOL DAY ONLY. 4%
ONLY DURING AUDITORY TRAINING 1%
NOT AT ALL. 1%

If you wear a hearing aid, how much benefit do you get from it?

ESSENTIAL. 55%
USEFUL. 30%
SOMEWHAT USEFUL 11%
MINIMALLY USEFUL 2%
NOT AT ALL USEFUL 1%

Figure 7. Sample items from the student questionnaire with distribution of observed responses.

CONCLUSIONS

These results indicate that even profoundly hearing-impaired students can achieve normal academic development. The subjects who were mainstreamed between the ages of three and six were decidedly the best performers. Students in this group obtained significantly higher scores than one or more of the later-mainstreamed groups on most of the measures collected for this study.

The subjects who were mainstreamed at age sixteen or later (including seven students who are enrolled in schools for the deaf) demonstrated the poorest performance. They obtained the lowest scores of the four groups on most measures. This is consistent with results reported by Allen and Osborn (1984), indicating that non-integrated (or in this case recently integrated) students do not perform as well as their integrated age mates.

The subjects mainstreamed during elementary grades and the subjects mainstreamed during junior high showed relatively few differences from students in the other groups. The differences that did exist between the two groups favored the elementary-aged group for auditory speech perception skills and speech intelligibility. However, in spite of their poorer auditory skills, the junior high group had a higher proportion of subjects achieving at or above the 8th grade level than did the group mainstreamed in elementary school.

Therefore, although the extreme groups appear to support the effectiveness of early mainstreaming for some children, there is no evidence from the vast majority of this sample that language or academic delays are associated with longer special education placement. On the contrary, data from the junior high group seem to suggest that extensive special education allows these students to succeed in the mainstream in spite of more severely impaired hearing and speech perception abilities.

Public Law 94-142 requires that handicapped children receive a free and appropriate education in the least restrictive environment, which often is interpreted to mean mainstreaming as early as possible. However, extensive examination of students who were mainstreamed at different points in their education experience suggests that, for orally educated, profoundly hearing-impaired children, special education throughout elementary school may improve their success rate in the mainstream. For these children, successful integration into regular classrooms is the result, not the cause, of well-developed language and reading skills. These children require intensive special education with trained professionals in order to develop adequate language skills for mainstreaming. The amount of special education required varies from child to child and is probably affected by a multitude of factors such as the child's residual hearing, intelligence, family support, aptitude for acquiring language, and skill of the child's teacher. One must be sensitive to evaluating these factors when helping families decide when to mainstream their hearing-impaired child.

REFERENCES

Allen, T. E., and Karchmer, M. A. In press. Communication in classrooms for hearing-impaired students: Student, teacher and program characteristics. In *Manual Communication in American Education,* ed. H. Bornstein. Washington, DC: Gallaudet University Press.

Allen, T. E., and Osborn, T. I. 1984. Academic integration of hearing impaired students: Demographic, handicapping and achievement factors. *American Annals of the Deaf* 129:100–113.

Berry, S. R. 1981. *Written Language Syntax Test.* Washington, DC: Gallaudet College Press.

California Achievement Test. 1977. Monterey, CA: CTB/McGraw-Hill.

Dunn, L. M., and Dunn, L. M. 1981. *Peabody Picture Vocabulary Test–Revised* (PPVT-R). Circle Pines, MN: American Guidance.

Dunn, L. M., and Markwardt, F. C. 1970. *Peabody Individual Achievement Test–Revised.* Circle Pines, MN: American Guidance.

Erber, N. P., and Alencewicz, C. 1976. Audiological evaluation of deaf children. *Journal of Speech and Hearing Disorders* 41:256–67.

Gates, A. J., and MacGinitie, W. H. 1965. *Gates-MacGinitie Reading Test.* Chicago: Riverside Publishing Company.

Gardner, M. F. 1979. *Expressive One-Word Picture Vocabulary Test.* Novato, CA: Academic Therapy Publications.

Gardner, E. F., Rudman, H. C., Karlsen, G. and Merwin, J. C. 1982. *Stanford Achievement Test* (17th edition). Cleveland, OH: Psychological Corporation.

Geers, A. E., and Moog, J. S. 1989. Factors predictive of the development of literacy in profoundly hearing impaired adolescents. *The Volta Review* 91 (2): 69–86.

Gittelman, D. A., and Popelka, G. R. 1987. The dynamic range configuration audiogram. *The Volta Review* 89:69–83.

Jensema, C. 1975. *The Relationship between Academic Achievement and the Demographic Characteristics of Hearing-Impaired Children and Youth* (Series R, No. 2). Washington, DC: Gallaudet University, Center for Assessment and Demographic Studies.

Kodman, F. Jr. 1963. Educational status of hard of hearing children in the classroom. *Journal of Speech and Hearing Disorders* 38:297–99.

Lee, L. L., and Koenigsknecht, R. A. 1974. *Developmental Sentence Scoring*. Evanston, IL: Northwestern University Press.

Libbey, S. S., and Pronovost, W. 1980. Communication practices of mainstreamed hearing-impaired adolescents. *The Volta Review* 82:197–213.

Monsen, R. 1981. A usable test for the speech intelligibility of deaf talkers. *American Annals of the Deaf* 126:845–52.

Moog, J. S. 1989. *The CID Phonetic Inventory*. St. Louis, MO: Central Institute for the Deaf.

Moores, D. F., and Kluwin, T. N. 1986. Issues in school placement. In *Deaf Children in America*, eds. A. N. Schildroth and M. A. Karchmer. San Diego, CA: College Hill Press.

Mullis, I. 1980. *Using the Primary Trait System for Evaluating Writing*. Princeton, NJ: Educational Testing Service.

Newcomer, P. L., and Curtis, D. 1984. *Diagnostic Achievement Battery*. Austin, TX: Pro-Ed.

Owens, E., Kessler, D., Teleen, E., and Schubert, E. 1985. *Minimal Auditory Capabilities Battery*–Revised Edition. St. Louis: Auditec.

Paul, P. V., and Quigley, S. P. 1990. *Education and Deafness*. White Plains, NY: Longman.

Peckman, C. S., Sheridan, M., and Butler, N. R. 1972. School attainment of seven-year-old children with hearing difficulties. *Developmental Medicine and Child Neurology*. 592–602.

Pflaster, G. 1980. A factor analysis of variables related to academic performance of hearing impaired children in regular classes. *The Volta Review* 82:71–83.

Quigley, S., and Thomure, R. 1968. *Some Effects of Hearing Impairment upon School Performance*. Urbana, IL: University of Illinois, Institute for Research on Exceptional Children.

Quigley, S. P., Steinkamp, M. W., Power, D. J., and Jones, B. W. 1978. *Test of Syntactic Abilities*. Beaverton, OR: Dormac.

Reich, C., Hambleton, D., and Houldin, B. K. 1977. The integration of hearing impaired children in regular classrooms. *American Annals of the Deaf* 122: 534–43.

Ross, M., Brackett, D., and Maxon, A. M. 1982. *Hard of Hearing Children in Regular Schools*. Englewood Cliffs, NJ: Prentice Hall.

Wechsler, D. 1981. *Manual for the Wechsler Adult Intelligence Scale–Revised*. New York: Psychological Corporation.

Winer, B. J. 1971. *Statistical Principles in Experimental Design*. NY: McGraw Hill.

Wolk, S., Karchmer, M. A., and Schildroth, A. 1982. *Patterns of Academic and Nonacademic Integration Among Hearing Impaired Students in Special Education*.

Series R, No. 9. Washington, DC: Gallaudet College, Office of Demographic Studies.

Woodcock, R. W. 1973. *Woodcock Reading Mastery Tests*. Circle Pines, MN: American Guidance Services.

Chapter • 17

Parents and Students Speak

Ruth R. Green

It has been said that "experience is the best teacher." If this is indeed the case, it is important to consider the experiences of parents whose children have been in mainstream educational settings and of the children themselves. Their personal accounts can reaffirm methods, elucidate areas for change, and help us reconsider our approach. Parents and children both are the experts of the mainstream process: their reactions and perspectives can either validate or call into question the mainstream placement decision.

Parents select educational options for their children depending upon what is available in their geographical area. In addition, the professionals with whom the parents have initial contact can shape their choices. We know that no one educational road is right for all hearing-impaired children. We also know that the experiences of those who have completed the journey will provide a perspective and will help us consider the obstacles and signposts along the way.

All the children in this chapter were educated in the mainstream. Each parent-contributor has a hearing-impaired child who was educated in the mainstream. The following questions were posed to parents:

When you first learned your child had a hearing impairment, what were your family's reactions?

What factors contributed to your selection of the educational program that your child first attended?

How do you feel about your decision?

What were the factors that contributed to your child's educational progress?

Did your child receive any support services while he or she attended school?

It was indicated that occasionally there are teachers who are concerned that parents are too directive. What strategies did you use to provide information to school personnel without creating antagonism?

What type of social experience did your child have?

Do you think a mainstream education has helped prepare your child for adult life? (How and why or why not?)

What recommendations would you make to other parents and to educators?

The following questions were posed to students:

What academic challenges did you face in the mainstream?

What support did you receive?

What were your social experiences? Were you involved with extracurricular activities?

How did other students relate to you?

What suggestions for changes would you make?

What recommendations would you give to teachers and to parents?

THE PARENTS SPEAK

Barbara Marlow-Murray (Mother)

Sherri Marlow (Daughter)   Date of Birth: 11/23/73. Junior, Edward R. Murrow High School, New York City.

When I first learned of Sherri's hearing impairment, my family refused to acknowledge her loss. It was particularly difficult for my parents, who spoke Yiddish at home and had to start to speak English to Sherri.

Sherri's hearing loss was diagnosed at the New York League for the Hard of Hearing. I wanted Sherri to become integrated into the hearing world and not be segregated from it, so I chose to have Sherri develop her oral/aural skills. I felt it was the right decision, and I feel happy with my decision. Several factors contributed to Sherri's educational success:

1. Her ability to concentrate and her drive to do well.
2. Early therapeutic settings—where she would work daily for an hour or more with me.
3. A good therapist at the New York League for the Hard of Hearing, who pushed me to constantly work with Sherri.
4. Good oral deaf adult role models, who instilled in me the confidence that I could develop Sherri's oral/listening skills.

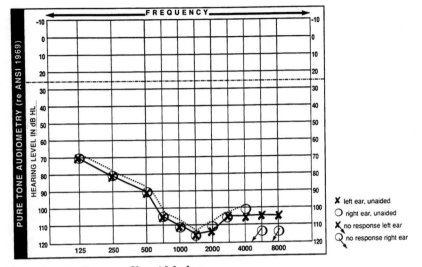

Figure 1. Audiogram: Sherri Marlow.

5. I always developed a positive relationship with Sherri's teachers, supervisors, and her peers.

Sherri received resource room help in school and speech and language therapy two hours weekly in addition to intensive language therapy at the New York League for the Hard of Hearing. I tried to keep school personnel informed and was active but not aggressive. I was active in the PTA.

Since Sherri didn't attend her neighborhood school but attended the public school in the district that had a resource room program for hearing-impaired students, it was difficult for Sherri socially. While she had hearing friends in school, they were not in the neighborhood and this limited out-of-school contacts. I think that, in spite of her social limitations, the mainstream experience expanded Sherri's horizons.

Parents need to be advocates for their hearing-impaired child and need to treat the child as a child first, then as a child with deafness. Educators need to give hearing-impaired children a chance. Recognize their individualities, love them, educate them, have high expectations for them.

Larry Avrin (Father)

Jeffrey Avrin (Son) Date of Birth: 5/2/72. Senior, Middletown High School North, New Jersey.

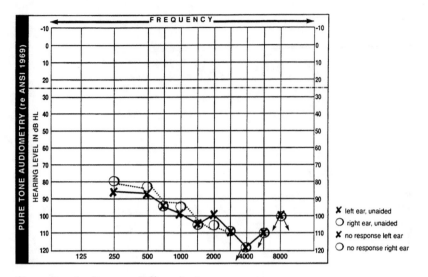

Figure 2.   Audiogram: Jeffrey Avrin.

When we first learned of Jeff's hearing impairment, my wife and I were in shock. We found it hard to believe and were angry. After a short time, we began to seek help. We desired to have Jeff learn to communicate orally and to function in the normal (hearing) world. As Jeff prepares for high school graduation and college, I feel that this was a correct decision.

The things that helped contribute to Jeff's success were his speech therapists, the language therapy program at the New York League for the Hard of Hearing, the academic support provided at his school, and his parents' persistence. In order to help his school better understand Jeff and his needs, we would arrange to meet with the teachers and to encourage open and free communication. Jeff's educational experiences have helped prepare him for the challenges ahead.

Social interactions have been difficult. While Jeff has attained Eagle Scout status, he has no real close friends.

To parents who learn that they have a child with impaired hearing, I would recommend that they become knowledgeable about services available, and that they participate in a parent support group. Above all, support but continue to push your child to practice his or her speech and remember that there is a light at the end of the tunnel.

To those educators who have hearing-impaired students but are unfamiliar with their special needs, I urge that they seek professional input. To professionals who are trained to work with hearing-impaired children, I encourage you to think about what you have done and continue to work to help more children.

Eve Spitzer (Mother)

Libbi Spitzer Kakon (Daughter)   Date of Birth: 8/26/69. Junior in college.

My daughter, Libbi, while attending college, is working as an assistant teacher in a class of developmentally delayed preschoolers and substituting in all grades (5 to 12). When we first learned of Libbi's hearing impairment, our reaction was one of disbelief and shock. With the support of the League, we decided to have Libbi attend a regular school with normal-hearing children. Our goal was to help Libbi learn to talk and be like everyone else. Because our family is ultra-orthodox, we would not consider anything other than her attending a Yeshiva (a religious Jewish School). I would make the same decision today.

I think Libbi's success was related to her ongoing speech and language therapy and non-stop incessant tutoring in all school subjects through 7th grade. Libbi's own love of books helped. She read and read and read. I feel that was a primary factor contributing to her educational progress. All of the help Libbi received was out of school. She received no help in school. To help the school personnel, I distributed pamphlets which the League publishes. School visits by the professional staff helped. I had a notebook which went between the teachers and myself on a daily basis. I showered them with praise (positive reinforcement).

Libbi had good social experiences. She was lucky, I think. Of

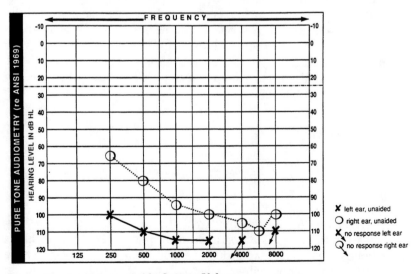

Figure 3.   Audiogram: Libbi Spitzer Kakon.

course, there were always exceptions, but, for the most part, her class-mates were helpful and caring. However, her social life was not the same as that of her peers. She had friends, even "best" friends, yet it was a different kind of relationship than those of other "best friends." She didn't spend long hours chatting with them, either in school or at home on the phone (which, incidentally, she uses with comparative ease). I have observed other hearing-impaired youngsters exposed to a similar type of upbringing as Libbi, undergoing the same kind of social experience. I get the feeling that "somehow they just don't fit in."

I think her mainstream experience has prepared her for adult life. The world out there is a *hearing world*—that's it, plain and simple. I believe a segregated education is not representative of the world "out there." I also feel that practice makes perfect, and by constantly asso-ciating with normal-hearing peers, communication skills are sharp-ened. I would tell other parents it's tough—but, rewarding. Reach out to others who can help you—parents and young adults who have done it, as well as the professionals. Sometimes, just sharing with an-other can help alleviate the anxiety. And, take one step at a time, one day at a time. Worrying doesn't help—take it from someone who knows.

As for the school personnel, try to put yourself into their shoes. I am referring to both parent and child. Please be understanding and "have a heart." The teacher's praise and recognition of the child's efforts is probably as important to the child as parental approval. So teachers, be lavish.

And to all: I, the very involved parent of a hearing-impaired child, now, young adult, am only just beginning to realize that I don't really comprehend the difficulties one encounters when one is hearing-impaired. As much as I thought I knew and felt, I really didn't. After all, nobody can actually put themselves in someone else's shoes. So be tolerant. The child with impaired hearing deserves all the praise you can give, and then some!

THE CHILDREN SPEAK

Darby Leigh   Date of Birth: 2/6/73. Junior, Dalton School, New York City.

I have never, and most likely never will, hear sounds in the same way as a hearing person. As a result, hearing people experience things every millisecond of the day that I never will. By the same token, I have experienced things and will experience things that no hearing person can.

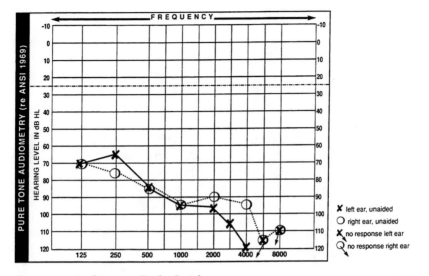

Figure 4. Audiogram: Darby Leigh.

My deafness makes me different, and that difference makes me strong. I seem to get respect from other people just for doing things a hearing person can do with ease. For example, watch television, use the telephone, listen to music, and so on. For whatever reason, I never think about the fact that I am doing something that would normally be difficult for someone who couldn't hear. In fact, I have never looked at myself as someone who was limited in any way, someone who couldn't do something that any other hearing person could do. I've always known that I was different, but even though people would intimate that I wasn't able to compete on the same level as hearing people, I would ignore them, or maybe I just didn't "hear" them.

I have always attended Dalton, a private hearing school. It has never been, and never will be, easy for me. I have experienced periods of rejection and isolation, but I have proven myself worthy of the privilege of attending this school by receiving grades as good as many of my hearing peers and better than most.

I have definitely survived the academic challenges of my school and life. Socially, I still feel though that I'm not accepted as a true equal, but, hey, that's their problem, they don't know what they're missing.

In addition to the social and academic challenges, music and athletics are important areas in a teenager's life. In spite of my profound hearing impairment, I learned to enjoy music and accomplished much more than just listening to different groups and types of musical entertainment. That may not seem like much, but it was once a seemingly unattainable, far away goal. The fact that one who can't hear had been trained and is now capable of hearing music, and to differentiate between fast and loud or slow and soft music, is a huge feat—a feat that is rightfully understood and respected by those who know me. I've had to spend seven or eight years of my Monday afternoons receiving training and therapy to hear and to speak. While this, indeed, was a drag for me at the time, it has built my character and taught me a lot about determination and perseverance.

My athletic accomplishments have been far greater than even I imagined they would be. For one thing, I never dreamed that playing football could be a possibility for me. The problems and negatives were many: the helmet wouldn't fit over my hearing aids, or that I wouldn't be able to hear the plays called in the huddle, or that my hearing aids would get broken when they were knocked around, and so on. My coach finally convinced me that there was some way around each one of these obstacles, and I'm now going to go into my fourth varsity football season next fall. All these problems slow me down and make me work much harder. I may experience more frustration than the other players, but that has helped build my character and make me a stronger person. I may not be a great player, but I play, and I'm part of the team, and that's more than most hearing people do. When the fall season ends and winter rolls around, I don't hibernate. Instead, I join the wrestling team. Wrestling demands so much from the participants, and the fact that oftentimes I can't hear the referee or my coach makes it all that much harder for me. I've stuck with it though and have never quit. Each time an obstacle confronts me, I accept it as a new challenge and learn to work around it. After the wrestling season is over, I take off my wrestling shoes and put on running sneakers for the track season. Here too, deafness creates problems, none that can't be solved though. Whenever I step on the football field, wrestling mat, or the track, my deafness forces me to act in a way that may be different from the other participants. Other spectators can see this difference, and they better recognize all the more effort that I've put into my playing and practice because of my deafness.

Being deaf doesn't mean you can't do something, being deaf only means that you have to work harder at what it is that you want to do. That working harder builds you as a person and makes you much more ready to face the next new challenge in your way. For those next new challenges never stop coming.

Anna Barenblatt   Date of Birth: 10/25/68. Senior, New York University, New York City.

My hearing loss was identified when I was eight months of age. I have always attended hearing schools. My mother helped me with my homework on countless nights, making sure that I absorbed and had not missed out on the daily essentials from school.

I have always relied on my lipreading skills in the classroom, but, when I went to college, I decided to take a course in sign language. I am able to obtain more from my courses through the use of an oral/sign interpreter. In addition, I have notetakers to augment my own notes. These support services have lessened the academic obstacles I had in my early school years, where I had virtually no special assistance.

In high school, a private school where I was the only student with impaired hearing, I was involved in extra-curricular activities, but the experience was painful. Although I was on the volleyball team, I was on the bench and rarely got to play because, as one of the coaches remarked, "You can't hear, that's why." When I confronted the coach and the athletic director, they merely brushed me aside and ignored the issue. I was stupefied at their unwillingness to support me in sports— wasn't that their job?

Soon after, I went to the local YMCA and took up fencing. There I received encouragement, support, coaching and, above all, sportsmanship. Here I am, five years later, as captain of the New York University's women's varsity fencing team. Our team is presently one of the top ranking fencing teams in the country. I, personally, have earned silver and gold medals in the individual category.

Teachers and students need to be more informed about the needs of students with deafness and should treat the student as an equal. Whenever possible, the student should take advantage of devices or

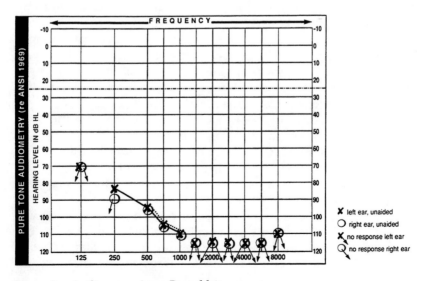

Figure 5.   Audiogram: Anna Barenblatt.

aids to ease the communication barrier, such as the FM system or other electronic equipment, oral/sign language interpreters, and notetakers.

I feel that ignorance and age-old prejudices imposed by society in general have put people with a hearing impairment in an unfair position. I am glad that many recent incidents coupled with strong advocacies (too numerous to count!) have helped debunk some myths about this disability. Also, we must give credit to technology, which has made it possible for some people with hearing impairments to be part of the mainstream.

In the meantime, attitudes must be reformed into acceptance. The general population should realize that it's the ability, not the disability, that counts.

George Oberlander, Jr., I.E. Date of Birth: 8/30/62. Mechanical Engineer.

My hearing loss was not diagnosed until I was almost 5 years old. Most people would probably feel that it was a disadvantage to be diagnosed so late. I feel, however, that the reason I lipread so well is because I had to rely on it as my only form of communication in my younger years. To illustrate how I communicated without a hearing aid when I was young, I can recall a story that my mother told me. One time she was talking to me while looking out the kitchen window. Not being able to understand her, I replied, "Turn around. I can't see what you're saying."

Being able to communicate without a hearing aid required more than just being able to lipread well. It also required the ability to anticipate what the other person was saying and to be able to obtain information via body language. For example, when my mother was talking to me and looking out the window, I obviously didn't hear her. I probably saw that her jaw was moving and determined that she was talking to me. I would say that more than 50% of what I receive as communication comes from anticipating what the other person is saying.

I wear two body aids because I feel that they help me the most. Some people wear behind-the-ear units because of cosmetics, and also because they believe that the aids are powerful enough for them to hear well. I have tried to wear behind-the-ear units, but I find that the body aids offer a much clearer sound for me, both in person-to-person communication and on the telephone.

I currently hold a Bachelor's Degree in Engineering Science. I studied at Hofstra University from September 1980 through May 1985.

I have gone to public schools all of my life. In elementary school, I was subjected to the "being picked on" syndrome experienced by kids

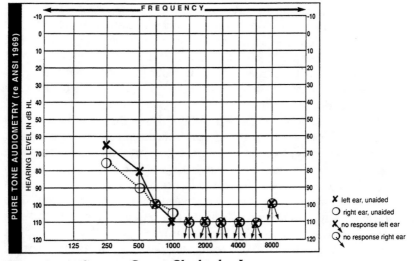

Figure 6.   Audiogram: George Oberlander, Jr.

with disabilities. I had a slow start, mostly because I was picked on, but also because I did not receive my first tutor until I was in the sixth grade. Up until that point, I relied on my teachers and my mother to fill in the blanks. Most of my teachers encouraged me and believed that I could succeed. I also had the support of a speech therapist who worked with me on vocabulary development and articulation three times a week. My speech therapist helped me to become more intelligible, but I am still not sure why I speak so well, since many hearing-impaired people with lesser hearing losses do not speak as well as I do.

In the fifth grade, I had a teacher who thought that I couldn't make it and recommended that I go to a school for the deaf. My mother argued strongly against this by using past report cards that showed that I had done well in previous grades, therefore, I remained in public school. This was the closest I ever came to going to a school for the deaf.

Social life in elementary school consisted of playing sports, both at school and at home. One of the things that I noticed was that when I played with a group of kids, I was considered different. However, if I played with someone one-on-one, then the disability was less noticeable, and I was just like anyone else. I attribute this difference to the kids jockeying for position and status in a group. At the time, I was mad at them for having a double standard, but now that I am older, I accept it as the way kids are. It had nothing to do with the fact that I was deaf, but more with the fact that I was different. In the long run, it made me a better, stronger person.

As I grew older and the kids matured, life moved away from playing sports to more social interactions, such as dances, parties, etc. Although it became easier for me to play sports with a group of people, it became harder for me to keep up with the social crowd, and so I spent much of my spare time in woodworking and power mechanic shops. I enjoy working with mechanical things and spent much of my high school years doing just that.

In middle school and in high school, I was fortunate because the Harrison School District realized that in order for me to succeed in a mainstream setting, I would need more support than I had received in elementary school. Therefore, they assigned a teacher of the deaf to work with me each day to fill in the information that I missed in class and to help my teachers make modifications in the classroom. This resource teacher was very helpful to me because, not only did she fill in the blanks, but she also gave me the skill and confidence to speak in front of people. Because of her and my parents, I was able to realize my potential, and I graduated from high school with a Regents Diploma.

I began my search for a college with Rochester Institute of Technology (RIT), because the National Technical Institute for the Deaf (NTID) was on the same campus. My intention was to go to RIT and use some of the services that NTID offered. When I went to visit the college, I was told that I would have to begin my college education learning sign language and attending classes for the deaf; I was appalled at this. Because of this, I did not go to RIT. I feel that, at that time, making me learn sign language would have been detrimental because my reliance on my hearing has helped me to be able to do many things that are needed in my high-paced professional job. This includes speaking on the telephone with clients and participating in meetings.

The next school that I looked at, and decided to attend, was Hofstra University on Long Island. Because my SAT scores were not good enough for me to be accepted into their engineering program, it was decided that I would begin in a division called New College. This was an alternative program designed to help any student, handicapped or non-handicapped, who needed extra assistance in college level reading, writing, etc. If I did well, then they would allow me to begin the engineering curriculum. I did do well and went on with my engineering studies in my second semester.

My college experience can be described in three words: "work, work, and work." In college, I was not provided with tutors. I was, however, provided with paid notetakers. Because I had taken my own notes in high school, I found it hard to use other peoples' notes. But after a period of time, I was able to adjust to a few notetakers that I kept semester after semester. In high school, notes were written on a blackboard and then you would recopy the notes into your notebook. College presented a unique twist, with me sitting in the classroom not taking notes but just trying to absorb the content of what the teacher was saying. Since I was spending so much time trying to understand the words, it was hard for me to comprehend what the teacher meant. Needless to say, my comprehension in the classroom was not very good. I made up for this by studying long hours and working with my friends. The biggest help, however, were the engineering professors at Hofstra University. They would give me all of the office time I needed and never made me feel out of place or that I was imposing on their time. In fact, one of them called me his "best customer." I probably would not have succeeded in getting my engineering degree if it was not for the time these professors gave me.

Looking back on everything, my challenges, my accomplishments, and my frustrations, there is nothing that I would change or do differently, not even having a fifth grade teacher who was more understanding of my needs. That teacher taught me that not everything would be handed to me on a "silver platter" and that to succeed, I would need to rely on myself, work hard, and make my own choices. I would only recommend that a handicapped person be taught that he or she should not expect other people to always make accommodations; it is as much the responsibility of the person with impaired hearing to make others feel comfortable with the handicap as it is for others to make him or her feel accepted.

I would recommend to teachers and to parents that they tell their students and their children that they *can* and not that they *can't*. I cannot emphasize enough the importance of this positive attitude.

A further recommendation for parents, who know their children better than anyone else, is to question the authority when a suggestion is made that they feel is not appropriate for their child. P.L. 94-142, The Education For All Handicapped Children Act, has given parents the right to be involved in planning their children's special education programs. Parents must take advantage of this right, be active participants in planning conferences, and become knowledgeable about the needs of their children.

[My portion of this chapter] is dedicated to Dr. Beatrice Spear, my teacher of the deaf, Mr. Irwin Rickler and Mrs. Enid Oberstein, my speech therapists, the teachers of the Harrison Central School District, all of the engineering professors at Hofstra University, my primary notetaker, James Veninger, and, most of all, to my parents who did not let me know the meaning of the word *can't*, as I go through life being a hearing deaf person.

CONCLUSIONS

As professionals, we have learned to assist hearing-impaired children by recommending appropriate amplification, developing speech and language skills, modifying curriculum, offering remediation, augmenting classroom instruction, reinforcing concepts, increasing vocabulary, and improving reading skills. As we review the comments of the contributors, we know that too little attention has been given to developing social interactions, age-appropriate social skills, and a sense of self-worth.

Parental involvement can be critical. Often, the parent needs to act as the ambassador: educating the teacher, providing information to peers, and helping the child to see himself or herself in a positive light. In addition, parents need to help the child become independent and learn to advocate for himself or herself. To assist in developing their assertiveness skills, hearing-impaired children should be included in the Individualized Education Program (IEP) meetings and should be helped to have a say in formulating the recommendations.

Each parent has reported on the need to develop and maintain positive relationships with school personnel. Adversarial actions do not engender the positive responses from teachers and educators that are needed to foster cooperation and to ensure that the child receives necessary academic support in the classroom.

Another theme echoed by both parents and children was that the mainstream educational experience helped pave the way for participation in the hearing world. Academic challenges were present, but each of the students developed strategies to meet the challenges. In addition, the determination to succeed and participate in a hearing world pervaded their entire educational and social experience.

To overcome some of the problems expressed in the area of social interaction, there is a need to look beyond academics. Classmates need to be provided with information about hearing impairment and the supports that are required to help the student with impaired hearing compensate for the disability. Shared information increases understanding. For example, one way for hearing classmates to develop increased understanding is to organize a speechreading contest in class. Such an experience often helps hearing peers realize the difficulties in language comprehension and places the student with impaired hearing in a positive light.

The strength(s) a hearing-impaired child possesses, whether in sports or crafts or any other area, can be used to build the child's self-image. Rather than being told, "You can't," hearing-impaired children—like hearing children—need to develop feelings of adequacy and self-esteem.

Many children with impaired hearing who are attending mainstream schools have more supports available to them now than they had in the past—resource rooms, itinerant teachers, interpreters, FM systems, and notetakers. In still too many instances, however, there is a continuing need to negotiate the entitlements for the child with impaired hearing. The IEP becomes the critical document in the negotiations, and everything the child requires to function in school should be detailed in it.

The young adults in this chapter all have attained a measure of success. Contributing to their success have been strong parental involvement and a determination to succeed. As Anna Barenblatt so aptly stated, "It's the ability, not the disability, that counts."

Chapter • 18

Overview and the Long View

Mark Ross

One of the steps I took as I prepared for the conference upon which this book is based was to visit the library at the American School for the Deaf. I spent some time reading a number of the initial volumes of the *American Annals of the Deaf*, dating from 1849. (This journal has the distinction of being the oldest continuously published journal in the United States.) I was looking for early references to the practice of mainstreaming, by whatever names the concept was known at that time. I did find some, which I review below, but I also found myself exposed to the pioneers in the field of education of the deaf in this country. I was impressed and very moved by these intelligent, articulate, and sensitive people who, except for the purely technical developments of the twentieth century, anticipated most if not all the insights, solutions, programs, and problems that we think we invented in this era. Another historical source was an article published in 1885 (Gordon 1885) that reviewed the practice of mainstreaming (not by that term) from 1815 to the time the article was published.

In the first section of this chapter, I present an overview of this literature, with a particular emphasis on insights and practices that still seem to be relevant. In the next section, the period immediately preceding Public Law 94-142 is reviewed. The major source for this section is a book edited in 1960 by Sir Alexander Ewing, based on the proceedings of an 1958 conference. I used this book as a text when I first started teaching in 1962. Reviewing it once again, I find it has held up very well in all the varied subject areas covered (which is either an indication of the slow pace of developments in the field of education of the hearing-impaired, or a tribute to the contributions of our colleagues of over thirty years ago—or perhaps both.)

A number of issues germane to the practice of mainstreaming in our current era are covered in the third section. I take advantage of having the last word in this volume to emphasize and expand on some issues already raised, basically from the perspective of some interesting research studies.

The "Mainstreaming Bill of Rights" is presented and discussed in the last section. My intention here is to distill the essential lessons presented in this book as they apply to the principles and practices of mainstreaming now and in the future.

THE EARLY TIMES

The controversy regarding regular education versus special education dates back to 1815 (Gordon 1885). At that time, the School Councilor of Bavaria wrote a forceful article condemning special institutions for the deaf as "useless" luxuries. Because he was, presumably, responsible for the educational budget in the province, one wonders if his attitude was not influenced, at least in part, by the relative cost of special, as opposed to regular, educational settings. If so, it would have been the first instance in the field of deaf education, but hardly the last, wherein an alternative placement was recommended under the guise of superior or "appropriate" education, when in fact the decision was motivated by budgetary considerations.

It was also about this time, in 1819, that John Arrowsmith wrote a book about the education of his "deaf and dumb" brother at home and at schools with hearing children. Evidently it was their mother who insisted that her deaf son be at home; she took responsibility for his education, working closely with his teachers at the local school to motivate and assist them in the child's education. This may be the first recorded instance of intense family involvement in the education of the affected child. Her hearing son—the author of the book—assisted her and later devoted himself to the education of deaf children: another possible "first" example of sibling involvement. He was the first to suggest explicitly that deaf children could, and should, be educated with hearing children. The book stimulated a great deal of interest, with some devotees attempting to replicate Arrowsmith's work while others severely criticized the approach. The book was reviewed by S. Porter (1849), who stated that subsequent experience with the Arrowsmith concept was "disastrous in every case." One should not ignore the fact that the reviewer represented the residential school concept then predominant in this country.

Large-scale integration of deaf children with hearing children was mandated by the educational authorities in France and Germany in the 1820s. This was an authoritarian time, and the "authorities" decided where and under what conditions deaf children would be educated. At one point, one hundred regular school programs in Germany accepted deaf children, with six integrated day programs in Bavaria alone. All that was necessary to manage these children in the regular schools, so the authorities believed, was for the teacher to "talk slowly and distinctly" and the children would begin to understand the motion of the lips and would be able to reproduce the sounds.

Many enthusiastic educators took up the challenge, and published their initial efforts, but not their subsequent experiences. However, by the mid-1800s a consensus developed; educating hearing-impaired children alongside hearing children was not successful. In 1858 the Government Inspector of the Education of Deaf Mutes in Western Prussia evaluated the integration efforts in Germany and declared the experiment a qualified failure. (Some children did benefit.) He wrote that the "hope that each deaf-mute could receive the necessary instruction at the local school in common with hearing children and without injury to the latter has been abandoned" (Gordon 1885). He also indicated that deaf children were a burden to regular teachers, made less progress than they had in residential schools, and wanted to return there. Presumably as a result of this report, the Ministry of Education in German withdrew its support for mainstreaming, and by 1882 only a few deaf children remained in regular schools. The experiences in France and England (the only countries reviewed in this report) were similar to Germany's. Reading these accounts of attempts at mainstreaming, one is impressed with their scope and seriousness; however, they lacked the array of support services that we now take for granted. Our colleagues of the past had a good idea, at least for some of the children, but the time was not right.

During the period when intense efforts to educate deaf children in the regular schools were widespread, educators developed a number of models and educational insights. They recognized the desirability of keeping deaf youngsters at home, and the potential linguistic and behavioral advantages of interacting with normal-hearing children. They also developed early management programs in regular schools with a later transfer to a special school, and vice versa. In-service training programs were provided for the regular teachers; better training for the special teachers was a great concern. Some programs had units in regular schools and partial mainstreaming opportunities for deaf children. Parent education was stressed, with instructions in using a natural language approach with deaf children. The distinction between *integration* and *assimilation* could be determined in how the children played with each other on the playground. It appears that the concern for the psycho-social welfare of hearing-impaired children has old roots.

There was an explicit recognition that some "successful" deaf children could understand speech when the speaker's lips were placed close to their ears. These people well understood the fact that degrees of hearing loss existed, with implications for a child's ability to develop and comprehend speech, they just did not have the tools to measure or exploit residual hearing. The difference between the performance of children with adventitious and congenital hearing loss was also well recognized.

Reading this literature was an enchanting experience. If a time travel machine could transport those educators to our time, or us to theirs, I am sure we would soon engage in animated debate about our different views and approaches, joined by a common mission to educate hearing-impaired children as best we could. In any generation, it seems, one can rarely find a more committed group of professionals than those who devote their lives to educating hearing-impaired children.

THE MIDDLE TIMES

In my historical review I rather arbitrarily skip about one hundred years and move the focus ethnocentrically to the United States. *Deaf* children were mainstreamed prior to this period (Numbers 1960), but rarely and then only after graduation from the special school. (*Hard-of-hearing* children, on the other hand, were routinely mainstreamed, but typically not very successfully.)

In the 1950s a variety of integration programs was offered to the children of Public School 47 in New York City (McLaughlin 1960). The programs were developed for children of different ages, needs, and residential districts. According to McLaughlin, the goal was to integrate children as early as possible, either in their local schools or in one close to P.S. 47. The children received special tutoring assistance in any case (somewhat more when the child was placed in a nearby school close to the special school). Teachers of the deaf were assigned permanently to some high schools and were able to offer daily assistance to the students. Staff members of P.S. 47 also were assigned permanently to the Audiology Clinic at Bellevue Hospital to assist in counseling the parents after the diagnosis of hearing loss and to provide information regarding educational possibilities for their child.

In another creative effort of that period, a team-teaching program was devised at P.S. 47 with twenty-five normal-hearing children and ten deaf children integrated in one class (McLaughlin 1960). After one year, both groups had improved academically more than expected, but the two groups did not really socialize. This was attributed to the sheltered experiences of the deaf group, who expected more attention than they received from the regular teacher. The program then was reorganized, with only two deaf children placed in each class. Although the teachers reported that both groups had gotten on well together, sociometric tests indicated that the hearing children did not really accept the deaf children. Another article in this same book cautioned that parents and teachers generally rate their children much more optimistically than is warranted by their performance (O'Conner 1960). This was true then, and is still a concern, which is why we insist on objective indices of a child's performance. Other reports of integrated programs are given in this same volume (Ewing 1960).

My own experience with integration dates from about this time. Based on my contacts with hearing-impaired children in a community speech and hearing clinic, there was never any question regarding the fact of mainstreaming. Most of the hearing-impaired children we saw were being educated, more or less adequately, in a regular school. Most of them were not what we would currently term "deaf" children. One prominent, and very knowledgeable educator of that time, defined children with 65 dB hearing losses or more in their better ear as "educationally deaf" (O'Conner 1960). In the pre-amplification period, certainly most of these children were functionally deaf; thanks to amplification, this is one area where we have made progress.

What was clear at that time, and has not changed since, is that appropriate educational placement and educational success require combined and intensive support of school staff and parents. Without the legal force of P.L. 94-142, clinicians and educators depended upon traditional modes of arranging appropriate programs for children. Most educators used their best professional judgments in making recommendations and providing services, and children whose parents did the most agitating were the ones who received the most attention, which is really not so different from the current situation.

RECURRING ISSUES IN MAINSTREAMING

A Question of Terminology

First it is important to agree on the terms we use to categorize children with hearing losses. We can preclude much diagnostic and placement confusion if we agree on the meaning of common terms used to label people with hearing losses (Ross and Calvert 1967; Wilson, Ross, and Calvert 1974).

When someone is labelled "deaf," it should mean that the person's communication *development* and current *primary* communication mode is visually based (either sign language or speechreading). Residual hearing (if any) is a secondary and supplemental sensory avenue; vision is the major channel for receiving information.

The term "hard of hearing" is used to convey the fact that the person's linguistic development is *primarily* auditorily-based, with vision serving as a secondary and supplemental channel. This person must *hear* in order to communicate and be educated. Hard-of-hearing people have much more in common with normal-hearing people than with those who are deaf, strange as this may seem.

"Hearing-impaired" is a generic term, used to refer to anyone with any type and degree of hearing loss. It is *not* a synonym for hard of hearing. The meaning of the term can be restricted by applying a descriptive adjective, such as mild, moderate, severe, or profound.

Some children appear to fall somewhere between hard of hearing and deaf. Paradoxically, these children often represent a therapeutic "success," in that they may have been taught, and have learned, to employ their residual hearing very well, in spite of average hearing losses in excess of 90 dB (the usual physiological, not functional, definition of the term "deaf"). Some of these children are essentially bi-sensory communicators (combining audition with vision for speech perception). Indeed, some may use an essentially bi-sensory mode for the *development* of language, grounded on the complementary sensory information provided by the auditory and visual channels.

PSYCHO-SOCIAL FACTORS

Three assumptions underlie the movement toward mainstreaming hearing-impaired children (Nolan and Tucker 1981):

1. Mainstreaming fosters social interactions with the "hearing world."
2. Mainstreaming provides hearing-impaired children with normal linguistic and behavioral models.
3. Mainstreaming offers access to wider curriculum possibilities than is possible in a special school.

In my opinion, one of the heartening emphases in recent mainstreaming efforts is the recognition that the psycho-social factor is at least as relevant as academic achievements. We have some evidence that academic and speech performance of mainstreamed children tends to be superior to comparable nonmainstreamed children (see below). We cannot make this statement with respect to the psycho-social status of mainstreamed hearing-impaired children. Reading the narratives by the parents and children in Chapter 17, one is struck by how heavily and poignantly this factor looms in the mind of the parents and in the experiences of the students.

As Northcott, Schwartz, and others have pointed out earlier, the placement of hearing-impaired children in a regular classroom is no guarantee of their acceptance by hearing children. In a very interesting study, Weisel (1988) used a multidimensional scale to investigate the attitudes of three groups of hearing students toward hearing-impaired students. One group of hearing students had daily opportunities to interact with the hearing-impaired students; the second group of hearing students were in the same school, but rarely, if ever interacted with them; the third group of hearing students was from a different school and never interacted with hearing-impaired children.

The results of the Weisel's (1988) study showed that the attitudes of hearing students toward the hearing-impaired students depended both on the degree of contact and the attitudinal dimension evaluated. Generally, it was found that subjects with a moderate degree of contact with the hearing-impaired (Group 2), expressed more negative attitudes than subjects in the other two normal-hearing groups. The moderate contact group met the hearing-impaired students in a segregated, group fashion, and not on a individual basis. This group seemed to interpret this situation as an expression by the authorities of biased sentiments toward the "special" students by virtue of their segregation. In turn this was interpreted by the hearing students as sanction for a derogatory approach toward disabled people. For this normal-hearing group, relations with the hearing-impaired children were category-based contacts, which can lead "to deindividuation and depersonalization of outgroup members" (Weisel 1988, p. 166).

No differences were found between the groups that had a high level of contact and those that had no contact. Children in the high-contact group were able to relate to the hearing-impaired children on an individual basis, and thus rid themselves of group stereotypes, whereas the children in the no-contact group evidently never had the occasion to formulate such stereotypes. *This study teaches us that we must try to arrange social and academic situations in the classrooms wherein children relate to each other on a personal basis.*

The social problems of mainstreamed children are not limited to just one country. Markides (1989) studied the friendship and association patterns of a large number of normal and hearing-impaired students in English secondary schools. All of the mainstreamed hearing-impaired children spent over eighty percent of their time in the regular classrooms; the normal-hearing children in the study were drawn from the same classrooms.

The results of the study were not very encouraging. Most of the hearing-impaired students considered another hearing-impaired student in the school as their best friend, in spite of the fact that the majority of the students in the class were hearing. Many more hearing-impaired than normal-hearing students did not have a best friend at school (perhaps because the hearing-impaired children were transported to a regional center, which was the neighborhood school for the hearing children). The main reason that the hearing students gave for not selecting a hearing-impaired student as a best friend related to speech intelligibility ("they talk funny"). The same pattern was observed on the playground. In contrast to the hearing group, the hearing-impaired students spent most of their time either alone or interacting with just one or two other children.

In reviewing his data and other studies, and integration practices generally, Markides (1989) concludes that the majority of hearing-impaired children in regular schools are:

> . . . fully participating members of the school community. They are coping with their lessons and are making good progress. It is also known, however, that others are not so fortunate. To varying degrees they feel excluded and ignored. The pace is too fast for them. They find difficulties with their lessons. They are floundering. They seek comfort and companionship among other hearing-impaired children. Their demeanour tends to be one of indifference, withdrawal and sometimes resentment. They tend to function as small but identifiable sub-groups within the hearing-impaired milieu of their respective schools. For them, integration in its broadest sense, is not working (p. 70).

Markides makes these conclusions as an advocate of mainstreaming, but recognizes that explicit steps need to be taken to improve the situation. Included in his recommendations is the need for more in-service training for the regular teachers, and better understanding by both teachers and hearing students of the complex and devastating nature of hearing loss. To this, I would add the implications of the Weisel (1988) study: the necessity for frequent, individualized interactions between hearing and hearing-impaired students. Although this does not ensure that "to know them is to love them," it does ensure the hearing students *will* know their hearing-impaired peers as unique people and not just as categories, which is not a bad lesson to apply, whatever the "category" in question.

Factors Related to Mainstreaming "Success"

There is no shortage of supposition on why some hearing-impaired children succeed in the mainstream and others do not. It seems that we all have our opinions—mine are below—but there is little hard research data to draw upon. One major effort was undertaken by Pflaster

(1980, 1981). Using academic performance as the criterion for defining "success," she evaluated 182 mainstreamed hearing-impaired children on 59 independent variables. Using an intercorrelational approach, she derived a number of key factors related to the academic performance of hearing-impaired children in the mainstream. Eleven factors emerged as statistically significant, but four of them accounted for most of the relationship to academic performance. These factors are:

1. *The suprasegmental components of a child's oral productions.* The acceptability of a child's speech depends more upon the quality and rhythmic components than upon articulation. In Markides (1989) study (reviewed above) the hearing children often accepted or rejected a hearing-impaired child based on the quality of the child's speech.

2. *The child's oral and written expressive language ability.* This should be a self-evident factor; a child hardly will be able to interact efficiently in a regular school without acceptable linguistic skills.

3. *The motivation of a child to succeed.* This includes such dimensions as effort, attitude, determination, and working at capacity.

4. *The child's oral and written receptive language skills.* The major dimensions in this factor are the children's abilities to speechread directions and questions.

Two of the eleven were considered central factors in that they were highly related to a number of the other factors. The first was receptive language, which was also one of the four major factors. It correlated highly with all the other linguistic factors. Simply said, the children who demonstrate the best language ability also function best academically in the mainstream. Not surprising, perhaps, but a necessary corroboration in research terms.

I was fascinated by the second central factor—communication attitude. Although this was not one of the four major factors listed above, statistical analysis showed that it related highly to six other factors, more than any other. Three of the factors it related to describe aspects of the child's personality (motivation, interpersonal behavior, and personal adjustment), and three describe linguistic dimensions (suprasegmentals, receptive language, and expressive language). As Pflaster (1981) puts it: "The emergence of a factor suggesting that the hearing-impaired child has a communicative attitude or set appears to be the single most important insight related to his or her successful integration" (p. 77). The personality that emerges is that of a child who actively desires to communicate by using spoken language. The child must be motivated and determined to succeed, with the prerequisite linguistic skills to enable him or her to do so.

If one rereads the three narratives by the mainstreamed hearing-impaired students (Chapter 17), one cannot but be impressed with how closely this research conclusion describes them. All of these students have excellent linguistic skills but, beyond that, their sheer determination to make it imbues their narratives. Where it came from and how it can be fostered are other questions. Whatever the answers, one can be certain that the parents play an important role.

MAINSTREAM PERFORMANCE: CAUSE OR EFFECT?

The accumulated weight of evidence clearly indicates that the academic performance of mainstreamed hearing-impaired children is superior to that of their segregated counterparts (Allen and Osborn 1984; Geers, this volume; Levitt, McGarr, and Geffner 1987; Ross, Brackett, and Maxon 1982; Schildroth and Karchmer 1986). This holds up even when the impact of such significant variables as hearing level and socio-economic status are eliminated (mainstreamed children tend to have better hearing and be of a higher socio-economic level). It is necessary to ask whether the children's superior performance is an effect of the mainstreaming or is the reason they were initially placed in a regular school setting. The truth, as is so often the case, is neither and both.

When local academic authorities come to make an initial placement decision for a preschool hearing-impaired child, their recommendation must clearly be influenced by the child's current communicative capacities. The children with relatively superior oral linguistic skills usually are placed in less restrictive educational settings than those with poorer oral language. If the relative difference in the children's performance is sustained as they proceed through their parallel academic tracks, the mainstreamed children will continue to demonstrate higher academic and linguistic achievements. Also, the "stars" in a more restrictive educational setting will tend to be mainstreamed sooner than their poorer achieving counterparts. After a few years, as one evaluates the relative performance of the two groups of children, clearly it will be the mainstreamed children who excel in academic performance scores. These initial and later placement decisions no doubt explain why the average performance of mainstreamed children is better than that of their peers in a segregated educational setting; however, I do not think that this explanation is the complete answer.

Except for a study by Reich, Hambleton, and Houldin (1977), which found a continued improvement in the children's performance the longer they were mainstreamed, no research data that I know of directly addresses this question. We do know that mainstreamed hearing-impaired children exhibit a wide range of abilities in all communicative dimensions (Levitt, McGarr, and Geffner 1987) that, in part, is related to whether or not the children received early training. Given these variations in the children's accomplishments, no single factor can explain the generally superior performance of mainstreamed hearing-impaired children over their more segregated counterparts. In my judgment, the mainstream placement in itself, and the conditions that obtain in such a setting, can serve as a stimulant to superior academic performance.

Educational expectations and standards generally are higher in mainstream settings than in segregated schools for the hearing-impaired. This is a consequence of the historically poorer performance in all academic and linguistic dimensions of hearing-impaired children compared to normal-hearing children. A regular classroom teacher does not know the extent of the performance gap that hearing-impaired children are "supposed" to display relative to their normal-hearing peers. Such a teacher would tend to interpret a particular hearing-impaired child's performance relative to the spread of accomplishments in the classroom. If a child with good intelligence, as measured by performance test scores, lags too much behind his or her normal-hearing peers, it becomes a cause for concern. The child is pressured to increase his or her performance; extra assistance is supplied (which should be done in any event); the parents are notified that the child's accomplishments are unsatisfactory, which can serve to raise their expectations; and, finally, the child absorbs the achievement norms of the class and may try to reach the other student's. All this undoubtedly makes for a stressful time for such a child, and it is vital to address this issue explicitly, but it can also make for a child whose academic and linguistic accomplishments are closer to normal-hearing children than of segregated hearing-impaired children.

THE IMPACT OF EARLY MANAGEMENT

The factors that support an appropriate and successful mainstream placement begin long before a child starts his or her formal education. The prerequisite for academic success is adequate linguistic skills, and these skills should be highly developed *before* a child starts school. This implies that parent-infant and preschool programs are a necessity, not an educational luxury, if hearing-impaired children are to be successfully educated in a mainstream setting. Although we have long recognized the theoretical need to provide early management programs, it is only in recent years that sufficient research evidence has accumulated to support this assertion.

Two recent studies investigated the accomplishments of several groups of children, some of whom were the recipients of early intervention programs and some of whom were not (Watkins 1987; White and White 1987). In both studies, the children who received home intervention training, particularly when this was combined with a later preschool program, scored higher on linguistic tests than control groups of hearing-impaired children who did not receive these services.

In another study, 120 ten- and eleven-year-old hearing-impaired children enrolled in schools for the deaf were followed for four years (Levitt, McGarr, and Geffner 1987). One of the major findings of this study was that the speech and language scores of those children who received their initial training prior to age three were better than the scores of those children who received it later. A few of the children who received early intervention scored below average. Most, however, scored above average. On the other hand, only a few of the children who did not receive early intervention scored above average; most scored below. The effects of hearing loss and socio-economic variables were statistically eliminated as possible explanatory factors in reaching this conclusion. The authors of this study point out that the relationship they obtained was correlational and not necessary causal. That is, there may be other intervening factors that are responsible for the obtained relationship.

What these three studies suggest is that whereas early intervention will not in itself guarantee later superior performance, the lack of it will almost certainly reduce the level of a child's potential performance.

THE MAINSTREAMING BILL OF RIGHTS

Hearing-impaired children should not be placed in the educational mainstream to sink or swim on their own. There are certain principles, practices, and prerequisites that can be applied to ensure, as much as humanly possible, that the children cannot only keep their heads above water, but that they can float with pleasure and success in the middle of the stream. The compilation of the necessary principles, practices, and prerequisites is what I term the "Mainstreaming Bill of Rights."

They are not original formulations. All can be found somewhere in the preceding chapters; indeed, evidence of their need goes back to the very first days of the mainstreaming concept. Our predecessors for the most part knew what had to be done, but because of technical and administrative limitations, they could not put these steps into practice. We, on the other hand, have the technical capability and the required administrative knowledge to institute successful mainstreaming of hearing-impaired children. What we lack is the social will and consensus to implement the concept successfully. Mainstreaming will be with us into the twenty-first century. The "Bill of Rights" outlined below can provide a conceptual framework for the successful mainstreaming of hearing-impaired children into the next century.

1. The physical placement of a hearing-impaired child in a regular classroom is not in itself a criterion of educational success. Mainstreaming refers to an educational placement, a more or less effective means through which we expect to reach our goals for some children. It is these goals—which must be explicitly defined—that justify the mainstream setting. If the goals can best be met in a non-mainstream environment, then this is where a child should be enrolled. *Appropriate* education is not always synonymous with the *least restrictive* setting. In other words, it is necessary to keep in mind the distinction between means (the educational experience) and ends (a child's accomplishments).

2. Mainstreaming is not a polar phenemonon. A child is neither fully mainstreamed nor fully segregated. Children can be appropriately mainstreamed for some academic and nonacademic activities and not for others. This does not imply that only the mainstream experiences are valuable and that the others are not. All, however, should be relevant to a child's abilities and needs.

3. The educational options in a mainstream setting must include a range of alternatives with objective criteria for placement in any option. Some children can be fully mainstreamed with only routine support services; others require a resource room as a home base. Some severely and profoundly hearing-impaired children employ, or should employ, a manual communication system; placement options in a regular school should also be available for these children.

4. A comprehensive assessment reflecting all facets of a child's behavior, performance, and status is always required. Informal observational impressions often provide as much information in describing a child as do formal tests. The overall assessment not only is used to plan an individualized education program, but is necessary to determine the suitability of a current or possible future educational placement. Yearly reevaluations are almost always necessary.

5. Mainstreaming is *always* an individual matter. Groups are never mainstreamed; only specific children, who may be part of a group, are mainstreamed. A program, therefore, must be designed to fit an individual child.

6. Psycho-social considerations are as important as academic and communication goals. Superior academic and communication performance, at the cost of an isolated, unhappy child, is too high a price

to pay. With sensitive educational management, psycho-social problems can be minimized or eliminated; they are not, in other words, an inevitable consequence of mainstreaming.

7. Support services are usually necessary; few hearing-impaired children in regular schools will realize their potential without these services. The particular ones required may, and probably will, change as the child progresses through school. The fact that a child is functioning at grade level justifies the continuation and not the elimination of support services.

8. The regular classroom teacher is the central educational figure for a mainstreamed hearing-impaired child and must play a significant role in any team planning efforts. The teacher should receive in-service training prior to the placement of a hearing-impaired child in the classroom. In-service training must continue for as long as the child remains in the classroom.

9. Involved professionals must define the essential educational services their students require and see that these services are available. Few schools can boast unlimited budgetary resources. This implies that the school staff must develop a system of educational priorities to ensure that the hearing-impaired students receive the most essential services.

10. Successful therapy and education are interactive processes. *Listen* to what children and parents are telling us. An approach that "prescribes," but does not respond to the stated or unstated needs of the parents and children, cannot be considered either pedagogically or humanistically appropriate.

SUMMARY

The roots of the concept of mainstreaming go back almost two centuries. There is an intrinsic appeal to the notion that hearing-impaired children should be educated alongside their normal-hearing siblings and peers. More is involved in their education, however, than our wishes to keep the children at home and somehow to make them "normal" through placement in a regular classroom. The educational challenge they present us is immense. Born with normal cognitive capacities and physical appearance, they typically enter a preschool or elementary program markedly delayed in their knowledge of the general culture's language. Early efforts by our predecessors to overcome this disparity and to mainstream hearing-impaired children were not generally successful.

Nevertheless, there is great merit to the concept of mainstreaming, provided we explicitly define our goals and make available educational options and the requisite supportive help. Our intent is to help the children feel "at home" in the mainstream. *Successful* mainstream experience broadens a child's social, educational, and vocational horizons. This permits children a wider range of choices as they go on to post-secondary education and to the demands of adult life. All educational options create a bias in later choices and decisions to some extent. As I see it, mainstreaming, because of the heterogeneous nature of educational experiences, is less limiting than a segregated educational placement (however necessary this may be for a minority of hearing-impaired children).

Those of us who advocate and recommend mainstreaming whenever possible need not make any apologies for our educational preferences. As we have seen, the practice has a long history. Our preference, however, is not and should not be the relevant consideration. *Appropriate education, and not mainstreaming, is the issue.* It is the children and their needs that must drive the educational process and their interests must be the focus of all our efforts. We can learn from the past and do better in the future.

REFERENCES

Allen, T. E., and Osborn, T. I. 1984. Academic integration of hearing-impaired students: Demographic, handicapping, and achievement factors, *American Annals of the Deaf* 129:100–113.
Ewing, A. 1960. *The Modern Educational Treatment of Deafness*, Manchester, England: Manchester University Press.
Gordon, J.C. 1885. Deaf-mutes and the public schools from 1815 to the present day. *American Annals of the Deaf* 30:121–43.
Levitt, H., McGarr, N., and Geffner, D. 1987. *Development of Language and Communication Skills in Hearing-Impaired Children*.ASHA Monograph #26, Washington, D.C.: American Speech-Language-Hearing Association.
Markides, A. 1989. Integration: The speech intelligibility, friendships and associations of hearing-impaired children in secondary schools. *Journal of British Association Teachers of the Deaf* (13)3:63–72.
McLaughlin, H. G. 1960. Integration of deaf children in hearing society. In *The Modern Educational Treatment of Deafness*, ed. A. Ewing. Manchester, England: Manchester University Press.
Nolan, M., and Tucker, I. G. 1981. *The Hearing-Impaired Child and the Family*. London, England: Human Horizons, Souvenier Press.
Numbers, M. E. 1960. Educational, vocational, and social experiences of graduates of Clarke School for the Deaf. In *The Modern Educational Treatment of Deafness*, ed. A. Ewing. Manchester, England: Manchester University Press.
O'Connor, C. D. 1960. Integration of graduates of the Lexington School for the Deaf in programs for the normally hearing. In *The Modern Educational Treatment of Deafness*, ed. A. Ewing. Manchester, England: Manchester University Press.

Pflaster, G. 1980. A factor analysis of variables related to the academic performance of hearing-impaired children integrated into regular classes. *The Volta Review* 82:71–84.

Pflaster, G. 1981. A second analysis of factors related to the academic performance of hearing-impaired children in the mainstream. *The Volta Review* 83:71–80.

Porter, S. 1849. Review of "Art of Instructing the Infant Deaf and Dumb", by J. P. Arrowsmith, published 1819. *American Annals of the Deaf* 2:117–19.

Reich, C., Hambleton, D., and Houldin, B. K. 1977. The integration of hearing-impaired children in regular classrooms. *American Annals of the Deaf* 122:534–43.

Ross, M., and Calvert, D. R. 1967. The semantics of deafness. *Volta Review* 69:644–49.

Ross, M., Brackett, D., and Maxon, A. 1982. *Hard of Hearing Children in Regular Schools*. Englewood Cliffs, NJ: Prentice-Hall, Inc.

Schildroth, A. N., and Karchmer, M. A. 1986. *Deaf Children in America*. San Diego: College-Hill Press.

Watkins, S. 1987. Long term effect of home intervention with hearing-impaired children. *American Annals of the Deaf* 132:267–75.

Weisel, A. 1988. Contact with mainstreamed disabled children and attitudes toward disability: A multidimensional analysis. *Educational Psychology* 8, No. 3:161–68.

White, S. J., and White, R. E. C. 1987. The effects of hearing status of the family and age of intervention on receptive and expressive oral language in hearing-impaired infants. In *Development of Language and Communication Skills in Hearing-Impaired Children*, eds. H. Levitt, N. McGarr, and D. Geffner. ASHA Monograph #26, Washington, DC: American Speech-Language-Hearing Association.

Wilson, G., Ross, M., and Calvert, D. R. 1974. An experimental study of the semantics of deafness. *The Volta Review* 76:398–414.

Index